Arterial Function in Health and Disease

To the memory of my friends
Donald A. McDonald and *Brenda M. Sargent*

Arterial Function in Health and Disease

Michael F. O'Rourke, M.D., F.R.A.C.P., F.A.C.C.
Associate Professor of Medicine, The University of New South Wales,
Medical Professorial Unit, St Vincent's Hospital,
Sydney, New South Wales, Australia

CHURCHILL LIVINGSTONE
EDINBURGH LONDON MELBOURNE AND NEW YORK 1982

CHURCHILL LIVINGSTONE
Medical Division of Longman Group Limited

Distributed in the United States of America by
Churchill Livingstone Inc., 19 West 44th Street, New York,
N.Y. 10036, and by associated companies,
branches and representatives throughout
the world.

© Longman Group Limited 1982

First published 1982

ISBN 0 443 021791

British Library Cataloguing in Publication Data
O'Rourke, Michael F.
   Arterial function in health and disease.
   1. Arteries.
   I. Title
   612 .133   QM191

Library of Congress Catalog Card Number 81-67825

Printed in Singapore by Kyodo Shing Loong Printing Industries Pte Ltd

Preface

Disease of arteries has become the modern scourge, accounting directly or indirectly for over 50 per cent of all deaths in the western world and a corresponding amount of acute and chronic ill-health. It behoves the physician who deals with arterial disease to understand normal function of arteries and the influence of disease on normal function, if his interventions are to be fully effective.

Despite the importance of arterial disease it is surprising that little emphasis is given to study of arterial function in undergraduate and graduate curricula. The medical student and practising cardiologist tend to see the arterial system as a distensible system of tubes receiving blood from the heart in spurts, and passing this on in a steady stream to the tissues of the body. This explanation, though correct in principle, is inadequate for the clinician who wishes to monitor the intra-arterial pressure wave, to explain wave contour in cardiac and arterial disease or to use a heart assist device intelligently. In contrast to the physician, the bioengineer sees a much more complicated system with immense problems in analysis and understanding, including varied geometric patterns of branching, non-uniform elasticity of arteries, non-linear wall properties, and anomalous viscosity of blood in smaller vessels.

With these differences in approach, it is hardly surprising that the advances which physiologists and bioengineers have made in the understanding of arterial function have not in the main been applied to clinical problems. Unfortunately a gulf has developed between the physician's simplistic ideas and the researcher's sophisticated method.

The purpose of this book is to try to bridge the gulf. Explanations will be given for phenomena frequently seen and dealt with in clinical practice in such a way as to make the more sophisticated articles and texts a little less formidable. The point should emerge that apparently complicated and esoteric approaches to the study of arterial function can provide more satisfactory, more complete, and simpler explanations than have hitherto been available.

1982   Michael F. O'Rourke

Acknowledgements

The idea of this book first arose in 1963 when the 'Goddess of Chance' cast me, as an impressionable postgraduate student, into the physiological laboratory of Michael Taylor at the University of Sydney, Taylor having just returned from his productive association with the late Donald McDonald in London. I saw then that the analytical approaches of McDonald and Taylor could throw fresh light on arterial function in disease – if only clinicians could understand their application and interpretation. Following 3 years with Taylor in Sydney – still scientifically the most exciting period of my life, I had the good fortune to work with Bill Milnor at Johns Hopkins, then Paul Korner, Darty Glover and John Hickie in Sydney. Data presented in the book were obtained in the departments of each of these men. The bulk of the book was written while I was on sabbatical leave at Harvard University in the Cardiovascular Division, of the Peter Bent Brigham Hospital with Tom Smith and Eugene Braunwald. I express thanks to all mentioned for facilities provided, and for support freely given. I offer particular thanks to the librarian and staff of the Countway Library, Harvard Medical School, where my office was located over a 12-month period in 1979–1980.

I cannot acknowledge adequately the source of ideas; these were developed in association with many, many persons. My stimulation from Michael Taylor was continued by Donald McDonald – that brilliant, human, but tragically misunderstood man, by Alberto Avolio and by many others. Substantial assistance with this book was given by many of my friends and colleagues – specifically Alberto Avolio, Barry Gow and Michael McGrath in Sydney, Walter Paulus, John Rutherford and Robert Sackstein in Boston, Joe Murgo in San Antonio, Wilmer Nichols in Gainsville, Chris Mills and Ivor Gabe at Midhurst, Derek Bergel in Oxford, Nico Westerhof in Amsterdam. I offer thanks to all these, and to others who also have allowed me to reproduce their illustrations.

Technical assistance was provided competently by my devoted assistant of many years, Kem Mang, and by my able secretary, Dinah Salmon and technician, Luke Fay. I enjoyed support from my clinical colleagues in the Cardiovascular Unit and Coronary Care Unit at St. Vincent's Hospital in Sydney where most of the clinical studies described herein were undertaken. Special recognition is due to senior members of the C.V.U. – Tony Seldon, George Hall and Harry Windsor and to Betty Walsh in C.C.U. Finally, I thank my dear wife, Margaret, and family – Matthew, John, Richard, Madeleine and Caroline for inspiration, assistance and forbearance, and my father who gave me the opportunity to enter a noble and immensely satisfying profession.

Contents

Orientation

The modern analytical approach to studies of arterial function began with the classic interdisciplinary work of the British physiologist Donald McDonald and mathematician John Womersley in the mid 1950s. These men showed through experimental measurement and theoretic calculation that the steady and pulsatile components of arterial pressure and flow waves can be considered quite separately and independently, as can the harmonic components of the compound waves. This approach will be followed and extended in this book.

The arterial system will be taken to have two distinct and separate functions – on the one hand to deliver blood at high pressure to bodily tissues, and on the other, to smooth the pulsations that result from intermittent cardiac ejection. The arterial system thus behaves as a **conduit** and as a **cushion**. These two functions can be dealt with independently through consideration of steady phenomena on the one hand, and oscillatory phenomena on the other. It can be shown that the main effects of arterial disease may be viewed in terms of how this affects one or other function – the conduit function by narrowing the vessel lumen, and the cushioning function by stiffening the vessel wall. It can further be shown that the functional effects of arterial disease are different; that disorder of conduit function affects the tissue or organ downstream while disorder of cushioning function has its principal ill effects on the heart upstream. The separation is thus:

Arteries as Conduits – mean pressure and flow, arterial narrowing, organ ischemia.

Arteries as Cushions – oscillatory components of pressure and flow waves, altered arterial distensibility, impaired cardiac function.

This book is divided into four parts. The first will consider general principles and physical laws concerning steady and pulsatile arterial phenomena, the techniques used for measuring these phenomena, and the justification for separating steady and pulsatile components of recorded waves. The second section deals with conduit function of arteries and the functional effects of arterial narrowing as caused by atherosclerosis. The third part of the book deals with analysis and interpretation of pulse waves, while the fourth part deals with clinical implications of altered cushioning function of arteries with ageing and in disease, as this affects the heart arteries and arterial pulse.

PART I

General Principles

1

Introduction

The systemic arterial system is a complex network of branching elastic tubes which at its origin receives blood in spurts from the heart, and at its multiple terminations passes this on as a steady stream into the arterioles and capillaries.

The conduit and cushioning functions of arteries were first referred to in 1628 by William Harvey in his classic book ' *De motu cordis et sanguinis in animalibus*'. Harvey described how cardiac systole caused passive distension of the systemic arteries whence blood was 'continuously, evenly, and uninterruptedly driven by the beat of the arteries into every member and part'. Harvey likened the arterial system to a distended bladder or glove which attenuated pulsations while distributing blood to peripheral organs through vascular conduits. In 1769 the English clergyman Stephen Hales described his measurements of

arterial pressure in dogs and horses, and his calculations of peripheral vascular resistance. Hales likened the cushioning function of arteries to the action of a large distensible reservoir. In the German translation of Hales' book, this was referred to as a *Windkessel* which was the large inverted air-filled dome of the contemporary fire engine (Fig. 1.1). This converted intermittent strokes of the water pump into a steady stream which could be directed at the seat of a fire. The term *Windkessel* is often used now in reference to the cushioning function of arteries.

Instruments used by Hales and later by Poiseuille, Ludwig and Faivre during the nineteenth century to measure intra-arterial pressure had very high inertia and so could not record arterial pulsations with any accuracy. Recordings obtained were of mean pressure with some pulsa-

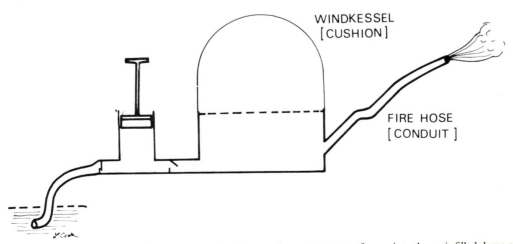

Fig. 1.1 The arterial system was likened by Stephen Hales (1769) to the comtemporary fire engine whose air filled dome or '*Windkessel*' acted as cushion, and whose fire hose acted as conduit. The Windkessel smoothed out the intermittent spurts from the pump so that water was delivered through the hose in a steady stream. The *Windkessel* represents arterial distensibility, the fire hose, the distributing arteries and the nozzle, the peripheral resistance

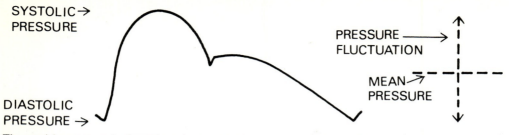

Fig. 1.2 The arterial pressure pulse (centre) can be described in terms of its highest and lowest values (systolic and diastolic pressures), or in terms of its mean value and the fluctuation of pressure around this mean

tile fluctuation. This pressure was used with assumed flow to infer vascular resistance. The first accurate measurements of pulsatile pressure were obtained by Otto Frank in Germany at the beginning of this century. Accurate optical manometers were introduced in the U.S.A. by Wiggers in 1924 and by Hamilton in 1934. It was not until 1942 that the first modern electromanometer was developed, and the early 1950s before these instruments were generally available. Intra-arterial pressure recordings have been taken from humans at diagnostic catheterisation or for monitoring purposes with increasing frequency since this time.

Most human data on arterial pressure have been obtained indirectly with the methods introduced by Riva-Rocci and Korotkov in the 1880s. Over the past 100 years, physicians, using these methods, have come to think of arterial dynamics, not in the same way as Harvey, Hales and Poiseuille, but in terms of the available measurements – in terms of systolic and diastolic pressure. These two values represent merely the limits between which arterial pressure fluctuates during a cardiac cycle (Fig. 1.2); no information is obtained on wave shape or mean pressure*. Ready availability of these values for systolic and diastolic pressure appears to have biased clinical thinking. In the past there has been a tendency for systolic pressure to be regarded as being determined by cardiac factors and diastolic pressure by arteriolar factors exclusively. Thus hypertension used to be defined entirely in terms of diastolic pressure. Only in the

last few years, as a result of actuarial reports and prospective epidemiological studies, has it become apparent that systolic pressure is as important, if not more important, than diastolic pressure in determining mortality from complications of hypertension.

A more complete understanding of arterial phenomena comes from a return to the approach of Harvey and Hales. Here one considers, not the systolic and diastolic pressure, but rather the mean pressure and the oscillation around this mean. Mean pressure is related exclusively to steady flow and the oscillation exclusively to pulsatile flow. This is the modern approach to interpretation of pulsatile arterial phenomena, introduced by McDonald and Womersley in the mid 1950s. Their work forms the basis of this book and will be referred to at length; it is discussed fully in the papers of each and in McDonald's two influential monographs.

To a clinician who is familiar with systolic and diastolic pressure, but not with mean pressure or with pulse waves expressed as a series of component harmonics, the approach suggested may seem foreign and uncomfortable. It is advanced on the basis of utility in separating steady flow (predominantly arteriolar and capillary) and pulsatile flow (predominantly arterial) events. It is based on sound physiological principles, and is hallowed by history. I do not suggest that systolic and diastolic pressures be disregarded, but rather that these be seen and appreciated for what they are:– the limits of arterial pressure fluctuation from beat to beat, with more complete information lying between these limits. As with anything, he who considers only two extremes can miss the truth of what lies between:– the man with his eyes on the sidelines misses the game in centrefield.

---

* Mean pressure is often calculated as being one-third of the value between diastolic and systolic pressure. This is reasonably accurate for peripheral arteries where the wave is peaked and triangular in shape. In central arteries the wave is less peaked and mean pressure is often closer to midway between the systolic and diastolic value.

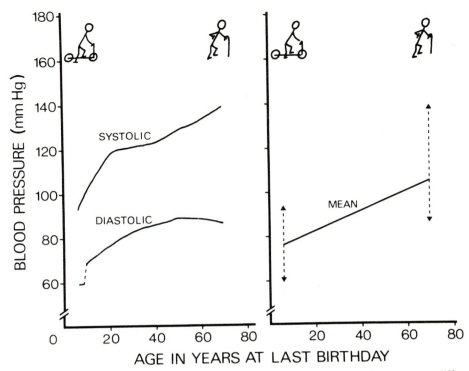

Fig. 1.3 Change in arterial pressure with age. The left panel shows average systolic and diastolic pressures at different ages as reported in the U.S. National Health Survey (DHEW Publication No (HRA) 78 – 1648 1977). The right panel shows the change in mean pressure and pulse pressure with age. Changes with age are most readily explained on the basis of altered cushioning function (decreased distensibility with greater pressure fluctuation) and altered conduit function (increased resistance with increased mean pressure) (See also Fig. 14.2, pp. 212–214)

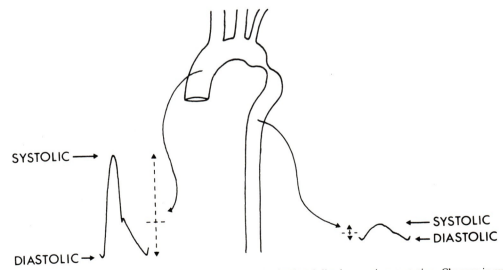

Fig. 1.4 Diagrammatic representation of arterial pressure waves proximal and distal to aortic coarctation. Changes in systolic and diastolic pressure are most readily explained on the basis of altered cushioning function (as this affects pressure fluctuation) and altered conduit function (as this affects mean pressure) (See also Figs. 13.1–13.4)

One does not have to understand harmonic analysis of arterial pulses to begin using McDonald's approach of separating mean from pulsatile events in studying arterial function. Three examples can be used to illustrate this.

Example 1. Changes in arterial pressure with aging have been known for many years (Fig. 1.3); systolic pressure increases appreciably while diastolic pressure increases but little during adult life. In the past, different explanations have been given for this, and much debate has ensued. When one looks at the same data from the point of view suggested, one does not ascribe any special importance to changes in systolic or diastolic pressure. Rather one infers a rise in mean pressure and increase in pulsation around this mean. One attributes increase in mean pressure to increase in vascular resistance as a consequence of decreased vascularity of body tissues, and increased pulsation to decreased arterial distensibility (see Ch. 14).

Example 2. Aortic coarctation results in increased mean pressure and increased fluctuation about this mean in the upper part of the body, but decreased mean pressure and decreased fluctuation around this mean in the lower part of the body. Sometimes, as in Figure 1.4, diastolic pressure may actually be lower in the upper part of the body above the coarctation than below. Such findings have in the past been interpreted to indicate increased peripheral resistance and arteriolar hypertension in the lower part of the body. The phenomenom is attributable to arterial pulsations being reduced more than mean pressure in the long and tortuous collateral arteries (see Ch. 13).

Example 3. Under normal circumstances both in experimental animals and in young healthy humans, there is considerable alteration in the contour of the arterial pressure wave between the ascending aorta and peripheral arteries (Fig. 1.5). Systolic pressure increases markedly while diastolic pressure falls. (The increase in systolic pressure can be as much as 25 mm Hg – hence one needs to specify the artery in which systolic and diastolic pressures are recorded.) Using the suggested approach one looks for a change in mean pressure and in pulse pressure between central and peripheral artery. One finds that mean pressure falls only slightly – perhaps by 1–2 mm Hg between the ascending aorta and brachial or femoral artery while pulse pressure increases by over 20 per cent. One can attribute the small change in mean pressure to energy losses associated with steady flow between the ascending aorta and peripheral artery, and the increased pulsation (as described in detail in Ch. 7) to pulse wave reflection.

The arterial system may be represented diagrammatically by the Windkessel and conduit, the former cushioning cardiac pulsations, and the latter transmitting blood to peripheral tissues (Fig. 1.6). This is of course an extreme simplification, since the two functions are not separated but are performed by the arterial system as a whole i.e. the conduits are cushions as well. However the proximal arteries, especially the proximal aorta are far more distensible than peripheral arteries and

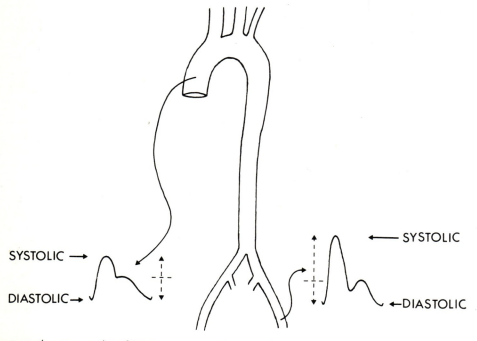

Fig. 1.5 Diagrammatic representation of pressure waves in the proximal aorta and in a peripheral artery. Differences in systolic and diastolic pressures in the two vessels are readily explained on the basis of slight fall in mean pressure and large increase in pressure pulsation. (See also Figs. 9.2, 9.3, 9.5)

WINDKESSEL

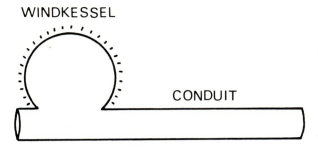

CONDUIT

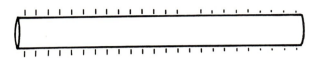

Fig. 1.6 The cushioning and conduit functions of the arterial system may be represented separately by a *Windkessel* and distributing tube (above), or by a single distensible tube (below) in which both functions are combined

are mainly responsible for cushioning flow pulsations.

There are other practical problems with the *Windkessel* model which make it incomplete and unsatisfactory for explaining arterial phenomena. In the *Windkessel*, pressure changes occur simultaneously in the distensible reservoir and in the distal conduit; this is not the case in life. In the *Windkessel* there is no amplification of the pulse wave as occurs in peripheral arteries. In the *Windkessel*, pressure falls exponentially during diastole; there is no secondary diastolic wave as usually seen in systemic arteries. The most realistic simple conceptual model of the arterial system is the distensible tube which joins the heart to the peripheral resistance; in this, cushioning and conduit functions are combined. With this simple model, one can still consider pulsatile and steady phenomena separately, but one can account for differences in pressure at different points at the same time, amplification of the pressure wave, and secondary oscillations in pressure and flow. This is the simple model proposed by Hamilton and Dow in 1939 and by McDonald and Taylor in 1959 to explain pressure wave contour in different arteries. Arterial models and physical principles underlying their use will be discussed in Chapter 4 and again in Chapters 9–11. It can be shown that the simple tube provides a surprisingly good representation of the whole arterial system. A minor modification will be introduced in Chapter 10 to account for differences in contour of pressure and flow waves in upper and lower limbs, and the heart's eccentric position in the body, closer to arterial terminations in the upper part of the body than to those in the lower part.

In a book on arteries, it is desirable to define what is meant by arteries, and to clarify how a simple tubular model can be taken to represent the whole arterial tree. The arterial system may be regarded as the network of tubes which joins the heart to the major resistance vessels. Most of the resistance to flow is in the arterioles (diameter 20–200μ) and capillaries, but smaller arteries (those less than 1000μ diameter) also constitute an appreciable part of the peripheral resistance. For practical purposes one can refer to the arterial system as ending in vessels of 200–1000μ, with vessels beyond being regarded as resistance vessels. In practical and anatomical terms it matters little where the arteries are taken to terminate in resistance vessels. The small arteries are very short (Table 1.1). Including or excluding vessels between 200–1000μ leads to little alteration in over-

Table 1.1. Dimensions of vessels, pressure drop along vessels, and resistance in segments of the mesenteric vascular bed of a dog. After Schleier (1918), from data of Mall.

Vascular Component	Diameter (mm)	Length (cm)	Pressure Drop (mmHg)	Resistance (Arbitrary Units)	Resistance/Length (Arbitrary Units)
Large artery	3	6	0.8	1.0	1.0
Medium arteries	1	4.5	3.2	4.0	5.3
Small arteries	0.6	3.9	7.4	9.3	14.3
	0.13	1.4	23.5	29.4	126
Arterioles (2)	<0.05	.46	20.7	25.1	338
Capillaries	0.004	.04	2.4	3.0	451

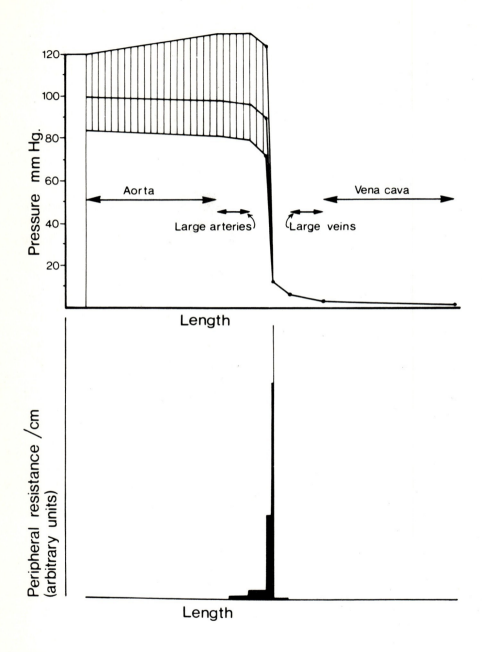

Fig. 1.7 *Top*: Change in mean pressure and in pulsatile pressure generated by the left ventricle, between the ascending aorta and vena cava. Mean pressure falls only slightly in the aorta and large distributing arteries whereas pulsatile pressure is augmented as a result of wave reflection. Mean pressure and pulse pressure fall precipately over a short length in the smallest arteries and in the arterioles as a result of the high resistance to blood flow that these vessels present
Bottom: Resistance in corresponding segments of the vascular bed. Figure prepared from data of Schleier (Table 1.1)

all length of the arterial system. Figure 1.7 helps to explain this point. This figure is similar to one shown by Milnor in Mountcastle's Textbook of Physiology, but is considered to be a more realistic representation of pressure and resistance changes in the systemic circulation because lengths of blood vessels are drawn to scale. Resistance changes in different vessels are calculated from Table 1. This figure emphasises that changes in resistance and pressure occur abruptly over a short length of the vascular tree. When resistance is expressed as a function of length i.e. resistance units per cm, one sees (as shown in the lower part of Figure 1.7), the abrupt change in resistance that occurs over a short length of the pathway between arteries and veins. It thus matters little for our purposes what one takes to be resistance vessels. Suffice is to say that the low resistance pathway through the arteries terminates in a high resistance over a short length. Our concept of the arterial system is the network of tubes proximal to the high resistance – i.e. graphically in the lower part of Figure 1.7 the space on the left of the 'wall'. The tubular model of the arterial system represents this space while the 'wall' itself, the peripheral resistance, represents the closed end of the tubular model.

One point must be made immediately about Figure 1.7. It represents the resistance in a network of vascular pathways where all component vascular pathways are the same length. This may appear to be unrealistic since the resistive vessels in different tissues are at different distances from the heart. As discussed in Chapter 9, the vascular bed in the lower part of the body behaves (when viewed from the proximal aorta) as though there were one region where vascular resistance increases suddenly; i.e. the vascular bed in the lower body behaves like a simple tube of finite length with the lower body resistance at its end. The length of this tube appears to be the average of all individual path lengths from descending aortic origin to individual resistance vessels in the lower part of the body. In other words the total peripheral resistance in the lower part of the body as seen from the proximal aorta appears to be 'lumped' at one point. The tubular model is thus a good representation of this part of the arterial system.

Figure 1.7 helps explain conceptually a number of fundamental points which will be described in more detail later. First, and most obviously, the very high resistance over a short length causes mean pressure to fall precipitously over this short length. Second, suddenly high resistance impedes pulsatile phenomena as well as steady flow so that amplitude of pulse pressure falls at the same time as mean pressure, resulting in steady flow through these resistance vessels. Third, arterial pulsations which cannot enter the high resistance vessels are reflected, and summate with pressure waves approaching the high resistance, so causing the pressure pulsation to be higher in peripheral than in central arteries. In these respects, the representation of resistance in the lower part of the figure is appropriate. The high resistance can be likened to a leaking sea wall. Water continually trickles through this wall while ocean waves bounce back and accentuate the amplitude of waves close to the wall.

REFERENCES

Faivre J 1856 Pathological physiology : experimental studies on the organic lesions of the heart. In: Ruskin A(ed) Classics in arterial hypertension 1956 Thomas Springfield 67–73

Frank O 1899 Die Grundform des arteriellen Pulses. Erste Abhandlung. Mathematische Analyse. Zeitschrift fur Biologie 37 : 483–526

Frank O 1905 Der Puls in den Arterien, Zeitschrift fur Biologie 46: 441–553

Hales S 1769 Statical essays. 3rd edition Wilson and Nichol London

Hamilton WF, Brewer G, Brotman I 1934 Pressure pulse contours in the intact animal. 1. Analytical description of a new high frequency hypodermic manometer with illustrative curves of simultaneous arterial and intracardiac pressure. American Journal of Physiology 107: 427–435

Hamilton WF, Dow P 1939 An experimental study of the standing waves in the pulse propagated through aorta. American Journal of Physiology 125: 48–59

Harvey W 1628 De motu cordis et sanguinis in animalibus. William Fitzer Frankfurt Translated by KJ Franklin 1957 Blackwell Oxford

Korotkov NS 1905 A contribution to the problem of methods for the determination of the blood pressure. In: Ruskin A (ed) Classics in arterial hypertension. 1956 Thomas Springfield p 127–133

Landis EM 1926 The capillary pressure in frog mesentery as

determined by micro injection methods. American Journal of Physiology 75: 548–570

Landis EM 1930 The capillary blood pressure in mammalian mesentery as determined by the micro injection method. American Journal of Physiology 93 : 353–362

Lilly JC 1942 Electrical capacitance diaphragm manometer. Review of Scientific Instruments 13 : 34–47

Ludwig C 1847 Contributions to the knowledge of the influence of the respiratory movements upon the blood flow in the arterial system. In: Ruskin A (ed) Classics in arterial hypertension Thomas Springfield 1956 p 61–66

McDonald DA 1955 The relation of pulsatile pressure to flow in arteries. Journal of Physiology (London) 127: 533–552

McDonald DA 1974 Blood flow in arteries. 2nd edition Arnold London

McDonald DA and Taylor MG 1959 The hydrodynamics of the arterial circulation Progress in Biophysics and Biophysical Chemistry 9: 107–173

Milnor WR 1974 The Circulation. In: Mountcastle VB (ed) Medical physiology. Mosby St. Louis p 839–1026

O'Rourke MF, Cartmill TB 1971 Influence of aortic coarctation on pulsatile hemodynamics in the proximal aorta. Circulation 44 : 281–292

Pickering GW 1968 High blood pressure. Churchill London 582–591

Poiseuille JM 1828 Recherches sur la force du coeur aortique. In: Ruskin A (ed) Classics in arterial hypertension. 1956 Thomas Springfield p 31–59

Rappaport MB, Bloch EH, Irwin JW. 1959 Manometer for measuring dynamic pressures in the microvascular system. Journal of Applied Physiology 14: 651–655

Riva–Rocci S 1896 A new sphygmomanometer. In: Ruskin A (ed) Classics in arterial hypertension 1956 Thomas Springfield 104–125

Schleier J 1918 Der Energieverbrauch in der Blutbahn. Pflugers Archives fur Gesamte Physiologie 173: 172–223

Schwartz CJ, Wethessen NT, Wolf S. 1980 Structure and function of the Circulation. New York Plenum

Steele JM 1941 Evidence for general distribution of peripheral resistance in coarctation of the aorta: report of three cases. Journal of Clinical Investigation 20: 473–480

Sugiura T, Freis E 1962 Pressure pulse in small arteries. Circulation Research 11: 838–842

Wiederhielm CA, Woodbury JW, Kirk S, Rushmer RF 1964 Pulsatile pressures in the microcirculation of the frogs mesentery. American Journal of Physiology 207: 173–176

Wiggers CJ, Baker WR 1924 A new unusual optical manometer. Journal of Laboratory and Clinical Medicine 10: 54–56

Womersley JR 1957 The mathematical analysis of the arterial circulation in a state of oscillatory motion. Wright Air Development Center, Technical Report WADC–TR 56–614

Womersley JR 1958 Oscillatory flow in arteries: the reflection of the pulse wave at junctions and rigid inserts in the arterial system. Physics in Medicine and Biology 2: 313–323

Zwiefach BW 1949 Basic mechanisms in peripheral vascular homeostasis Transactions third conference, Josiah Macy Foundation 13–52

2

Arterial waves

Information on arterial function is gained from measurement and interpretation of arterial waves. The waves one needs consider are the pressure wave, the diameter wave, the pressure gradient wave and the flow wave. These vary considerably in contour and in relative content of mean and pulsatile components. Each is repeated with the regularity (or irregularity) of the heart beat. Each is displayed graphically as the measured parameter plotted against time. This chapter deals with these waves, general principles of interrelationships, methods of measurement, and the principles of accurate measurement. Details of relationships will be dealt with in chapters 9 and 11.

DESCRIPTION OF ARTERIAL WAVES

Pressure waves

Figure 2.1 shows pressure recorded simultaneous-ly in the proximal aorta, abdominal aorta and femoral artery of a dog. In the proximal aorta the systolic pressure peak is followed by the incisura, caused by aortic valve closure; during diastole there is a secondary wave followed by a steady fall in pressure. As pressure is measured progressively further from the heart, a number of changes become apparent. The foot of the wave is delayed; amplitude of the wave increases considerably even though mean pressure falls slightly; the incisura becomes less prominent and the diastolic wave becomes more apparent.

These are the basic features of arterial pressure waves and the changes seen in the distal aorta and peripheral lower body arteries. As described in Chapters 7 and 9, wave reflection is largely responsible for these alterations in pressure wave contour. Other mechanisms, and the differences seen under different conditions, will be dealt with in Chapter 7 and 9. At this stage one might note in

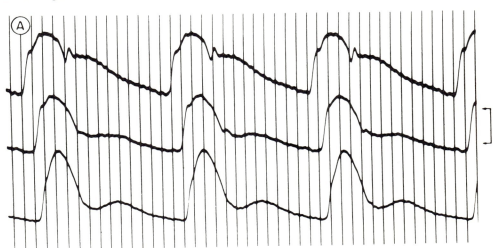

Fig. 2.1 Pressure waves recorded in the aortic arch at the root of the brachiocephalic artery, (upper trace), abdominal aorta (middle trace) and femoral artery (lower trace) in a dog. From O'Rourke (1967)

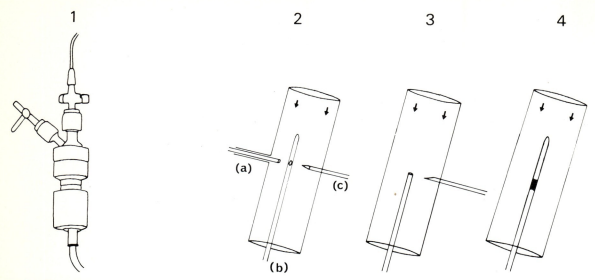

Fig. 2.2 Technique of pressure measurement.
1. Strain-gauge transducer connected by a saline-filled catheter to the point of measurement.
2. Measurement of lateral pressure:
   a with an end-hole catheter inserted through a side branch of an artery;
   b with a side-hole catheter inserted through a peripheral vessel;
   c with a needle inserted directly through the vessel wall, and with the bevel facing across the direction of flow.
3. Measurement of impact pressure with an end-hole catheter inserted through a peripheral artery or with a needle inserted through the arterial wall, and with the bevel rotated to face into the direction of flow.
4. Measurement of lateral pressure with a Millar catheter mounted transducer

comparing pressure with other waves, that the pulsatile fluctuation represents about 30 per cent of mean pressure in the proximal aorta and 40 per cent or so of mean pressure in the iliac artery.

With the usual measuring technique, (Fig. 2.2), pressure is measured at right angles to the arterial wall. As be discussed in Chapter 8, pressure energy, at high flow velocity is converted into kinetic energy so that lateral pressure falls in relation to end-on or impact pressure. This is the basic mechanism for genesis of the anacrotic and bisferiens pulse (Ch. 17) in aortic valve disease. In the absence of valvular stenosis and in the absence of arterial constriction (as might be caused by a cuff-type electromagnetic flow transducer) peak flow velocity is relatively low (less than 80 cm sec^{-1}), and there is no appreciable difference between pressure measured end-on or side-on to the direction of flow.

Diameter waves

Diameter waves appear almost identical to the arterial pressure wave (Fig. 2.3). Conceptually this is what one would expect; the pressure pulsation acting laterally on the arterial wall causes a like change in diameter. There are however a number of subtle differences. The diameter pulsation is only three to eight percent of mean diameter and so is considerably smaller than the ratio of pulsatile to mean pressure. The other two differences become apparent when one compares the details of pressure and diameter pulsations at high recorder speed, or plots instantaneous pressure against instantaneous diameter on the two axes of an oscilloscope (Fig. 2.3). Here one appreciates that there is a delay of diameter behind pressure (which is due to internal viscosity of the arterial wall), and that the relationship between pressure and diameter is not linear, with the arterial wall becoming less compliant as pressure increases.

Linear methods of analysis are sometimes used to describe the relationship between distending pressure and arterial diameter. These must be applied with caution and on the assumption that they describe properties at a certain mean pressure as a result of small changes of pressure and diameter about this mean value.

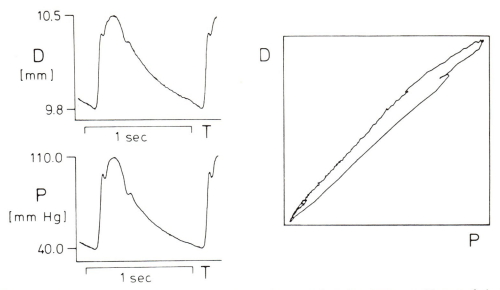

Fig. 2.3 Diameter (above) and pressure (below) waves recorded simultaneously from the common carotid artery of a human subject. The figure at right shows instantaneous diameter (ordinate) plotted against instantaneous pressure (abscissa). From Summa (1978)

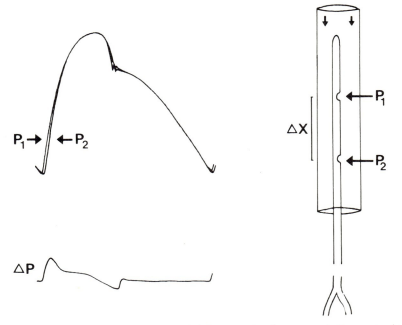

Fig. 2.4 Diagrammatic representation of pressure waves recorded from two sites 5 cms apart in the proximal aorta of a human subject together with (below) the differential pressure between the two sites as recorded by a differential manometer

Pressure gradient waves

It is apparent from Figure 2.1 that there is a difference in pressure between two parts of an artery at the same instant in time. This results from the finite time taken for the pulse to travel from one point to the other. The pressure gradient may be measured by subtracting instantaneous pressure at one point from instantaneous pressure at the other point, or, more conveniently, from use of a differential manometer. As would be expected, the differential pressure wave recorded from points 5 cm apart has a very low amplitude (Fig. 2.4). Differential pressure is rarely recorded by clinicians except across a stenosed valve or along a narrowed artery. Pressure gradient along a normal artery is mentioned here for the sake of completeness, to illustrate the effect of finite wave velocity on pressure measured simultaneously at two points close together in an artery and to make a basic point which has confused many. It is the pressure (or energy) gradient which generates flow, not the absolute pressure. Blood moves from .one point in a cylindrical artery to another as a result of a pressure (energy) gradient. It is the tiny differential pressure gradient which one can only just measure which is responsible for blood flow along the aorta. In contrast to pressure and diameter waves, the pulsatile component of this differential pressure wave is relatively large, being 20 or so times (i.e. 2000 per cent) the mean component (Fig. 2.4). Before introduction of the electromagnetic flow catheter for clinical studies, flow waves were actually calculated from this differential pressure using the known inertial and viscous properties of blood and physical properties of the arterial wall (Womersley 1955, McDonald 1955, 1960, Fry 1959).

Flow waves

Figure 2.5 shows flow waves recorded in the ascending aorta and in its major branches. In the ascending aorta, blood spurts forward during systole, with peak flow achieved in the first third of systole. There is some backflow with closure of the aortic valve. During diastole there is no apparent flow, retrograde flow into the coronary arteries usually being too small to detect in the ascending aorta. Unlike pressure and diameter, but like pressure gradient, the pulsatile component of the arterial flow wave is much greater (around four times greater) than the mean component. In the descending aorta and peripheral arteries, peak forward flow occurs as expected during systole, but there is quite frequently an appreciable secondary flow wave in diastole, preceded by a negative flow wave. At the origins of the descending thoracic aorta and brachiocephalic artery, these secondary flow oscillations are seen to be reciprocal (Figs. 9.6, 9.7) with backflow in the brachiocephalic artery corresponding to forward flow in the descending aorta, and forward diastolic flow in the brachiocephalic artery corresponding to backflow in the descending thoracic aorta. As described in Chapters 7 and 9 these secondary flow fluctuations are a consequence of reflection and re-reflection of the cardiac impulse from reflecting sites in the upper and lower parts of the body.

The flow wave is the longitudinal movement of blood in an artery over the cardiac cycle. One gets no sense of flow from inspecting an artery or measuring pressure within it. The pressure wave measured at the junction of the brachiocephalic artery and descending aorta shows no greater diastolic wave than in the ascending aorta where blood is virtually stationary during diastole. Likewise, when blood flow in an artery is obstructed, the pressure wave upstream is little changed from when the artery was patent and gives no information as to the absence of blood flow within the artery. To gain information from the pressure wave on flow into the vascular bed downstream one needs to know the input impedance of that particular vascular bed. As described in Chapter 8 this is determined by the properties of the whole vascular bed downstream, and can be measured by relating corresponding steady and pulsatile components of pressure and flow waves recorded in the artery of supply.

MEASUREMENT OF ARTERIAL WAVES

It is not appropriate here to describe details of conventional or newer instruments. These are dealt with elsewhere. Excellent descriptions of instruments in current clinical use are given in Fry 1960, Shirer 1962, Wetterer 1962, Gabe 1972, Bergel 1972, Mills 1972, Roberts 1972, Reneman 1974, McDonald 1974, Murgo 1975, Murgo et al 1977 while exciting new innovations are described in many recent articles (e.g. McAlpin et al 1976, Kalmanson and Veyrat 1979), and in the proceedings of many recent conferences (Anliker 1978, Kolin 1978, Kenner and Hinghoffer-Szalkay 1981). This treatise is concerned with waves that can be recorded accurately and can be calibrated

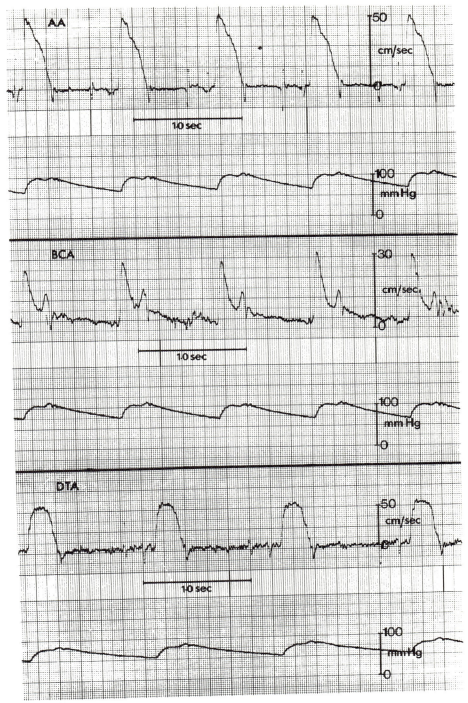

Fig. 2.5 Flow waves recorded with pressure at short time intervals apart in the brachiocephalic artery (centre) ascending aorta (above) and descending thoracic aorta (below) of a kangaroo. Similar flow waves are seen in man (Fig. 8.25) and in other mammals (Figs. 9.6, 9.7) Note the similarity of pressure waves in the three arteries but the dissimilarity of flow waves.

precisely. Passing mention only will be made of non invasive techniques for measuring pressure, flow and diameter (see Busse et al 1978, Pasch et al 1975). Important as these are in clinical practice, they have found little value to date in basic cardiovascular research. Their future clinical value (which is substantial) will doubtless be based on calibration against the signals measured directly and invasively, that are considered here.

Pressure

In the past, the most reliable and popular method of pressure measurement has been the strain gauge manometer (Fig. 2.2) connected through a catheter to the site of pressure measurement. Lateral pressure (i.e. pressure side-on to the direction of flow) may be measured either by inserting an end hole catheter through a side branch of the artery, by inserting a needle through the vessel wall with the bevel at right angles to the direction of flow, or through the side opening of a catheter inserted from a peripheral artery (Fig. 2.2). Impact or end pressure is measured (Fig. 2.2) either through the end opening of a catheter inserted from a peripheral artery or through a needle inserted through the vessel wall, and whose bevel is rotated to face into the direction of flow (O'Rourke 1968). The advantage of an external transducer with connecting catheter is that the manometer itself is relatively robust and inexpensive. The disadvantage is that ability to record pulsatile pressure faithfully is degraded by the catheter system and its attachments – particularly when the catheter or connections are long or narrow, or when their walls are soft or when air bubbles become trapped in any part of the system. This problem is considered below under 'dynamic accuracy'. The miniature catheter mounted strain gauge manometers (Murgo and Millar 1972, Murgo 1975, Murgo et al 1980) are being used increasingly in clinical studies. Their high dynamic accuracy (with resonant frequency > 1000 Hz) enables details of pressure waves to be measured with great precision. Their drawback is expense and relative fragility.

Pressure gradient

Differential pressure (Fig. 2.4) between two points may be measured through a double lumen catheter with ports 3–5 cm apart by two carefully balanced manometers, or by a differential manometer. Alternatively, differential pressure may be measured by use of a multi sensor catheter with two strain gauges mounted a known distance apart (Murgo 1975, Murgo et al 1980). Because differential pressure is of such small amplitude, great care must be taken in filling manometer catheter systems (if these are used) and in balancing the two manometers.

Diameter

Changes in arterial diameter may be measured by calipers attached to the arterial wall (Gow 1966, Bergel 1972, Kolin 1978), by ultrasonic techniques (Arndt 1969, Hokanson et al 1972, Barnes et al 1976) or from the shadows cast by light or X-rays beamed on the vessel wall (Bergel 1972, Busse et al 1979, Wetterer et al 1977) (Fig. 2.6). There has been considerable variation in values of arterial diameter measured by different workers, using different techniques, and so considerable difference in values of arterial distensibility derived from simultaneous measurements of diameter and pressure. Concern has been expressed as to how much an external or internal caliper may load an artery, and how much an external ultrasonic transducer may distort the vessel. (Busse et al 1979, Gow 180). Pulsatile diameter changes of arteries are quite small and still cannot be measured with the same degree of accuracy as pulsatile pressure.

Flow

In the past, many techniques were used to measure phasic blood flow. At this time, the electromagnetic flowmeter has been highly refined and has become the preferred technique (Mills 1972, McDonald 1974, Murgo et al 1977, 1980). The principle of action is that of electromagnetic induction. A magnetic field is induced within the artery at right angles to the direction of flow. Blood, a conductor of electricity, cuts across this magnetic field and sets up at right angles (i.e. in a third dimension) a potential difference which is proportional to the velocity of flow. This is amplified and displayed as the flow signal. Electromagnetic flow transducers are available as cuffs to be applied to the outside of a surgically-exposed vessel (see Wetterer 1962, Kolin 1978), or as a catheter (Mills and Shillingford 1967, Murgo 1975) for measurement of blood flow from within the vessel (Fig. 2.7). The cuff transducers are ideal for operative measurement of blood flow, and for recovery experiments in conscious animals. The catheter flowmeters have found greatest use in humans during diagnostic catheterisation.

Frequency response of these instruments is determined by carrier frequency and output filter (Gessner and Bergel 1964, O'Rourke 1965, Goodman 1966) and is usually quite adequate for accurate recording of phasic flow detail. Frequency response of ultrasonic flowmeters has not been evaluated in the same way as the electromagnetic, and these instruments have not gained popularity for accurate registration of pulsatile flow.

The Doppler ultrasonic flow transducer has been used in many experimental studies. This is

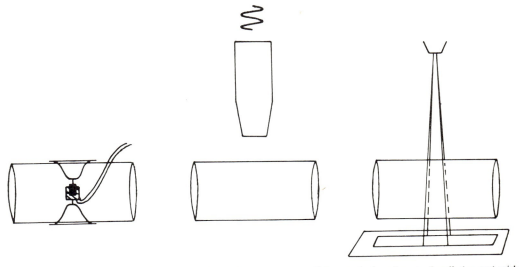

Fig. 2.6 Measurement of pulsatile arterial diameter (left) with an electrical caliper attached to the vessel wall, (centre) with an ultrasonic transducer, and (right) from the shadow cast by light or X-rays.

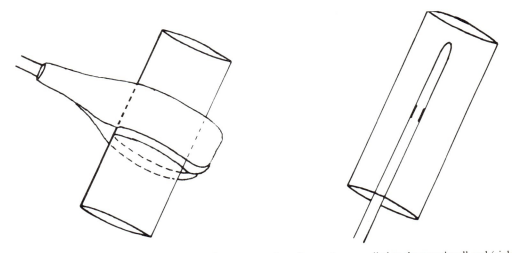

Fig. 2.7 Measurement of pulsatile flow (left) with an electro-magnetic cuff transducer applied to the vessel wall and (right) with an electromagnetic catheter advanced from a peripheral artery

applied as a cuff to a surgically-exposed vessel. Flow velocity is measured from the change in frequency of ultrasound which results from the movement of blood. The Doppler instrument has been very useful for studies of unrestrained animals where radio-telemetery is utilised. For accurate registration of flow wave contour, this instrument is less than ideal, because of dynamic inaccuracy, apparent sensitivity ot minor alteration in velocity profile, and inability with the earlier instruments to distinguish between forward and backward flow (Roberts 1972, Reneman 1974).

New applications of ultrasonic techniques carry great promise. Recent advances include the Echo-Doppler Velocimeter which permits simultaneous and non-invasive measurement of diameter and relative velocity (Kalmanson and Veyrat 1979; Safar et al 1981). Advances in electromagnetic techniques include reintroduction of the external field intra vascular electromagnetic flowmeter system, (McAlpin et al 1976) and combination of electromagnetic sensors with diameter (Kolin 1978) or pressure transducers (Murgo 1975).

ACCURACY OF PRESSURE, DIAMETER, AND FLOW RECORDINGS

The objective of recording is to obtain an exact facsimile of the pressure change, diameter change, or flow change that is occurring in the artery. To the extent that this is not achieved, a measuring error exists. Measuring errors are inevitable with any system. One's aim in taking recordings is to be aware of possible sources of error, to know the limitations of the system in use, to keep errors as small as possible, and to make interpretations only within the range of accuracy of recorded events (see Fry 1960, McDonald 1974).

Errors may arise in any part of the full recording system – in the catheter (if one is used) which connects the experimental recording site to the electrical transducer, the transducer itself, the electrical processor and amplifier, and the graphic recorder. In testing for accuracy, the whole system should be evaluated.

There are three aspects of recording accuracy (Fry 1960):– the static accuracy, the dynamic accuracy, and the physiological reactance.

Static accuracy refers to accuracy in measuring slowly varying changes in pressure, diameter or flow. It implies two qualities – stability and uniqueness; stability of baseline and of calibration factor, and ability to measure the same signal with the same accuracy no matter how it is applied. Static accuracy is checked by observation for baseline drift over a prolonged period of time and by application of known steady calibrations of increasing, then decreasing magnitude. For pressure, calibration is performed with a column of mercury, for diameter, with a vernier or micrometer or with cylinders of known width. Flow calibration is performed *in vitro* by passing blood or physiological saline (which usually generates the same signal (O'Rourke 1965) at known velocities through the cuff transducer or over the flow catheter. Flow calibration can be performed *in vivo* when the flow transducer is on or in the ascending aorta or main pulmonary artery, by measuring cardiac output simultaneously with the Fick or thermodilution technique and relating this value of flow to the mean value of the aortic or pulmonary artery flow wave, and taking zero flow to be the integrated flow signal during diastole (Bergel and Milnor 1965). Each instrument should be calibrated over the range of pressure, diameter or flow which is to be measured in life to ensure that calibration factor remains constant – i.e. that recordings are taken within the linear range of the instrument.

Static accuracy will be present if there is no baseline drift and if all points on the calibration curve fall along the same straight line. Despite sophistication of modern instruments, baseline drift and calibration changes may occur during the course of an experiment. The careful worker will check baseline and calibration before and during the course of each experiment.

Dynamic accuracy refers to fidelity in measuring events which vary with time. This embraces two components – noise and dynamic response. Noise is the rapidly-varying signal that arises from various experimental and instrumental sources and which usually bears no relationship to the event being measured. Noise may result from imperfect contact of the transducer, or from electrical components within the recording system, or from electrical interference with other instruments. Noise limits the extent to which a signal can be amplified. Dynamic response refers to the accuracy with which the system records an event which changes rapidly with time. This can be determined by analysing the system response when it is driven with a known input wave. The dynamic response is analogous to the response of a 'hi-fi' musical recording system and is expressed in the same way – as a graph of modulus and phase response plotted against frequency (Fig. 2.8). The 'hi-fi' music enthusiast is interested in precisely the same information as the cardiovascular researcher – accurate reproduction of compound waves, and so of their component harmonics – over a wide frequency range in order that there will be negligible distortion of recorded sound. The 'sound buff' wishes to span the range of 30–30,000 Hertz (cycles sec^{-1}). The researcher would be happy indeed to have an accurate signal to 30 Hz. As described later (Ch. 6) most of the

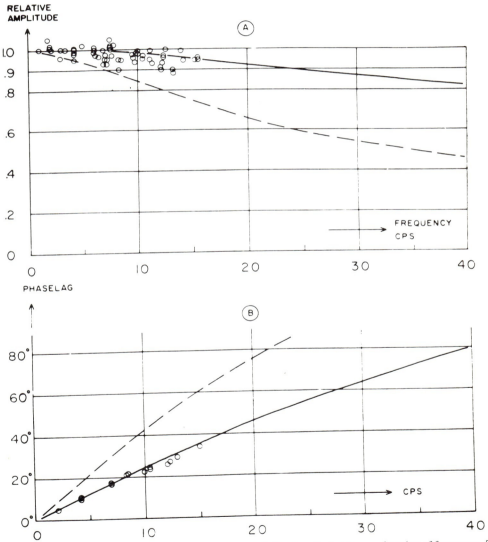

Fig. 2.8 Amplitude response (above) and phase lag (below) of a gated sine wave flowmeter as a function of frequency. The circles represent the results of hydraulic determinations at the 'high' filter switch setting and the solid line represent the electrically determined response at this setting. The dotted lines represent the electrically determined response at 'medium' filter setting. From Gessner and Bergel (1964)

energy in arterial pressure, flow, and diameter waves is in the harmonic components up to 15 Hz. Dynamic response without distortion up to at least 15 Hz is therefore desirable.

Dynamic response of a manometer system can be determined by imposing a sinusoidal pressure oscillation on the catheter tip, then comparing output signal to input signal as frequency is increased from say 1–15 Hz. The response can be expressed (Fig. 2.8) as modulus (amplitude of output signal ÷ amplitude of input signal) and phase (delay of output signal after input signal) as a function of frequency. A more convenient approach to obtain the same frequency response graph is the pressure – step or 'pop' test of Hansen and Warburg, (1950) (McDonald, 1974). In this, a steady pressure is applied to the catheter tip by inflating a balloon attached to the catheter tip. Pressure is abruptly dropped by rupturing the balloon with a pin or lighted match. From the oscillations in output pressure signal which result, one can calculate (as described in Appendix 1) the damped natural frequency and damping factor, and from this, the frequency response graph of modulus and phase plotted against frequency. When determining dynamic response of a manometer system, it is important that the whole system be tested as it is used in an experiment or clinical study. It is pointless (and misleading) to record only the frequency response of the transducer or of the transducer attached to a different catheter assembly.

One might add parenthetically that dynamic response of many catheter assemblies as used for clinical diagnostic studies is extremely poor. This is attributable to the multiple connections and long catheters which are used for the sake of convenience, together with failure to expel air bubbles which tend to adhere at connecting points. Most clinicians are not aware of these problems or of the ensuing distortion of pressure waves – particularly sharp inflections such as end-diastolic pressure – which result (Patel et al 1965, Schostal et al 1972). One does not need a Millar catheter to record pressure waves accurately. Quite satisfactory recordings have been and can be obtained with conventional fluid-filled catheters when fundamental principles are adhered to in their preparation and use.

Dynamic response of diameter-measuring and flow-measuring instruments cannot conveniently be performed with the step or 'pop' test. A sinusoidal input must be applied at different frequencies to the transducer, then output signal compared to input in modulus and phase. For the electromagnetic flowmeter it has been established that the electrical filter is the only source of instrumental dynamic inaccuracy (Gessner and Bergel 1965, O'Rourke 1965, Goodman 1966). Hence, the electrical dynamic calibration given by the manufacturer for a given filter setting suffices for all transducers. Most modern flowmeters have been designed to give a flat amplitude response (output amplitude ÷ input amplitude) and a linear phase delay (which implies the same absolute time delay) up to 15 Hz. Thus there results a flow signal which is delayed by around 10 m sec but is undistorted with respect to flow components up to this frequency.

In discussing dynamic accuracy and frequency response it is impossible to avoid the analogy to music and of components of the pulse to components of musical waves. We are happy to consider these in terms of harmonics or overtones and to think of musical waves in the frequency rather than in the time domain. It is just as logical (when the heart is beating regularly) to consider components of arterial pressure, flow, and diameter in the same way. This concept is extended in Chapters 6–11.

Physiological reactance refers to the unwanted effect of the recording transducer or catheter on the physiological event being measured. For pressure recording, the presence of a large catheter in a small vessel will distort the recorded pressure. For diameter, presence of a heavy or stiff transducer on a small vessel will attenuate the output signal. For flow, an inappropriately large catheter or inappropriately small cuff will distort the flow signal. There can also be interaction of physiological reactance when more than one parameter is being measured. For instance the electromagnetic flow cuff may not distort flow but may alter the velocity profile downstream so that the manometer tip is in the centre of a high velocity jet, where addition (if pressure is measured end-on to the direction of flow) or subtraction (if pressure is measured side-on) of a kinetic energy component will distort the recorded pressure wave (see p. 118).

One cannot eliminate physiological reactance but one can minimise the inaccuracies which result, by awareness of its existence. One aims to have the effects of physiological reactance within the unavoidable noise level of the instrument.

ARTEFACT IN RECORDINGS OF ARTERIAL WAVES

Artefacts are legion and arise from many sources. The most troubling artefact is that which is associated with the heart beat and so affects the shape of each recorded wave in the same way. Sources of artefact are often obvious and correctable, such as movement of a catheter outside a blood vessel, or obvious and uncorrectable, such as sudden movement of a catheter within the chambers of the heart as the heart contracts. Artefacts in pressure recording often result from intermittent kinking of the catheter or from presence of a thrombus which acts as a valve at the tip of the catheter. A catheter from which blood cannot readily be drawn cannot be relied upon to transmit an accurate pressure wave. Artefacts in diameter recording may result from tethering of the vessel wall or from movement of the transducer so that it is not aligned at right angles to the vessel wall. Artefact in flow may result from movement of the flow catheter within the artery or from imperfect contact between the cuff and arterial wall throughout the cardiac cycle. Flow artefact can also result from alteration in magnetic field strength caused by the presence of ferrous metal in the region of the transducer, from inadequate earthing, or from 'pick-up' of the electrocardiographic signal by the transducer's electrodes (Wetterer 1962). Any unexpected finding in recordings of arterial pressure, flow or diameter waves should be attributed to artefact until this can be excluded.

One of the most potent sources of apparent artefact in pressure recording, when this is being measured together with flow, is the interconversion of pressure to kinetic energy at high flow velocity. This results in lateral pressure being reduced at peak flow velocity with respect to end-on or impact pressure. Consideration of this subject will be deferred until chapter 8 since it raises the important but still contentious issue of whether impact or lateral pressure should be related to flow in determination of vascular impedance and resistance.

REFERENCES

Anliker M 1978 Diagnostic analysis of arterial flow pulses in man. In: Baan J, Noordergraaf A, Raines J(eds) Cardiovascular system dynamics Cambridge (Mass) MIT Press 113–123

Arndt JO 1969 Uber die Mechanik der Intakten A carotis communis Des Menschen unter verschiedenen Kreislaufbedingungen. Archives Kreislaufforschg 59: 153–197

Barnes RW, Bone GE, Reinerston J, Slaymaker EE, Hokanson DE, Strandness DE Jr 1976 Noninvasive ultrasonic carotid angiography: prospective validation by contrast arteriography. Surgery 80: 328–335

Barnett GO, Greenfield JC Jr., Fox SM 1961 The technique of estimating the instantaneous aortic blood velocity in man from the pressure gradient. American Heart Journal 62: 359–366

Bergel DH 1972 The measurement of lengths and dimensions. In: Bergel DH Cardiovascular fluid dynamics. Academic Press London p. 91–115

Busse R, Bauer RD, Schabert A, Summa Y, Bumm P, Wetterer E 1979 The mechanical properties of exposed human common carotid arteries in vivo. Basic Research in Cardiology 74: 545–554

Busse R, Pasch TH 1978 Ultraschall-Doppler-Diagnostik der Extremitatenarterien 1. Physiologie, Pathophysiologie, Diagnostik In: Ultraschall-Doppler-Diagnostik in der Angiologie. Kriessmann A, Bollinger A (eds) Georg Thieme Verlag Stuttgart p. 1–8

Fry DL 1959 Measurement of pulsatile blood flow by the computed pressure gradient technique, IRE Transactions on Medical Electronics ME6 259–264

Fry DL 1960 Physiologic recording by modern instruments with particular reference to pressure recording. Physiological Reviews 40: 753–788

Gabe IT 1972 Pressure measurement in experimental physiology. In: Bergel DH (ed) Cardiovascular fluid dynamics. Academic Press London p. 11–50

Gessner U, Bergel DH 1964 Frequency response of electromagnetic flowmeters. Journal of Applied Physiology 19: 1209–1211

Goodman AH 1966 Electronic dynamic calibration of electromagnetic flowmeters. Journal of Applied Physiology 21: 933–937

Gow BS 1966 An electrical caliper for measurement of pulsatile arterial diameter changes in vivo. Journal of Applied Physiology 21: 1122–1126

Gow BS 1980 Circulatory correlates: vascular impedance, resistance and capacity. In: Bohr D and Somlyo D (eds)

Handbook of Physiology Section 2 The cardiovascular system Vol 2 vascular smooth muscle, American Physiological Society Maryland p. 353–408

Hansen AT, Warburg E 1950 A theory for elastic liquid containing membrane manometers. Acta Physiological Scandinavica 19: 306–332

Hokanson DE, Mozersky DJ, Sumner DS, Strandness DE Jr 1972 A phase-locked echo tracking system for recording arterial diameter changes in vivo. Journal of Applied Physiology 32: 728–733

Kalmanson D, Veyrat C 1979 Echo-Doppler velocimetry in cardiology. In: Hwang NHC, Gross DR, Patel DJ Quantitative cardiovascular studies p. 689–714 University Park Baltimore

Kenner T, Hinghofer-Szalkay H 1981 Cardiovascular system dynamics: models and measurements. Plenum (IN PRESS)

Kolin A 1978 New approaches to electromagnetic measurement of blood flow and vasomotion without recourse to surgery. In: Bauer RD and Busse R The arterial system, Springer Berlin 122–150

McAlpin RN, Kolin A, Stein JJ 1976 The external field intravascular electromagnetic flowmeter system as applied to standard arteriographic catheters and conscious humans. Catheterisation in Cardiovascular Diagnosis 2: 23–37

McDonald DA 1955 The relation of pulsatile pressure to flow in arteries. Journal of Physiology, (London) 127: 533–552

McDonald DA 1974 Blood flow in arteries, 2nd edn London Arnold

Mills CJ 1972 Measurement of pulsatile flow and flow velocity. In: Bergel DH (ed) Cardiovascular fluid dynamics Academic Press London p. 51–90

Mills CJ, Shillingford JP 1967 A catheter tip electromagnetic velocity probe and its evaluation. Cardiovascular Research 1: 263–273

Murgo JP 1975 Multisensor cardiac catheterisation: new methods to study cardiovascular dynamics in man. Proceedings 28th ACEMB p. 503

Murgo JP, Giolma JP, Altobelli SA 1977 Physiologic signal acquisition and processing for human hemodynamic research in a clinical cardiac catheterisation laboratory. Proceedings of the IEEE 65: 696–702

Murgo JP, Millar H 1972 A new cardiac catheter for high fidelity differential pressure recordings. 25th ACEMB Bal Harbour Florida p. 303

Murgo JP, Westerhof N, Giolma JP, Altobelli SA 1980 Aortic input impedance in normal man: relationship to pressure waveshapes. Circulation 62: 105–116

O'Rourke MF 1965 Dynamic accuracy of the electromagnetic flowmeter. Journal of Applied Physiology 20: 142–147

O'Rourke MF 1967 Pressure and flow waves in systemic arteries and the anatomical design of the arterial system. Journal of Applied Physiology 23: 139–149

O'Rourke MF 1968 Impact pressure, lateral pressure and impedance in the proximal aorta and pulmonary artery. Journal of Applied Physiology 25: 533–541

O'Rourke MF 1981 Vascular Impedance: a call for standardisation. In: Kenner T, Hinghoffer-Szalkay Berlin Plenum (in press)

Pasch TH, Bauer RD, Busse R 1976 Determination of arterial input impedance spectra from non-invasively recorded pulses. Basic Research in Cardiology 71: 229–242

Patel DJ, Mason DT, Ross J Jr. Braunwald E 1965 Harmonic analyses of pressure pulses obtained from the heart and great vessels of man. American Heart Journal 69: 785–000

Reneman RS (ed) 1974 Cardiovascular applications of ultrasound. American Elsevier New York

Roberts C (ed) 1972 Blood flow measurement. Sector London

Safar ME, Peronneau PA, Levenson JA, Toto-Moukouo JA, Simon A 1981 Pulsed doppler: Diameter, blood flow velocity and volumic flow of the brachial artery in sustained essential hypertension. Circulation 63: 393–400

Schostal SJ, Krovetz LJ, Rowe RD 1972 An analysis of errors in conventional cardiac catheterisation data, American Heart Journal 83: 596–603

Shirer HW 1962 Blood pressure measuring methods. IRE Transactions on Biomedical Electronics 9: 116–125

Strandness DE, Sumner DS 1975 Hemodynamics for surgeons. New York, Grune and Stratton p. 21–46

Summa Y 1978 Determination of the tangential elastic modulus of human arteries in vivo. In: Bauer RD, Busse R (eds) The arterial system. Springer Berlin p. 95–100

Thompson JE, Garrett WV 1980 Peripheral-arterial surgery New England Journal of Medicine 302: 491–503

Verdouw PD, Lancee CT, Krauss XH, Hugenholtz PG 1978 New invasive techniques in cardiology: multiple sensors. In: Baan J, Noordergraaf A, Raines J (eds) Cardiovascular System Dynamics. Cambridge (Mass) MIT press p. 543–552

Wetterer E 1962 A critical appraisal of methods of blood flow determination in Animals and Man. IRE Transactions on Biomedical Electronics 9: 165–173

Wetterer E, Busse R, Bauer RD, Schabert A, Summa Y 1977 Photoelectric device for contact-free recording of the diameters of exposed arteries in situ. Pflugers Archives 368: 149–152

Womersley JR 1955 Method for the calculation of velocity, rate of flow and viscous drag in arteries when the pressure gradient is known. Journal of Physiology (London) 127: 553–563.

3

Physical properties of blood and arteries

The properties of the whole arterial system are a consequence of arterial geometry and of the physical properties of arterial walls and contained blood. Physical laws and principles which involve these are discussed in Chapter 4. Effects of differences in vascular geometry are considered in Chapter 11. It is proposed here to consider the properties themselves – the viscosity and density of blood and the distensibility and viscoelasticity of the arterial wall.

VISCOSITY

Concept and history

Fluid viscosity was first described by Issac Newton in his Principia Mathematica, as *defectus lubricatis* – a defect of slipperiness or type of internal friction between adjacent laminae of moving fluid (McDonald 1974). Hales' classical book 'Statical Essays containing Hemostatics' was published in 1733, shortly after Newton's death. His earlier book 'Vegetable Status' had been published under Newton's authority as President of the Royal Society (Hales 1727, Manuel 1968). It is interesting that the idea of peripheral vascular resistance that Hales conceived was dependent on a property of blood that his colleague had first described. There was little further application of the concept of viscosity to circulatory phenomena for over 100 years when the French Physician Poiseuille published in 1842 his studies of liquid flow in narrow tubes and established that flow depends on a constant related to viscosity and on the fourth power of the radius (see Ch. 4). Progress during the present century continued with the development of viscometers (Hess 1911, Hatschek 1928), with the observation by Hess that blood has anomalous viscous properties, and with emergence of the discipline of rheology as the study of deformation and flow of solids and liquids. Excellent recent reviews of this subject are given by Bayliss (1962), Merrill (1969), La Celle and Weed (1971), McDonald (1974), Chien (1975), and Schmid-Schönbien (1976). Clinical interest in blood viscosity has increased following identification of diseases characterised by plasma protein abnormalities, and whose clinical features are attributable to abnormally high blood viscosity in small blood vessels (Wells, 1970) and of a mechanical technique (plasma exchange) that can promptly alleviate these symptoms. In addition, demonstration of impaired blood flow with increased viscosity in borderline as well as definite polycythemia (Humphrey et al 1979), has given new respectability to old therapies – the lancet and the leech.

Measurement of viscosity

Viscosity of a fluid is measured by relating shear stress to shear rate when the fluid is moving in concentric or parallel laminae. The unit of viscosity is the poise (after Poiseuille) which is 1 dyne sec cm^{-2}. (A liquid has a viscosity of 1 poise if a shearing force of 1 dyne cm^{-2} needs to be applied between two surfaces separated by 1 cm of the liquid in order to maintain a velocity difference of 1 cm sec^{-1} between the two surfaces). Water has a viscosity of 0.01 poise at about 20°C.

The two principal types of viscosity measuring device are the capillary tube and rotational viscometer. The capillary tube viscometer is the simplest instrument. In this, viscosity is measured from the time taken for a known pressure to force a given volume of the fluid through the tube. Viscosity of this fluid is usually expressed relative to that of water, but the instrument can be calibrated in absolute terms. The disadvantage of this system is that it is unsuitable for measurement of viscosity of suspensions – such as blood – because of axial streaming of the component particles (the Fahraeus Lindqvist effect – see below), because of sedimentation of particles, and because rate of shear is not constant over the cross section of the capillary tube.

The rotational viscometer has been designed to apply an almost uniform rate of shear across the fluid tested. The most popular instrument is the cone in plate viscometer. In this, viscosity is determined at different shear rates (altered by changing speed of rotation) from torque required to spin a cone separated from an opposing plate by a thin layer of the fluid.

Homogenous fluids show a constant relationship between shear stress and shear rate i.e. their viscosity is constant at all shear rates. These fluids are said to be newtonian (after Newton). They obey the laws stated by him in the *Principia*. Water is a newtonian fluid; so is serum; blood is not.

Blood viscosity

General

Blood viscosity depends on the separate contributions of plasma and of cellular elements, and on the interaction between cellular elements and plasma proteins. Red cells are far more numerous than leucocytes and platelets. These latter elements provide an impediment to blood flow when they adhere to vessel walls; they assume importance in determining viscosity only when abnormally abundant – as in leukemia. Under normal circumstances the red cells and plasma proteins are the major determinants of blood viscosity.

Viscosity of plasma is usually around 1.6 times that of water. Viscosity is higher than water on account of its component macro molecules – the plasma proteins, particularly the high molecular weight globulins and fibrinogen. The viscosity of plasma without fibrinogen is constant at different rates of shear i.e. it is a Newtonian fluid. With fibrinogen, viscosity increases slightly at low shear

rates because the long macro molecules tend to adhere.

The contribution of red cells to blood viscosity is discussed in a number of recent reviews (La Celle and Weed 1971, Chien 1975). Schmid Schönbein (1976) gives a fascinating account of functional and teleological considerations of red cell size, shape and content. Containment of hemoglobin within the red cell results in the minimal (asymptotic) value of blood viscosity being just over twice that of plasma – about 3.5 – 5cP. This value is relatively low on account of the high degree of deformability of the red cells. The fact that red cell deformability is an important factor in normal blood flow is obvious when one considers that average red cell diameter in man of $7 \mu m$ is greater than average capillary diameter (around $5 \mu m$) (Wells 1970).

Presence of red cells in blood is responsible for its non newtonian behaviour – the dependence of whole blood viscosity on rate of shear (Fig. 3.1). Below 50 sec^{-1}, viscosity of whole blood rises steeply; above this value viscosity is relatively constant, decreasing only slightly with increasing rate of shear. The high viscosity at low shear rates is

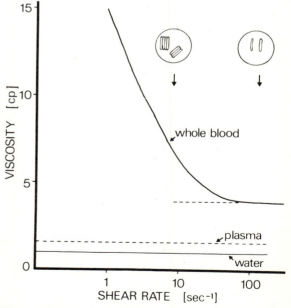

Fig. 3.1 Relationship between viscosity (ordinate) in centipoise (cP) and shear rate (abscissa) for water, plasma, and whole blood with hematocrit 45%. Inset is shown diagrammatically the form of red cells at 1 and 100 sec^{-1}

dependent on high molecular weight proteins in plasma, being far less pronounced when these are removed from blood, and far more pronounced when present in abnormal amounts (McGrath and Penny, 1976, 1978) (Fig. 3.2). This property of blood is readily explained on the basis of reversible aggregation of red cells at low shear rates – such aggregation being facilitated by the high molecular weight globulins. Above 100 sec^{-1}, red cells are completely separate and move either as biconcave disks or as 'parachute' forms (Fig. 3.1, Chien 1975). This slight further fall in viscosity over 100 sec^{-1}, is attributable to further deformation of the red cells, with more assuming the 'parachute' shape.

Increase in red cell content leads to increase in the asymptotic and shear-dependent values of blood viscosity (Fig. 3.2). The relationship between viscosity and hematocrit is non-linear (but almost linear when viscosity is plotted on a logarithmic scale, as in Fig. 3.3). Viscosity is nearly doubled with increase in hematocrit from 40 to 50% (Fig. 3.3).

Viscosity of blood – as of other fluids – is increased when temperature decreases (Fig. 3.2). This effect is quite appreciable, with an increase in viscosity of approximately 25 per cent when temperature falls from 37° to 25°C (Merrill et al 1963, Rand et al 1964, McGrath and Penny 1978).

NORMAL BLOOD VISCOSITY

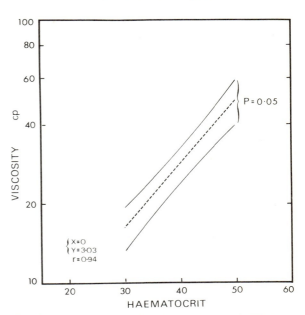

Fig. 3.3 Semi-logarithmic plot of the relationship between hematocrit and blood viscosity, measured at a shear rate of 0.18 sec^{-1} and temperature of 35°C. The linear regression line and tolerance limits for p = 0.05 are shown. From Mc Grath (1974)

Effects of blood viscosity on pressure/flow relationships

When the effects of autoregulation are abolished in a vascular bed, and the bed is perfused with saline or with plasma, there is a linear relationship between arteriovenous pressure difference and blood flow (Whittaker and Winton 1933, Bayliss 1962, Fig. 3.4) This is what one would expect with Newtonian fluids. When however the bed is perfused with blood, the relationship becomes non-linear at low flow rates. (Fig. 3.4). This is attributable to the non-newtonian properties of blood with increasing viscosity at low shear and low flow rates. Such non-linear pressure/flow relationships have been noted in other vascular beds, with flow becoming infinitesimally small at relatively high pressures, particularly when arteriolar tone is high, and calibre, narrow, (Burton 1962). Such behaviour has been attributed by Burton to critical closing pressure of arterioles. While this may be the case, very high blood viscosity at

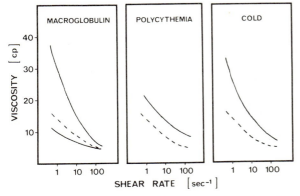

Fig. 3.2 Effects of altered macroglobulin level, polycythemia, and cold on blood viscosity at different shear rates.
Left: Dotted line, normal blood; lower line – macroglobulin removed from normal blood; top line – blood from patient with macroglobulinemia
Center: Dotted line, normal blood; solid line, blood from patient with polycythemia
Right: Dotted line, normal blood at 37°C; solid line, normal blood at 20°C

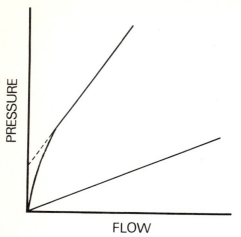

Fig. 3.4 Relationship between pressure gradient (ordinate) across a vascular bed, and flow (abcissa) through the bed. Lower line – perfusion with plasma. Upper line – perfusion with blood. Dotted line shows intercept on pressure axis of straight section of upper line

very low shear rates could cause a similar effect. There is still contention as to whether blood has a yield stress under some circumstances – whether blood behaves as a solid below a given stress, and as a fluid above. Presence of a yield stress for blood could also account for a pressure flow curve showing a positive intercept on the pressure axis (Whitmore 1968).

The pressure gradient/steady flow curve for blood in Figure 3.4 raises another point that may be considered here. Resistance of a vascular bed is calculated from individual points on such a curve. The concept of resistance assumes that steady pressure gradient across the bed and flow are linearly related – i.e. that the relationship is linear and passes through the origin. It is quite clear that this is not the case and that the inherent non linearity must be considered in interpreting values of resistance calculated from single values of pressure and flow.

There is one unusual property of blood that affects its viscosity in narrow tubes (less than 300 μm diameter) and in a vascular bed. This was first demonstrated and explained by Fahraeus and Lindqvist (1931) who showed that apparent viscosity of blood (viscosity relative to that of water) is lower in narrow tubes, and in a vascular bed, than when tested in other viscometers. In a vascu-

lar bed, a given pressure gradient created a higher flow than would have been expected from measurements of blood viscosity in conventional viscometers. They attributed this to axial streaming of red cells, so that cellular content was lower at the edge of the tube where (with a parabolic velocity profile) most shear was taking place. Thus, functional resistance to flow was determined mainly by the cell-poor peripheral part of the blood stream in these small vessels. This obviously desirable phenomenon – referred to as the Fahraeus Lindqvist effect – has been confirmed repeatedly (Chien 1975, Schmid Shönbein 1976) and has been shown to depend on the easily deformable properties of the red cells. It is not seen when red cells lose their deformability – as in spherocytosis.

Hyperviscosity syndromes in clinical practice

Blood viscosity is increased in conditions characterised by increased numbers of red cells (polycythemia), by decreased deformability of red cells, or by abnormal macroglobulins (Wells 1970, McGrath 1981, McGrath and Penny 1976). Abnormalities of or increased numbers of red cells increase the asymptotic value of viscosity (above 50 sec[1]) whereas plasma globulin abnormalities have their greatest effect on viscosity at shear rates below 50 sec[1]. Shear rates in all blood vessels are usually in excess of this figure (Whitmore 1968). Shear rates are lowest in venules and veins, particularly when blood flow is decreased by other factors, such as arteriolar vasoconstriction associated with cold. Clinical features of hyperglobulinemias are attributable to hyperviscosity and sludging of blood in venules and veins, with resulting impaired tissue blood flow. As might be expected, these features are often most apparent in the extremities, and in cold weather where increased viscosity due to lowered temperature potentiates the effect of red cell aggregation on viscosity. The problems also tend to be self perpetuating with increased viscosity causing impaired tissue flow, and impaired flow causing further increase in viscosity. The clinical features of these conditions are alleviated – often dramatically –, though temporarily, by plasma exchange (Isbister 1979). Primary red cell abnormalities – decreased deformability and increased numbers – affect predominantly the asymptotic value of blood viscosity, rather than the value at low shear rates. Clinical features due to hyperviscosity appear to be related to increased resistance in arterioles, with hypertension and decreased organ flow. These features are alleviated by bleeding (in polycythemia) and by alteration of cellular rigidity where this is possible.

Blood viscosity in arteries

It appears that the anomalous properties of blood (increased viscosity at low shear rate, Fahraeus Lindqvist effect) are not relevant to consideration of pulsatile pressure/flow relationships under normal conditions in arteries where calibre is wider, and peak flow, greater than in vessels in which such viscous properties become apparent. This was the conclusion reached by Taylor (1959, 1960) from his calculations based on experimental data of Kumin (1949), and of Kuntz and Coulter (1967) on the basis of experimental studies. This subject is discussed further by McDonald (1974). Also as discussed by McDonald (1974), it is difficult to know how to handle the shear-dependent properties of blood in large arteries when shear rate is low across most of the vessel for most of the cardiac cycle (because velocity profile is flat) and where there may be no blood flow at all during diastole. It appears however that cell aggregation and consequent increased blood viscosity are not seen in arteries where flow is pulsatile.

It is probably reasonable under normal conditions to use the asymptotic value of blood viscosity (3.5–5cP) in calculations of pulsatile blood flow in arteries, and a slightly lesser value (due to Fahraeus Lindqvist effect) in the smaller vessels of a whole vascular bed.

BLOOD DENSITY

Happily, the value of blood density is very close to that of water and varies little with changes in hematocrit or plasma protein concentration. The value used in calculations for this book is 1.05 g cm^{-3} (McDonald 1974).

ARTERIAL DISTENSIBILITY

An obvious feature of arteries is that they are distensible, so that the artery expands passively during systole, and shrinks passively during diastole. So obvious is this, and so constant with each beat of the heart, that one would expect the concepts and interpretation of arterial distensibility to be simple and straightforward, and free from substantial controversy. Unfortunately this is not the case and the subject can be very confusing. Confusion arises from a number of sources including terminology, indices used for description of arterial distensibility, non-linear elastic properties of any artery, non-uniform elastic properties of different arteries, difficulties in accurate measurement of arterial diameter, relaxation in muscle of excised arteries, retraction of excised arteries, the differing effects of smooth muscle on wall elasticity and arterial diameter, and viscosity of the arterial wall. The account to be given here is a simplified one. More detailed recent accounts include McDonald (1974), Roach (1977), Bergel (1978), Dobrin (1978), Patel and Vaishnav (1980) and Gow (1980).

Structure of the arterial wall

The distensibility of arteries depends predominantly on the elastic fibres within the arterial walls. Other components of the wall – collagen fibres, smooth muscle cells, and non-fibrous mucoprotein matrix also contribute to the elastic properties, particularly in the smaller vessels. The relative composition of different components in the arterial wall depends on location:– the central arteries (especially the proximal aorta) contain a higher proportion of elastin, and the peripheral arteries more collagen and smooth muscle.

In the proximal aorta, elastin is arranged in concentric sheets or lamellae within the media. Histological texts usually show these elastic lamellae as wavy lines. This appearance is a consequence of the artery being fixed for examination when unstretched; when the artery is fixed while distended at physiological pressures, these lamellae are straight (Wolinsky and Glagov 1964, 1967). In the aorta the thick elastic lamellae appear to form concentric plates which are separated by smooth muscle cells together with collagen and elastic fibrils embedded in mucoprotein. The fibrils and cells are orientated in an oblique pattern between the circumferentially arranged lamellae. The elastic fibrils reach across obliquely to join adjacent elastic lamellae. The smooth muscle cells are attached to the elastic fibrils and to the thicker elastic lamellae. The collagenous fibrils reach between the elastic fibrils in a concentric pattern which has a helical pattern of small pitch. Such an arrangement (Wolinsky and Glagov 1964) explains the elastic properties of the aorta with stress being distributed between the elastic lamellae through the interconnecting elastic fibrils at physiological distending pressures, and being applied to the less extensible collagenous fibrils at higher distending pressures (Roach and Burton 1957). The aortic adventitia has few elastic fibrils; its collagenous fibres are arranged in loose bundles without any consistent alignment. It is generally assumed that the adventitia plays little part in the mechanical properties of the arterial wall over the physiological range.

In peripheral arteries, the elastic lamellar structure of the aorta is lost. Elastic sheets remain as the internal and external elastic laminae which separate the media from intima and adventitia respectively. The media is made up predominantly of muscle cells with smaller, thinner elastic fibrils and thicker, more numerous collagen fibres. Orientation of the fibres and muscle cells appears to be similar to that in the proximal aorta (Bloom and Fawcett 1968, Robertson 1977, Rhodin 1980).

Chemical studies of arterial composition corroborate the histological features (Harkness and McDonald 1955, Cleary 1963, McDonald 1974). Most of the wall is water; half of the dry weight is collagen or elastin. In the proximal aorta the ratio of elastin to collagen is approximately 70:30, but in the distal aorta the ratio reverses and in peripheral arteries it is close to 40:60 (Fig. 3.5). Chemical treatment of arteries was performed by Roach and Burton (1957) to dissolve differentially the elastin and collagenous components of the wall in reaching the conclusions, noted above, that elastin predominantly determiness distensibility at low and normal pressure, and collagen at very high pressures.

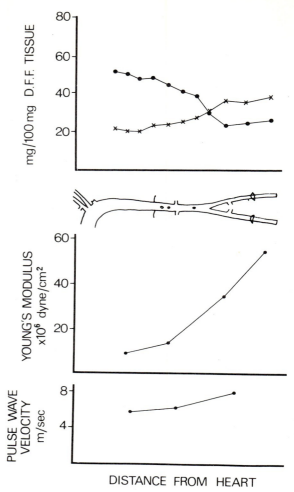

Fig. 3.5 Change in chemical content and in physical properties between central and peripheral arteries.
Top: Elastin content (closed circles) and collagen content (crosses) of arteries between the proximal thoracic aorta (left) and femoral artery (right) of a 22 year old man. Values are in mg/100 mg dry fat free tissue (after Cleary, 1963)
Center: Young's modulus of segments of proximal thoracic aorta, abdominal aorta, iliac artery and femoral artery of young human subjects (after Learoyd and Taylor, 1966)
Bottom: Pulse wave velocity over the thoracic aorta, abdominal aorta and iliac artery of young human subjects (after Learoyd and Taylor, 1966)

Implications of the 'two phase' content of the arterial wall are discussed by Wolinsky and Glagov (1964). These include high distensibility over the physiological range of arterial pressures, high tensile strength at abnormally high pressures, and protection of the collagen fibres against yield and rupture at points of possible structural defects through presence and alignment of the elastic fibrils. These properties of the arterial wall and the further contribution of smooth muscle are of obvious relevance in the pathogenesis of aneurysms and arterial degeneration and will be discussed in Chapters 12–14.

Measurement of distensibility

Arteries are referred to as being 'elastic'. In using this term one must immediately introduce two caveats. A perfectly elastic body is one which obey's Hooke's law '*Ut tensio, sic vis*' (as the extension so the force). Arteries are not perfectly elastic; the stretch/strain diagram is concave towards the pressure axis (Fig. 3.6), with small changes of pressure at low distending pressure causing relatively large extension, and similar changes at high distending pressure causing relatively little stretch. This is attributed to the different loading of different components of the arterial wall. The artery is said to have non-linear elastic properties. This term (non-linear elasticity) should not be confused with the term 'non-uniform elasticity' which refers not to the properties of an artery at one point, but to the decreasing distensibility of the arterial system between the proximal aorta and peripheral arteries (Taylor 1967). The second caveat is in the term itself. The biologist is apt to

consider 'increased elasticity' to mean 'increased distensibility' but the 'increased elasticity' really means 'more rigid'. A 'more elastic' material has a higher Young's modulus; it is less deformable. To avoid confusion it is better not to talk in terms of altered elasticity but rather in terms of greater or lesser distensibility.

Distensibility of an arterial segment is measured from the change in radius, diameter or circumference induced by a change in lateral pressure. This is best expressed in terms of the Young's modulus, the standard term for extensibility in the physical sciences. Young's modulus is a theoretic concept and refers to the stress that must be applied to a material to induce 100 per cent elongation. No material has uniform elastic properties over such a range so that Young's modulus is measured from small changes in pressure and elongation.

Young's modulus only applies strictly to materials which are homogeneous and have a constant relationship between stress and strain – i.e. that obey Hooke's law. As explained, arteries do not obey Hooke's law, being less distensible at high pressures and more distensible at low pressures. When Young's modulus or any index of distensibility is given for an artery, it refers to the relationship between small stress and small strain at a given mean pressure. The implication is that the arterial wall obeys Hooke's law over small pressure and diameter changes; different Young's moduli will be calculated at different mean pressures and diameters.

If say, the descending thoracic aorta of a human were found to have a radius of 1.0 cm and a wall thickness of 0.1 cm, and to be distended 10 per cent by a pressure pulse of 120/80 mmHg, then an incremental Young's modulus at this mean pressure can be calculated as follows:–

Change in pressure = $40 \times 0.1 \times 980 \times 13.6 = 5.332 \times 10^4$ dyne cm^{-2}

Change in wall tension = $5.332 \times 10^4 \times 1.0$ dynes (From La Place's law)

This altered wall tension is applied to a strip 0.1 cm thick, so that total wall tension = 5.332×10^5 dyne cm^2

This produces extension of 10 per cent

∴ Tension for 100% extension = 5.332×10^6 dyne cm^{-2}

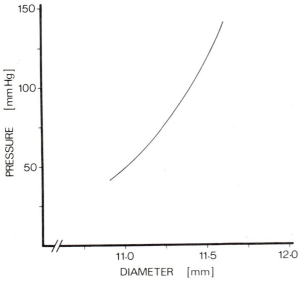

Fig. 3.6 Non-linear relationship between distending pressure and arterial diameter (after Busse et al, 1979)

and so Young's modulus = 5.332×10^6 dyne cm^{-2}

When dealing with cylindrical structures such as arteries, it is often more convenient to express distensibility directly in terms of pressure change and diameter change. The most popular such index is Peterson's pressure/strain modulus (Peterson et al 1960), usually referred to as Ep. This takes no account of wall geometry (absolute diameter and wall thickness). It describes the pressure required for (theoretic) 100 per cent increase in diameter.

$$Ep = \triangle p \times \frac{D}{\triangle D}$$

For the same artery as described above
$\triangle p = 40$ mmHg = 5.332×10^4 dyne cm^{-2}
This causes 10 per cent distention
$\therefore$ For 100% distention, Ep = 5.332×10^5
dyne cm^{-2}

Distensibility of different arteries

Values of Young's modulus and Ep for different arteries are given in Table 3.1. These all vary between the theoretic value for pure elastin and that for pure collagen, with modulus and Ep of the proximal aorta being lowest and that of peripheral arteries highest, some four times that in the proximal aorta. This is what one would expect on the basis of differences in histological structure and chemical content. As discussed in the next chapter, arterial distensibility is the major factor in determining pulse wave velocity. Pulse wave velocity increases progressively between the central aorta and peripheral arteries. Figure 3.5 shows changes in chemical content, Young's modulus and pulse wave velocity between central and peripheral arteries. Implications of these changes

in structure and function between arteries close to and far from the heart have been analysed by Taylor (Taylor 1967, 1969 a,b) and will be discussed in Chapter 10.

Contribution of smooth muscle to arterial distensibility

It was once considered that smooth muscle plays no significant role in the mechanical properties of arteries (Torrance and Schwartz 1961). This was based on the finding that elastic properties were similar before and after paralysis of smooth muscle with potassium thiocyanate. More recent and precise studies however have shown that smooth muscle tone does contribute to the elastic properties of the wall, and that drugs or chemicals that stimulate or relax muscle tone do appreciably alter Young's modulus.

Findings are confusing since these interventions alter arterial caliber as well as distensibility. It is generally agreed that at the same transmural pressure, the relaxed vessel has a higher elastic modulus (i.e. is less distensible) and the constricted vessel has a lower elastic modulus (i.e. is more distensible), (Dobrin and Rovick 1969, Gow 1972, 1980, Cox 1976, Bergel 1978). Controversy has arisen when comparisons were made at the same strain, (Dobrin and Rovick 1969, Dobrin (1978), Gow 1980). The most recent appraisal suggests that at the same strain, the same conclusions apply as for pressure – i.e. that the relaxed vessel is less distensible, and the constricted vessel more distensible (Gow 1980). Alterations in arterial distensibility and diameter caused by change in arterial smooth muscle tone may explain a number of matters presently under close clinical investigation –

Table 3.1: Young's modulus, pressure/strain modulus (Ep), and pulse wave velocity in experimental animals and young human subjects. From a variety of sources, summarised by McDonald (1974)

SITE	YOUNG'S MODULUS (dyne cm^{-2})	'Ep' (dyne cm^{-2})	PULSE WAVE VELOCITY (cm sec^{-1})
Ascending Aorta		$(.34-1.47) \times 10^6$	400–500
Descending Thoracic Aorta	$(3.0-9.4) \times 10^6$	$(.40-1.55) \times 10^6$	400–700
Abdominal Aorta	$(9.8-14.2) \times 10^6$	$(1.54-2.40) \times 10^6$	550–850
Iliac Artery	$(11.0-35.0) \times 10^6$	$(2.76-9.62) \times 10^6$	700–800
Femoral Artery	$(12.3-55.0) \times 10^6$	$(1.69-3.26) \times 10^6$	800–1,300

the apparently high characteristic aortic impedance in patients with heart failure, the apparent reduction of aortic impedance by vasodilator drugs, and the subtle beneficial effects of these drugs that cannot be attributed to arteriolar or venular dilation (Pepine et al 1978). This is discussed further in Chapters 10 and 16.

Apart from this effect on arterial distensibility, smooth muscle contributes much to arterial viscosity – that property of the arterial wall which is responsible for the delay between applied pressure and resulting diameter change. Stimulation of smooth muscle results in greater delay of arterial diameter change after applied pressure change, indicating increased viscosity of the wall (Gow 1980).

ARTERIAL VISCOSITY

All components of the arterial wall contribute to its viscosity. However because of their bulk and consistency, muscle and gelatinous mucoprotein undoubtedly play the major role. Arterial viscosity

results in a small but definite lag of pulsatile diameter change behind applied pressure, and hysteresis when pressure and diameter are plotted against each other on the X and Y axes of an oscilloscope screen (Fig. 2.3). An inevitable consequence of this viscosity is that for a given pressure change, the diameter change will be less under dynamic conditions than under static conditions. In other words, arterial viscosity contributes to the frequency-dependence of Young's modulus (Bergel 1961a,b). A further consequence is that wave velocity (which is determined by arterial viscoelasticity) is also frequency-dependent. Fortunately these effects are very small and Young's modulus determined under dynamic conditions at physiological frequencies is rarely more than 10–20 per cent greater than determined under static or near static conditions (Bergel 1961a,b). The major effect of wall viscosity is to dampen the arterial pulse wave; this effect is similar in magnitude to that caused by viscosity of blood within the vessel (Taylor 1966). Detailed discussion of arterial viscosity is included in Bergel (1961a,b, 1972, 1978) and Gow (1980).

REFERENCES

Apter JT, Marquez E 1968 Correlation of visco-elastic properties of large arteries with microscopic structure. Circulation Research 22: 393–404.

Bauer RD, Busse R, Schabert A, Summa Y, Wetterer E 1979 Separate determination of the pulsatile elastic and viscous forces developed in the arterial wall in vivo. Pfluger's Archives 380: 221–226

Bayliss LE 1962 The rheology of blood. In: Handbook of Physiology, American Physiological Society, Washington D.C. Section 2 Circulation Vol. 1 Ch 8. p 139–150.

Bergel DH 1961a The static elastic properties of the arterial wall. Journal of Physiology (London) 156: 445–457

Bergel DH 1972 The properties of blood vessels. In: Fung YC (ed) Biomechanics Prentice Hill, New Jersey p 000

Bergel DH 1978 Mechanics of the arterial wall in health and disease. In: Bauer RD, Busse R (eds) The arterial system Springer Verlag Berlin 3–14

Bergel DH, Schultz DL 1971 Arterial elasticity and fluid dynamics Progress in Biophysics and Molecular Biology 22: 1–36

Bloom W, Fawcett DW 1968 A textbook of histology. Philadelphia Saunders p. 272–279

Burton AC 1962 Physical principles of circulatory phenomena. Handbook of Physiology American Physiological Society Washington DC Vol 2 Circulation No. 1 85–106

Busse R, Bauer RD, Summa Y, Korner H, Pasch TH 1976 Comparison of the viscoelastic properties of the tail artery in spontaneously hypertensive and normotensive rats. Pfluger's Archives 364: 175–181

Busse R, Bauer RD, Schabert A, Summa Y, Bumm P, Wetterer E 1979 The mechanical properties of exposed human common carotid arteries in vivo. Basic Research in Cardiology 74: 545–554

Chien S 1975 Biophysical behaviour of red cells in suspensions. In: Surgenor D Mac N (ed) The red blood cell 2nd edn, Ch. 26. New York, Academic Press p. 1031–1133

Chien S, Usami S, Taylor HM 1966 Effects of hematocrit and plasma proteins on human blood rheology at low shear rates. Journal of Applied Physiology 21: 81–87

Cleary E 1963 A correlative and comparative study of the non-uniform arterial wall. M.D. Thesis, University of Sydney

Cox RH 1976 Arterial wall mechanics and composition and the effects of smooth muscle activation. American Journal of Physiology 230: 462–470

Cox RH 1976 Effects of norepinephrine on mechanics of arteries in vitro. American Journal of Physiology 231: 420–425

Dintenfass L 1962 Considerations of the internal viscosity of red cells and its effect on the viscosity of whole blood. Angiology 13: 333–344

Dobrin PB, Rovick AA 1969 Influence of vascular smooth muscle on contractile mechanisms and elasticity of arteries. American Journal of Physiology 217: 1644–1651

Dobrin PB 1978 Mechanical properties of arteries. Physiological Reviews 58: 397–460

Fahey JL, Barth WF, Solomon A 1965 Serum hyperviscosity syndromes. Journal of the American Medical Association 192: 464–467

Fahraeus R, Lindqvist T 1931 Viscosity of blood in narrow capillary tubes. American Journal of Physiology 96: 562–568

Gow BS 1972 Influence of vascular smooth muscle on the visco elastic properties of blood vessels. In: Bergel DH (ed) Cardiovascular fluid dynamics. Academic Press New York p.65–110

Gow BS 1980 Circulatory correlates: impedance, resistance and capacity. In: Bohr DF, Somlyo AP, (eds) Handbook of Physiology, Section 2 The cardiovascular system, Vol. 2 Vascular smooth muscle, American Physiological Society Maryland p. 353–408

Gow BS, Hadfield CD 1979 The elasticity of canine and human coronary arteries with reference to postmortem changes. Circulation Research 45: 588–594

Hales S 1727 Vegetable statics. Republished 1961 London Scientific Book Guild

Hales S 1769 Statical essays. 3rd edition Wilson and Nichol, London

Hallock P, Benson IC 1937 Studies on the elastic properties of isolated human aorta. Journal of Clinical Investigation 5: 595–602

Haynes RH, Burton AC 1959 Role of the non-Newtonian behaviour of blood in hemodynamics. American Journal of Physiology 197: 943–950

Humphrey PRD, Du Bouly GH, Marshall J, Pearson TC, Ross-Russell RW, Symon L, Wetherley-Mein G, Zilkha E 1979 Cerebral blood flow and viscosity in relative polycythemia. Lancet 2: 873–878

Isbister J 1979 Plasma exchange: a selective form of bloodletting. Medical Journal of Australia 2: 167–173

Kuntz AL, Coulter NA Jr. 1967 Non-Newtonian behaviour of blood in oscillatory flow. Biophysical Journal 7: 25–36

La Celle PL, Weed R 1971 The contribution of normal and pathologic erythrocytes to blood rheology. Progress in Hematology 7: 1–31

Learoyd M, Taylor MG 1966 Alterations with age in the viscoelastic properties of human arterial walls. Circulation Research 18: 278–292

Manual FF 1968 A portrait of Isaac Newton. Harvard Cambridge

McDonald DA 1974 Blood flow in arteries. 2nd edn Arnold London

McGrath M 1974 A correlative study of haemorheological, Immunological and clinical parameters in disorders of blood flow. M.D. Thesis University of N.S.W.

McGrath M 1981 Blood viscosity in macroglobulinemia, multiple myeloma and polycythemia. In Dintenfass, L and Seaman, GVF (eds) Blood viscosity factors in heart disease, thromboembolism and cancer. In press

McGrath MA, Penny R 1976 Paraproteinemia. Blood hyperviscosity and clinical manifestations. Journal of Clinical Investigation 58: 1155–1162

McGrath MA, Verhaeghe RH, Shepherd JT 1980 the physiology of limb blood flow. In: Juergens JL, Spittell JA Jr, Fairburn JF Peripheral vascular diseases. Philadelphia Saunders p. 83–105

Merrill EW 1969 Rheology of blood Physiology Reviews 49: 863–887

Merrill EW, Gilliland ER, Cokelet G 1963 Rheology of human blood near and at zero flow: effects of temperature and hematocrit level. Biophysical Journal 3: 199–213

Merrill EW, Cokelet GC, Britten A, Wells RE 1963 Non-Newtonian rheology of human blood – effect of fibrinogen deduced by subtraction. Circulation Research 13: 48–55

Murphy JR 1967 The influence of pH and temperature on some physical properties of normal erythrocytes and erythrocytes from patients with hereditary spherocytosis. Journal of Laboratory and Clinical Medicine 69: 758–775

Nygaard KK, Wilder M, Berkson J 1935 The relation between viscosity of the blood and the relative volume of erythrocytes (hematocrit value). American Journal of Physiology 114: 128–131

Osserman EF 1979 Plasma cell dyscrasias. In: Beeson PB, McDermott W, Wyngaarden JB Cecil's Textbook of Medicine Saunders Philadelphia p. 1852–1867

Patel DJ, Janicki JS, Carew TE 1969 Static anisotropic elastic properties of the aorta in living dogs. Circulation Research 25: 765–779

Patel DJ, Vaishnav RN 1980 Basic hemodynamics and its role in disease processes. Baltimore University Park

Pepine CJ, Nichols WW, Conti CR 1978 Aortic input impedance in heart failure. Circulation 58: 460–465

Peterson LH, Jensen RE, Parnell J 1960 Mechanical properties of arteries in vivo. Circulation Research 8: 622–639

Rhodin JA 1980 Architecture of the vessel wall. In: Bohr DR, Somlyo AP, Sparks HV (eds) Handbook of Physiology Section 2 The cardiovascular system. Volume 2 Vascular smooth muscle American Physiological Society Maryland p. 1–31

Roach MR 1977 Biophysical analysis of blood vessel walls and blood flow. Annual Review of physiology 39: 51–71

Roach MR, Burton AC 1957 The reason for the shape of the distensibility curves of arteries. Canadian Journal of Biochemistry and Physiology 35:681–690

Robertson AL 1977 The pathogenesis of human atherosclerosis. In: Gross HL, Fites LL (eds) Atherosclerosis Kelamazoo Upjohn P. 38–41

Schmid-Schönbein H 1976 Microrheology of erythrocytes, blood viscosity, and the distribution of blood. flow in the microcirculation In: Guyton A, Cowley AW (eds) International Review of Physiology. Cardiovascular physiology II, Volume 9 Baltimore University Park P. 1–62

Schmid-Schönbein H, Fischer T, Driessen G, Rieger H 1979 Microcirculation. In: Hwang HC, Gross DR, Patel DJ (eds) Quantitative cardiovascular studies. Baltimore University Park P. 353–418

Schwartz CJ, Wethessen NT, Wolf S. 1980 Structure and function of the Circulation. New York Plenum

Solomon A, Fahey JL, 1963 Plasmaphoresis therapy in macroglobulinemia. Annals of Internal Medicine 58: 789–800

Stehbens WE 1979 Hemodynamics and the blood vessel wall. Thomas Springfield

Taylor MG 1966 The input impedance of an assembly of upon its oscillatory flow Physics in Medicine and Biology 3: 273–290

Taylor MG 1966(b) The input impedance of an assembly of randomly branching elastic tubes. Biophysical Journal 6: 29–51

Taylor MG 1967 The elastic properties of arteries in relation to the physiogical functions of the arterial system. Gastroenterology 52: 358–363

Taylor MG 1969 The optimum elastic properties of arteries. In: Wolstenholme GE, Knight J (eds) Ciba Foundation symposium on circulatory and respiratory mass transport, Churchill London P. 136–147

Taylor MG 1969 Arterial impedance and distensibility. In: Fishman AP, Hecht HH (eds) The Pulmonary Circulation and Interstitial space, The University of Chicago Chicago p. 341–354

Torrance HB, Schwatz 1961 The elastic behaviour of the arterial wall. Journal of the Royal College of Surgeons of Edinburgh 7: 55–60

Wayland H 1967 Rheology and the microcirculation. Gastroenterology 52: 342–355

Wells R 1970 Syndromes of hyperviscosity. New England Journal of Medicine 283: 183–186

Wells RE Jr, Merrill EW 1962 Influence of flow properties of blood upon viscosity – hematocrit relationships. Journal of Clinical Investigation 41: 1591–1598

Wetterer E and Pieper HP 1953 Ueber die Gesamtelastizitaet des arteriellen Windkessels und ein experinmentelles Verfahren zu ihrer Bestimmung an lebenden Tier. Zeitschrift fur Biol. 106–23

Whitmore RL 1968 Rheology of the Circulation. Pergamon Oxford

Whittaker SRF, Winton FR 1933 Apparent viscosity of blood flowing in the isolated hindlimb of the dog and its variation with corpuscular concentration. Journal of Physiology London 78: 339–369

Wolinsky H, Glagov S 1964 Structural basis for the static mechanical properties of the aortic media. Circulation Research 14: 400–413

Wolinsky H, Glagov S 1967 Alamellar unit of aortic medial structure and function in mammals. Circulation Research 20:. 99–000

Wolinsky H, Glagov S 1969 Comparison of abdominal and thoracic aortic structure in mammals. Deviation of man from the usual pattern Circulation Research 25: 677–686

Wolinsky H 1970 Comparison of medial growth of human thoracic and abdominal aortas. Circulation Research 27: 531–538

4

Physical principles and circulatory models

POISEUILLE'S LAW FOR STEADY FLOW

In 1842 the French physician J.M. Poiseuille reported his studies of fluid flow through small glass capillary tubes. Poiseuille had earlier developed methods for measuring the arterial pressure pulse. Poiseuille's later studies were done in order to understand better the factors which determine perfusion of peripheral tissues. He showed that fluid flow in these tubes varied inversely with length of the tube, directly with pressure difference between the two ends of the tube and directly with the fourth power of the tube's radius. His results were expressed by the formula:–

$$Q = \frac{K.P.D.^4}{L}$$

where Q = volume flow, P = pressure along the tube, D = diameter, L = length of the tube and K is a constant.

The form of Poiseuille's law as we now know it was determined from theoretic solution of viscous liquid flow in a cylindrical tube by Hagenbach in 1860 (McDonald 1974), as

$$Q = \frac{(P_1 - P_2).\pi.r^4}{8.\mu.L}$$

where r = radius of the tube and μ is viscosity in poises. The term $\frac{\pi}{128.\mu}$ is Poiseuille's constant K.

The conditions under which Poiseuille's law strictly applies are apparent in the way it is derived from theoretical principles (McDonald 1974). These are:
1. The tube under study is a cylinder which does not branch and does not taper

2. The tube is rigid so that diameter does not change with distending pressure
3. The tube is long compared with its inlet length
4. Flow is laminar and there is no turbulence and no secondary flow
5. Flow is steady and so not subject to accelerations or decelerations
6. The fluid is homogenous and so has no anomalous viscous properties
7. The fluid does not slip at the wall

The only one of these conditions which is fulfilled in the circulation is number 7. None of the rest strictly apply. Vessels do branch, they do expand, length of individual branches is short, some disturbed blood flow does occur during part of the cardiac cycle at least in the larger vessels, flow is pulsatile in arteries, blood is non-homogeneous and does have anomalous viscous properties in very small vessels and at very low shear rates (Ch. 3).

There seems to be every reason to expect that Poiseuille's Law would have no relevance to the circulation. And yet it has! In each individual small resistance vessel, blood flow is steady, and laminar. Blood viscosity is constant in these vessels (though of lower magnitude than in the larger vessels). Other things being equal, blood flow is determined almost exclusively by changes in arteriolar calibre, and small changes in arteriolar calibre cause large changes in blood flow. Poiseuille's law is implied when one relates steady blood flow through an artery to mean arteriovenous pressure gradient across its vascular bed, then expresses this relationship as resistance and attributes changes in resistance to alterations in arteriolar calibre.

This concept has found general acceptance

(Green and Rapela 1964, Levy 1979) even though as discussed in the last chapter, it fails to consider other factors that can disturb a linear relationship between arteriovenous pressure gradient and flow under some circumstances i.e. -autoregulation caused by altered arteriolar calibre, critical closure of blood vessels and increased viscosity of blood when flow is extremely low.

WOMERSLEY'S SOLUTION FOR PULSATILE FLOW

Poiseuille's Law was developed for individual capillary tubes where apparently limiting conditions apply and yet has been found relevant and useful in describing steady blood flow through a whole vascular bed at whose input pressure and flow are markedly pulsatile. It is therefore not surprising to find that similar considerations for pulsatile flow are useful in characterising pulsatile pressure/flow relationships in large arteries. This has been demonstrated by John Womersley for a single cylindrical tube similar to that used by Hagenbach in deriving the theoretical solution of Poiseuille's Law. Starting with the general Navier-Stokes equations of motion, and using the same conditions as Hagenbach (except of course restrictions 2 and 5), yet still allowing for steady flow, Womersley showed that the relationship between both steady and pulsatile components of flow in a segment of artery are to a first approximation, linear, and so can be described as longitudinal impedance. Womersley derived longitudinal impedance theoretically, and showed that from this and measured pressure gradient, pulsatile and steady components of flow in an artery can be calculated. His derivation for the steady component of flow was identical to that of Hagenbach. Womersley's calculations further permitted him to predict velocity profiles for pulsatile flow in arteries. He predicted that velocity profiles in the larger arteries of dogs, sheep and man at usual heart rates would be essentially flat.

Womersley's theoretic predictions for pulsatile flow in arteries have been repeatedly confirmed under experimental circumstances - for values of longitudinal impedance, for calculation of flow from

differential pressure and for details of velocity profile across an artery (Fry 1959, Greenfield and Fry 1965, Fry and Greenfield 1964, Ling and Atabek 1966, Reuben et al 1970, McDonald 1974). Womersley's work (Womersley, 1955a, 1957, 1958) was performed in collaboration with Donald McDonald in the mid 1950s. His detailed papers are unintelligible except to experienced mathematicians, but have been interpreted in detail by McDonald (McDonald 1960, 1974). The all too brief interdisciplinary collaboration of these two men, both now deceased, stands as a milestone in the field of cardiovascular physiology.

Womersley's derivation of longitudinal impedance as the relationship between flow and *differential pressure* in an artery (which is discussed further in chapter 6) led to the even more useful concept of input impedance being introduced to describe the relationship between flow and *absolute pressure*. This concept was developed by McDonald's pupil Michael Taylor in a series of theoretic and experimental studies (Taylor 1957a, b, 1959a, b, 1965a, b, 1966a, b, 1967, 1969, McDonald and Taylor 1956, 1959). These were based on Womersley's theoretically-derived solution to the equations of motion and indicated likewise that non-linearities in the relationship between pressure and flow are extremely small. As described below and in chapter 8 multiple subsequent studies of vascular impedance under experimental conditions in animals and in human clinical studies have confirmed this to be the case (O'Rourke and Taylor 1966, 1967, Noble et al 1967, Bergel et al 1966, Dick et al 1968, Westerhof et al 1979, Murgo et al 1980).

The work in this area has yielded a series of unexpectedly favourable dividends: Poiseuille's equation, though apparently quite inapplicable to a vascular bed has proved useful in describing and interpreting steady pressure/flow relationships as vascular resistance; the more general solution to the equations of motion as derived by Womersley has disclosed that pulsatile pressure/flow relationships in arteries can be regarded as linearly related, so simplifying their analysis and opening the way to use of longitudinal impedance in the study of vascular segments, and input impedance in the study of whole vascular beds.

VASCULAR RESISTANCE AND THE EQUIVALENT ELECTRICAL MODEL

For steady flow through the systemic circulation or part thereof, the vascular tree can be represented by the simple electrical network in Fig. 4.1(a) where R is the resistance. Direct current (which corresponds to flow) and steady voltage (which corresponds to mean pressure) are related by Ohm's Law.

Current (Flow) = Voltage (Pressure) ÷ Resistance

This electrical model is overly simplistic of course because it does not take into account auto-regulation, critical closure, and altered viscosity of blood at low flow rates. Yet it is widely used and has been found helpful in characterising resistive properties of a vascular bed. It will be utilised here with the knowledge that there are limitations to its application. The point to be made in passing is this – there is as much if not more potential for nonlinearity in this hallowed relationship than in the more sophisticated models that describe pulsatile pressure/flow relationships.

It is fortunate indeed that this model does not represent the systemic circulation. If it did, flow would occur only during systole. During systole, pressure would rise to a very high level which would be determined entirely by the peripheral resistance (and of course left ventricular ejection). During diastole, pressure would be at right atrial level and coronary arteries could not be perfused. This model (Taylor 1965a) has the heart connected directly to the arterioles; there is no arterial system. This model is useful for describing the relation between the steady component of pressure and flow but totally unrealistic in representing the whole circulation. The arterial system adds *reactance* – through the distensibility of arterial walls (which can be represented by electrical capacitance) together with the density of blood within them (which can be represented by electrical inductance) (Spencer et at 1958, Remington 1963). To describe the properties of arteries one must add capacitance and inductance to the electrical model; properties of this model then become frequency-dependent and need to be described in the same way as electrical circuits with these components – as electrical impedance.

VASCULAR IMPEDANCE AND ELECTRICAL MODELS OF THE SYSTEMIC CIRCULATION

The next most simple model of the vascular system comprises resistance and capacitance – the former as before representing peripheral resistance and the latter representing arterial distensibility. The hydraulic equivalent of this model is the *Windkessel* (Frank 1899, 1905) (Figs. 1.1, 4.1(b)).

As in the pure resistive model, the resistance provides the only pathway for steady electrical current across the circuit. Energy is lost only in the resistance as current flows through this. The capacitance (C) stores electric charge only; at a given voltage with steady current flow its charge is constant. It is only when applied voltage changes that electric charge moves into or out of the capacitance. Thus in this circuit, the behaviour for D.C. (steady) voltage is exactly the same as in the purely resistive model. It is only when applied voltage changes that presence of the capacitance becomes apparent. For an oscillating voltage, the capacitor stores some of the electric charge so that it does not all pass through the resistor. Thus this circuit's opposition to oscillating voltage is lower than that of the purely resistive circuit; how much lower will obviously depend on how quickly the voltage is altered, and on the size of the capacitor in relation to the size of the resistor. The opposition to current flow in A.C. circuit theory is called Impedance, which is expressed as a graph of modulus and phase plotted against frequency (Fig. 4.2). The impedance of this model falls with increasing frequency by an amount that depends on the relative size of resistance and capacitance. Likewise impedance phase (the delay between applied voltage and current) falls from zero at zero frequency – where the resistive properties of the circuit dominate —— to $-90°$ at an infinitely high frequency (where the capacitative properties of the circuit dominate).

As discussed in Chapters 7–9, this model (which corresponds to a *Windkessel*) though better than the resistive model is still quite unsatisfactory for describing arterial behaviour. The first objection is that it neglects the mass or density of blood and the energy stored by blood as momentum when it is set into motion. This can be added to

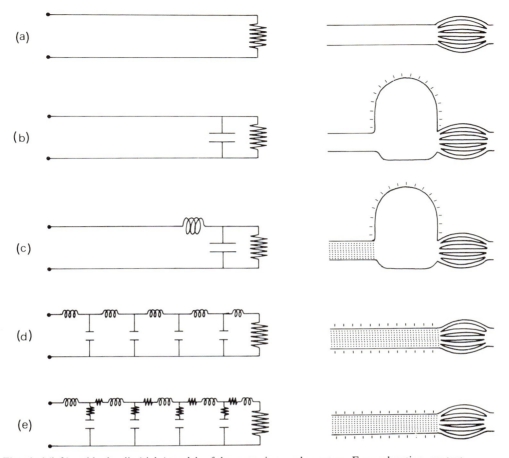

(a)

(b)

(c)

(d)

(e)

Fig. 4.1 Electrical (left) and hydraulic (right) models of the systemic vascular system. For explanation, see text

the previous circuit as an electrical inductance. Like a capacitor, an inductance stores electrical charge only (but in the form of an electrical field); it does not dissipate electric charge. Like a capacitor its presence in a circuit is only relevant when applied voltage is changing – it does not alter the resistive properties of the circuit for direct current. Unlike a capacitor however it opposes rather than assists changes in applied voltage, and the phasic relationship between applied voltage and current is the opposite of the capacitance. These are precisely what one would expect from the effects of density in a hydraulic model. Thus in all respects, the electrical inductance represents the effects of blood mass (Fig. 4.1(c)).

In a circuit which comprised resistance and inductance (L) only, impedance would increase above the resistive value with increasing frequency and phase would rise progressively to approach + 90° at high frequencies (voltage preceeding current – see Fig. 4.2). When in an electrical circuit, both inductance and capacitance are combined with resistance, the resulting impedance depends on the magnitude of each. In the whole arterial system, the effects of arterial distensibility outweigh the effects of blood density; thus in the arterial model, capacitance is large with respect to inductance, and input impedance modulus falls with increasing frequency and impedance phase falls from 0° to almost −90° at high frequencies (current leading applied voltage). The present discussion refers to models of the whole systemic circulation including arterioles as resistance and arteries as reactance. (Longitudinal impedance which relates differential pressure in an arterial segment to arterial flow shows effects of blood mass dominant, with impe-

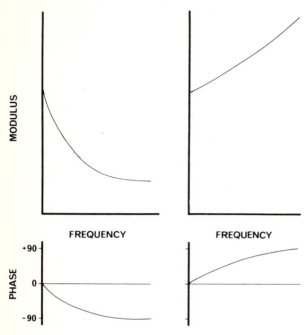

Fig. 4.2 Electrical impedance, expressed as modulus (amplitude of sinusoidal voltage divided by amplitude of sinusoidal current) (top) and phase (delay of sinusoidal current after sinusoidal voltage) (bottom), for an R.C. circuit (resistance and capacitance) (left), and for an L.C. circuit (resistance and inductance) (right)

dance modulus increasing with frequency, and differential pressure preceding blood flow (Womersley 1957b, McDonald 1974)).

But this model (Fig. 4.1(c)) is still not realistic. It includes the effects of arterial elasticity and blood density but takes these both to be lumped at the one point. One would record in this system two different voltage and current waves – one proximal to the inductance, and one distal. It is known however that in the arterial system, the foot of pressure and flow waves is progressively delayed in more peripheral arteries and that the contour of waves changes progressively and markedly. These changes result from the elastic properties of arteries and inertial properties of blood being distributed along the arterial system. A sudden step in pressure or flow at the aortic valve does not simultaneously distend the whole arterial system nor set all the blood in motion. Rather a wave is generated that travels over the whole arterial system at a finite velocity.

A more realistic model of the arterial system is

that shown in Figure 4.1(d) where blood mass in different arteries is represented by a large number of inductances in series, and arterial distensibility by a large number of capacitances in parallel. As before, the model terminates in a single terminal resistance. This system displays finite wave velocity and progressive alteration of voltage and current waves between input and terminal resistance. Though more complicated than the purely resistive and simpler resistive and reactive models, the same considerations still apply – the terminal resistance determines the behaviour to steady current and the network of capacitors and inductances determine the opposition to oscillating current.

This model can be further improved. There is nothing in the first four models to account for energy losses associated with arterial pulsations, nor the small fall in mean pressure which occurs before flow pulsations are completely attenuated. Allowance can be made for this by having small resistors in series with the capacitors, and other small resistors in series with the inductances (Fig. 4.1(e)). The first represent the viscous properties of the arterial walls (which as described on page 31 are responsible for diameter fluctuations lagging behind applied pressure) and the second, the viscous properties of blood in the large arteries.

The hydraulic equivalent of the last two models is an elastic tube filled with liquid and having an almost completely closed end. The end of this tube corresponds to the terminal resistance, the length of the tube to the number of capacitors and inductances, and the regional wave velocity in the tube to the relative value of capacitance to inductance at each point. Since there is a finite wave velocity and finite terminal resistance, in these electrical and hydraulic models, the possibility of wave reflection at the terminal resistance arises. For both hydraulic and electrical models, the effects of wave reflection at the terminal resistance will only be absent at the input if (a) the elastic tube is infinitely long (in the electrical model there are an infinite number of capacitors and inductances) or if (b) terminal resistance to steady flow (or D.C. current) is as low as the impedance of the tube to oscillating flow (or A.C. current). In the absence of wave reflection at the input of elastic tube or electrical network, the modulus of input

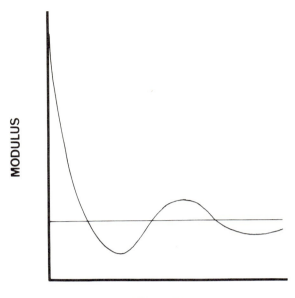

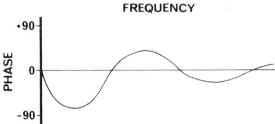

Fig. 4.3 Electrical impedance at the input of an electrical transmission line model such as Fig. 4.1 (d,e). In the absence of wave reflection modulus and phase are constant. In the presence of wave reflection, modulus and phase show marked fluctuations

impedance would remain almost constant and impedance phase near zero with increasing frequency (Taylor 1965a, 1966a, McDonald 1974) (Fig. 4.3). Impedance in the absence of wave reflection is called characteristic impedance. When however the effects of wave reflection are apparent at the input, impedance modulus and phase fluctuate about the values of characteristic impedance, with minima and maxima of modulus and zero phase crossing at frequencies that depend on the apparent length of the network or tube, and the wave velocity (O'Rourke and Taylor 1966). This subject has been fully explored by Taylor in his studies of arterial models (Taylor 1957–1969). For the simple tubular model, successive maxima and minima of modulus and successive zero crossings of phase will occur at multiples of the frequency at which

the first minimal value of modulus occurs. This subject is pursued further in Chapter 7.

Electrical models are very useful in giving a conceptual idea of circulatory function and in studying impedance characteristics. Models of the whole vascular tree as described by Noordergraaf and Westerhof are physically bulky and require awkward rewiring when changes of vascular properties are to be studied. When this level of complexity is reached, further studies are best done with mathematical models in a digital computer, as described by Taylor, Avolio (1976, 1980) and others (Wemple 1972, Caro et al 1978, Anliker 1978, Kenner 1978, 1979, Oddou 1978).

HYDRAULIC AND MATHEMATICAL MODELS OF THE SYSTEMIC CIRCULATION

The simplest hydraulic model of the systemic circulation is the Windkessel (Fig. 1.1) which is represented in electrical terms by the R.C. (resistor and capacitor) circuit (Fig.4.1(b)). This has already been discussed and found wanting because arterial distensibility is taken as 'lumped' at the one point, blood density is ignored, there is no provision for finite wave velocity and no possibility of wave reflection or of any diastolic pressure or flow fluctuation. The model is of historical importance however because of its initial inference by Harvey and its description by Hales and because it was the basis of early attempts to measure stroke volume from the arterial pressure pulse. Early work by Frank and others in Germany and by Hamilton, Remington and colleagues in the U.S.A. in the days before cardiac catheterisation, was directed at deriving something that could not be measured (cardiac output) from a parameter (arterial pressure) that could. As shown by Remington and associates (Remington et al 1948) human arterial distensibility is so variable and the effects of wave reflection so unpredictable that the *Windkessel* model is of little value in predicting cardiac output from arterial pressure.

The next hydraulic model of the arterial system is the simple distensible tube with the proximal end representing the aortic valve and the distal end, the lumped peripheral resistance (Fig.

1.6.). This is represented by the models in Figure 4.1(d) and (e). Such models were suggested by Otto Frank (1905) to explain diastolic pressure fluctuations as reflected waves, by Remington, Alexander, Wood and others, and notably by Hamilton and Dow to explain reflection in terms of 'standing waves' (Hamilton and Dow 1939, Alexander 1953, Remington 1963). The concept of 'standing waves' in arteries was soundly rebuffed by McDonald, Taylor, and others (McDonald 1974, McDonald and Taylor 1959) on the basis of the 'standing wave' requiring 100 percent reflection and zero attenuation – which obviously was impossible. An accommodation between the two camps – championed at the time by two forceful and testy personalities, John Remington on the one hand and Donald McDonald on the other – was suggested by me in 1967 (O'Rourke 1967b) only to incur the tolerant but substantial wrath of both.

Work performed by O'Rourke and Taylor (1967) suggested that the systemic circulation could be represented by an asymmetrical T tube whose short and long arms behave respectively like the apse and nave of a cathedral, with reflection and re-reflection of the pulse at both ends. Other work (McDonald 1968, 1974, Avolio et al 1976, O'Rourke and Avolio 1980) has provided further support for this general concept of the arterial system. This will be discussed in more detail in Chapters 8 and 9.

Most studies of pulsatile phenomena in arteries have shown definite evidence of wave reflection, and tubular models have been used to explain this. There has been debate as to whether the end or ends are closed (the present consensus is that they are closed) and what a closed end represents (Alexander 1953, Remington 1963, McDonald 1974). Even recent studies attempt to explain the closed end in terms of some particular characteristic of the distal aorta (Westerhof et al 1978) whereas I argue strongly (see chapters 7–9) that available evidence points to this representing the resultant of peripheral arterioles and not branching points in the aorta or major arteries.

Another application of a tubular model should be mentioned. Frank (1930) has suggested use of this model and of the 'water hammer' formula:–

$$\bar{V} = \frac{\bar{P}}{\rho.c}$$

(where $\bar{V}$ is stroke volume, $\bar{P}$ is pulse pressure, ρ is density, and c is pulse wave velocity), for calculating stroke volume from aortic pressure. As discussed in Chapter 7, this assumes that there is no wave reflection at all and that the amplitude of pulse pressure is determined exclusively by stroke volume and by the local properties of the ascending aorta. Because of definite and obvious wave reflection under most circumstances, this overestimates stroke volume. However, in the presence of generalised vasodilation and hypotension, when wave reflection is low, this gives a useful approximation to stroke volume. In a recent twist of this same theme, Bourguignon and Wagner (1979) suggested that aortic pressure might be calculated from ventricular ejection, measured by isotopic methods. As with the water hammer formula, this fails totally to consider wave reflection, and so is susceptible to large errors.

The most authoritative studies on hydraulic tubular arterial models are those of Michael Taylor (1957b, 1959b, McDonald and Taylor 1956, 1959). Because of the difficulty in constructing and testing such tubular models, and because of the ease in dealing with mathematical models, there has been little interest in further development of such studies over the past ten years.

In contrast to hydraulic models there have been numerous recent studies on mathematical models of the systemic circulation. Segments of books and reviews have been devoted entirely to these models (Caro et al 1978, Kenner 1978, 1979, Anliker et al 1978).

Possibly the most realistic and useful mathematical models have been those developed by Taylor as an extension of his earlier work on hydraulic and electrical analogs (Taylor 1965b, 1966a, b). Taylor showed that a peripheral vascular bed could be represented in a computer by a randomly-branching network of tubes which terminate in values approximating the peripheral resistance. When realistic values of arterial length, radius, and visco-elasticity were used, together with known values of blood viscosity and density, it was found that the whole branching network behaved as though there was only one incompletely closed end which represented the resultant of all individual terminal resistances – i.e. it behaved like a simple tube. Input impedance of this assembly was virtually identical to that determined from pressure and flow waves at the input of the femoral vascular bed. Changes brought about by reducing peripheral reflection coefficient from 80% to zero were identical to those determined experimentally following intra-arterial injection of a potent vasodilator, and changes brought about by increasing reflection coefficient to 95 per cent were identical to those determined experimentally during extreme vasoconstriction of the vascular bed (O'Rourke and Taylor, 1966, Chapter 8).

Taylor proceeded further with this model to show that the whole systemic circulation could be so represented, but that the best results were obtained when the fore and hind parts of the body were represented by two separate networks with different average distances to peripheral reflecting sites. Taylor also showed that pressure wave transmission and amplification in such a network was virtually identical to that in systemic arteries (Taylor 1966b). With this model, Taylor was able to examine separately the effects of different types of branching, different degrees of elastic nonuniformity, and differences in blood and wall viscosity.

Taylor's modelling was extended by Avolio (Avolio 1976, Avolio et al 1976, Avolio 1980) who used measured lengths of arteries and known branching arrangements to simulate the arterial system of man and different mammals, and virtually identical computational techniques. Results were very similar to those measured in different animal types and in man (Avolio et al 1976, O'Rourke and Avolio 1980), and as discussed further in Chapters 8 and 9, aid explanation and interpretation of experimental and clinical studies.

PULSE WAVE VELOCITY

Values of pulse wave velocity were given in chapter 3 where the relationship between wave velocity and arterial distensibility was inferred. Finite wave velocity was pointed out as a property of electrical transmission line models (with multiple L.C. networks) and of elastic tubes, but to be an impossibility in the Windkessel.

Finite velocity of the arterial pulse was first referred to by Erasistratus in 280 B.C. (see Aperia, 1940) and is a well known and fundamental property of the arterial system. It is the basis of pulse

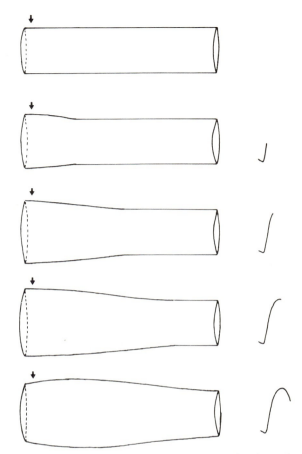

Fig. 4.4 Shape of a distensible tube before and at four intervals in time after injection of fluid into the mouth of the tube. The pressure wave in the mouth of the tube (indicated by the arrow) is shown inset at right. See text for further explanation

wave reflection. It is desirable to have a proper conceptual idea of what this is.

When the left ventricle begins to eject, a small quantity of blood passes into the ascending aorta; this causes a pressure to rise and the wall to distend. During the first few milliseconds of ventricular ejection this sharp rise in pressure (which develops later into the foot of the pressure wave at this point) is confined to a short segment of the proximal aorta; pressure is higher here than in the next segment downstream. The disturbance (as the foot of the pressure wave) passes on to the next segment, then to the next, and on to the next, while all the time pressure continues to rise in the proximal segment as a result of continuing ventricular ejection (Fig. 4.4).

Pulse wave velocity is measured from the time

difference between the foot of pressure waves recorded simultaneously at known distances apart along an arterial segment. Under normal circumstances this ranges from 4 m sec^{-1} in the ascending aorta to 12 m sec^{-1} in the femoral artery.

The speed of travel of any disturbance in a physical system depends on the elasticity and density of the medium in which it travels. Issac Newton first determined this for the speed of sound in air as

$$c = \sqrt{\frac{K}{\rho}}$$

where K is the volume elasticity and ρ the density of air. The relationship between arterial elasticity and wave velocity was first explored by Thomas Young around 1808 (Laird 1980). As Laird and McDonald (1974) point out, Young's contribution to physics is remembered as his modulus of elasticity, but it is generally forgotton that he was a physician, and that his early studies were directed at explaining arterial behaviour. Young calculated wave velocity as

$$c = \sqrt{\frac{\triangle P}{(\triangle V/V)\rho}}$$

where ρ is density and $\triangle P$ is the change of pressure required to increase volume of an arterial segment by $\triangle V$ above its initial value V. (This is similar to Peterson's pressure/strain modulus Ep (p. 30). (For a short, tethered arterial segment, the numerical values are identical). Wave velocity is now often calculated directly from Young's Modulus of the arterial wall as

$$c = \sqrt{\frac{E.h}{2.r.\rho}}$$

where E is the elastic (Young's) modulus of the wall, h is wall thickness and 2.r is internal diameter. This equation is frequently used and is referred to as the Moens-Koeteweg equation, having originally been derived by these two men (McDonald 1974). These formulae can be used as follows:–

1. What is pulse wave velocity in a segment of thoracic aorta in which a 40 mm Hg change in pressure causes a 10% change in diameter and no longitudinal extension i.e. a 20% change in volume?

$$c = \sqrt{\frac{40 \times 980 \times 1.36}{1.05 \times 0.10}}$$
$$= 504 \text{ cm sec}^{-1}$$

2. What is pulse wave velocity in a segment of thoracic aorta whose Young's Modulus is 5.33 $\times 10^6$ dyne cm^{-2} and ratio of wall thickness to internal diameter is 0.05?

$$c = \sqrt{\frac{5.33 \times 10^6}{1.05 \times 20}}$$
$$= 504 \text{ cm sec}^{-1}$$

Because of its relationship to arterial distensibility and wall thickness, pulse wave velocity increases between central and peripheral arteries, with increasing distending pressure, with age, and in arterial degenerative disease (Bramwell and Hill 1922, Bergel 1978, O'Rourke et al 1968). Implications of this are discussed in Chapters 9, 10, 12, 13, 14, 16.

It is clear that pulse wave velocity is fast in relation to arterial dimensions. In a normal sized man, no arterial termination is further than 1.5 metres from the aortic valve. At an average wave velocity of 8 Msec^{-1}, the wave will reach this furthest point in 0.188 sec and if reflected will return to the heart in 0.376 sec. Since heart period is usually around 0.5–1.0 sec, it is clear that the effects of wave reflection will be seen within the same pulse that generates the reflected wave.

One might speculate why pulse wave velocity is normally within the range given in Table 3.1. The upper limit is set by the timing of reflected waves. If wave velocity were high, the reflected wave would return during systole, and so (as discussed further in Ch. 9) increase left ventricular systolic pressure and so increase myocardial oxygen demands and reduce stroke volume. If pulse wave velocity were low – say for the first example given above, 200 cm sec^{-1} instead of 500 cm sec^{-1}, arterial distensibility would have to be more than 6 times greater. Were this the case, small changes in mean pressure as with exercise would be associated with gross billowing of the arterial system and so with temporary loss of blood into the grossly distended arteries. This matter is discussed by Taylor (1965a) in a perceptive review of teleological considerations in arterial design. Another problem that might develop with very low pulse wave velocity, is the possibility of this being exceeded by flow velocity from the ventricle. Flow velocity in the ascending aorta is normally less than 100 cm sec^{-1} (peak). Should peak flow velocity exceed regional pulse wave velocity, pressure would build up in that segment of the aorta faster than it could be dissipated, and longitudinal shock waves would result. Such a mechanism (which resembles that for an aeroplane when it first exceeds the speed of sound) may underly the genesis of aortic ejection clicks and 'pistol shot' sounds when aortic flow velocity is increased in aortic valve incompetence.

The complicated topic of apparent phase velocity (or apparent wave velocity) will not be discussed in this book. As described, wave velocity was measured from the foot of the pressure wave, which is not affected by wave reflection. If one tried (as one does with Fourier analysis) to measure wave velocity of different components of the pulse which are altered by wave reflection, one would find this to be different at different frequencies and to behave (when expressed as a function of frequency) in much the same way as modulus of input impedance. Those interested in this topic are referred to McDonald's (1974) monograph and other publications (McDonald and Taylor, 1959, O'Rourke 1967, Milnor et al 1969).

TURBULENCE IN ARTERIES

Assumption of laminar or streamline flow underlies the concept of linearity as assumed in application of Poiseuille's Law, and use of arterial impedance for characterising vascular properties. As discussed at length by McDonald (1974) this appears to be the case in all but the largest vessels, and even in these, disturbed flow appears to be present only during a short part of the cardiac cycle. McDonald considered that in experimental animals at least, one could assume laminar flow and so apply linearised analytical techniques. Doubtless the same applies to normal man. However, clinicians deal frequently with flow across stenotic valves or through narrowed arteries, or into dilated or irregular arteries; flow that is sufficiently turbulent to cause vibration of the

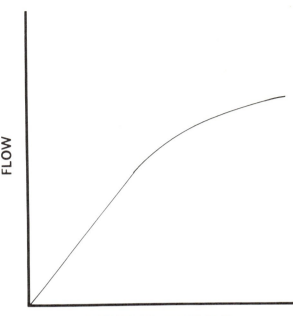

Fig. 4.5 Relationship between flow (ordinate) and pressure gradient (abscissa) of a newtonian fluid in a simple tube. With onset of turbulence the linear relationship between pressure and flow is disturbed

arterial wall and to be perceived as a cardiac or vascular murmur. The presence of such murmurs denotes that turbulence is present, that energy is being lost in secondary flows, and hence that one cannot apply the analytical techniques that have hitherto been described. Physicians are of course particularly interested in these patients and in understanding how the altered flow and pressure patterns related to the underlying disease. In approaching this subject one can only be qualitative, or at best, semiquantitative.

It has been shown that as turbulence occurs in a pipe, the normally linear relationship between pressure and flow is disturbed such that further increments in pressure gradient cause correspondingly lower increments of flow (Fig. 4.5). The onset of turbulence in a tube frequently occurs when the Reynold's number exceeds 2000. Reynold's number Re is calculated from the formula

$$Re = \frac{v.D.\rho}{\mu}$$

where v is flow velocity in cm/sec, D is diameter in cm, ρ is density in g/cm^3 and μ is viscosity in poises. Once turbulence occurs, it is impossible to predict what the relationship will be between pressure and flow – all one can say is that flow will be less than predicted from pressure/flow relationships at lower flow rates. Reynold's number was shown to predict onset of turbulence in a long smooth tube. Turbulence will occur earlier if the tube is irregular, or if fluid enters it in a jet. For the blood circulation Reynold's number is useful for stressing the dimension D (McDonald 1974). At a given flow velocity, turbulence is more likely to occur in a wide than in a narrow tube. This is the probable basis of systolic aortic turbulence and the systolic aortic murmur in aortic sclerosis.

TORICELLI'S ORIFICE FORMULA FOR CARDIAC VALVULAR AND ARTERIAL STENOSES

In attempting to explain the pressure drop and energy losses across valvular and arterial stenosis, Gorlin and Gorlin (1951) introduced the orifice formula. Gould and colleagues subsequently applied the same principles to arterial stenoses (Gould 1978, Gould et al 1978, Brown et al 1977). The orifice formula bears some resemblance to Bernouilli's Theorem which will be considered next. It is important to realise that these are quite different. The orifice formula applies to flow of a viscous fluid through an orifice and out in a jet, within which energy is lost and a pressure gradient results. Bernouilli's Theorem applies to an inviscid fluid that flows in streamlines through tubes of different diameter, within which energy is interconverted between potential and kinetic, but no energy is lost.

Since the orifice formula is frequently used by clinicians, but is often not well understood, and since its basis is relatively simple, a brief account will be given here. The model is shown in fig. 4.6. In this one assumes that there is no energy lost above or within the orifice but that all energy is lost in the jet and its associated vortices downstream. This energy can be measured as kinetic energy in the jet as:–

$$\tfrac{1}{2}.\rho.v^2$$

or as the potential energy loss across the jet as:–

$$\rho.g.h$$

where ρ is density of blood, v is linear velocity in cm sec^{-1}, g is gravitational acceleration 980 cm sec^{-2} (which is needed in all calculations to convert pressure in cm H$_2$O to dyne. cm^{-2}). Since pressure is measured in mm Hg, h (which in Fig. 4.7 is $P_1 - P_2$) must be multiplied by 1.36. Linear velocity v can be expressed as volume flow V (ml/sec) divided by cross sectional area of the jet A (cm^2). Since kinetic energy loss is equal to potential energy loss,

$$\tfrac{1}{2}.\rho.(\tfrac{V}{A})^2 = \rho \times 980 \times 1.36 \times (P_1 - P_2)$$

On rearrangement, and cancellation of ρ,

$$V = A\sqrt{(P_1 - P_2) \times 1333 \times 2}$$

and $A = \dfrac{V}{36.5\sqrt{P_1 - P_2}}$

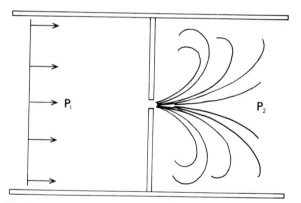

Fig. 4.6 The effect of a narrow orifice on flow through a tube. Energy is lost within and beyond the orifice as a result of viscous resistance within the jet and in the vortices downstream

Other constants are sometimes introduced into the orifice formula to account for narrowing of the jet beyond the orifice. The orifice formula will be referred to again (Ch. 5) in relation to arterial stenoses. At this point it may be noted that in the presence of such an orifice, pressure difference is related to the square of flow and not directly to flow itself, as in laminar flow through a cyclindrical tube.

BERNOUILLI'S THEOREM

$$h_1 - h_2 = \frac{v_2^2}{2g}$$

This was introduced by Daniel Bernouilli in the eighteenth century to explain interconversion of potential and kinetic energy as an inviscid liquid flows through a series of differently sized tubes (Fig. 4.7). Since the fluid is inviscid (has no viscosity), there are no energy losses along the tube, and so at all points along the tube, the sum of potential and kinetic energy components is the same. Thus, in Fig. 4.7 at point A, energy per gram of liquid is

$$\rho gh_1 + \tfrac{1}{2}\rho v_1^2$$

and at point B,

$$\rho gh_2 + \tfrac{1}{2}\rho v_2^2$$

Since there are no energy losses, these are equal, so that:–

$$\rho gh_1 + \tfrac{1}{2}\rho v_1^2 = \rho gh_2 + \tfrac{1}{2}\rho v_2^2$$

and

$$(v_2^2 - v_1^2) = 2g(h_1 - h_2)$$

If the tube is very wide at A, v_1 will be very small, and v_1^2 so small that it can be ignored. In this case the difference in pressure between A and B is given by:–

Like so many of the formulae described here, this is not strictly applicable to the circulation – because in this case, blood is considered to be inviscid. The effects of viscosity however are negligible over short distances in relatively wide tubes when streamline laminar flow is retained. Therefore Bernouilli's Theorem is relevant to arterial phenomena.

The first implication of Bernouilli's Theorem is that pressure difference does not always determine flow. This is apparent from Figure 4.7 where fluid runs from B to C against a pressure gradient. It is really the *energy* gradient that forces blood from one point in the circulation to another; when flow is related to pressure or pressure gradient, one assumes that kinetic energy is small (or similar) at both points, so that the measured pressure difference represents energy gradient.

The second implication of Bernouilli's Theorem is that the measured lateral pressure wave will alter when flow velocity is high, with lateral pressure at peak velocity being lower than it would be if blood had no mass or if under experimental circumstances pressure were measured end-on to the direction of flow. (Measuring pressure end-on to the direction of flow converts kinetic to potential

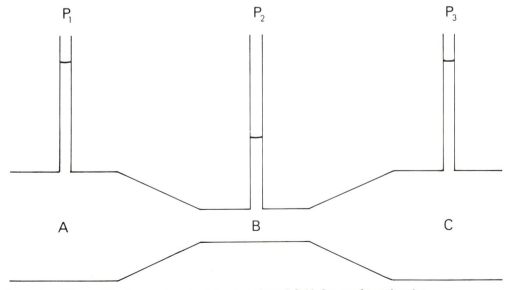

Fig. 4.7 Illustration of Bernouilli's theorem in an ideal (i.e. non viscous) fluid. See text for explanation

energy so that total energy is measured as pressure.) This indeed is the case. At peak flow velocity of 100 cm sec^{-1}, as is often recorded in the ascending aorta, one would expect a decrease in lateral pressure of $\frac{100 \times 100}{2 \times 1333}$ or approximately 4 mm Hg. Such changes in the lateral pressure wave have been recorded (O'Rourke 1967a), as have even greater differences in side-on as compared to impact pressure waves at higher velocities. (At 200 cm sec^{-1}, the predicted difference is about 16 mm Hg). These considerations raise the question as to whether end-on (impact) or lateral pressure should be related to blood flow in calculation of vascular impedance. Surprisingly, this matter remains controversial. The theory of impedance makes no provision for kinetic energy. Electrical models have nothing to mimic kinetic energy. It is thus tempting to ignore kinetic energy in measurement of impedance. Many, probably most, workers have done just this. Certainly under most conditions where peak flow velocity is relatively low there is little difference between impact and lateral pressure waves, so it makes little difference as to whether flow is related to impact or lateral pressure. However, when peak velocity is high, as in exercise or in the presence of arteriovenous shunts the reduction in lateral pressure may be sufficient to cause impedance modulus to be markedly underestimated (O'Rourke 1967a). The apparent reduction in pulmonary vascular impedance noted by Hopkins et al (1979) in arteriovenous shunt can be explained entirely on this basis. After much debate, Michael Taylor and I used impact pressure in our first and subsequent joint work on vascular impedance. We consider it proper to relate flow to a measure of energy difference across a vascular bed, and believe that this energy difference will be underestimated, sometimes substantially, by use of lateral pressure. This matter is discussed again in Chapter 9, and in O'Rourke 1980 (a), 1981.

EXTERNAL VENTRICULAR WORK

Mechanical energy imparted to blood by the heart may be calculated from pressure and flow in the ascending aorta and pulmonary artery. Evans and Matsuoka (1915) were the first to measure steady external left ventricular work, in Starling's laboratory. Using his heart – lung preparation, they calculated the potential and kinetic components respectively as:–

$$W = (P \times C.O. \times \rho) + \left(\frac{C.O. \times \rho \times \left(\frac{C.O.}{A} \right)^2}{2} \right)$$

Total Steady External L.V. Work/Min = Potential + Kinetic Work/Min, where P is mean arterial pressure, C.O. is cardiac output, ρ is blood density, A is cross sectional area of the tube linking ventricle to Windkessel and of course g is 980 cm sec^{-2}.

These workers (Evans and Matsuoka 1915, Evans 1918) found that kinetic energy was a sizeable proportion (3–28 per cent) of total external left ventricular work. Katz (1927) regarded this as an artifact and attributed it to the narrow calibre of and subsequently high velocity in the tubing which connected ventricle to *Windkessel*. His own subsequent work and that of others (Katz 1931, Remington and Hamilton 1947, Prec et al 1949) showed that kinetic energy is a small proportion (less than five percent) of external left ventricular work under experimental conditions. It is acknowledged however that in consequence of low pulmonary arterial pressure and correspondingly low potential energy, kinetic energy accounts for a larger proportion of right ventricular work (Bergel and Milnor 1967).

As discussed earlier, when pressure is measured end-on to the direction of flow, blood is brought to rest at the catheter tip and kinetic is converted to potential energy. Thus, in measuring pressure end-on to the direction of flow, there is no need to calculate kinetic energy separately, since total steady external ventricular work per beat is given by the formula:–

Total Steady External Work = P$_{impact}$ × C.O.

All these foregoing considerations assume that linear velocity is constant across the cross section of the vessel where pressure is measured – i.e. that the velocity profile is flat. As already discussed, there is good theoretical and experimental evidence that this is the case in the aorta and pulmonary artery of larger experimental animals, and in man.

External ventricular work is referred to here as *steady* external ventricular work, because as measured by Evans and Matsuoka it was calculated from mean values of pressure, flow, and velocity. Katz (1931) pointed out that this underestimates the true value. For the potential component of external heart work, the value obtained from integrating the product of pressure and flow over the whole cycle is greater than the value obtained from the product of integrated pressure and integrated flow. Likewise the integral of $\frac{1}{2}.m.v^2$ over the whole cycle exceeds the value given by $\frac{1}{2}.m.$ (average velocity)^2. Thus the pulsatility of cardiac ejection adds an extra component to steady external ventricular work over and above that originally calculated by Evans and Matsuoka. Therefore:—

Total External Ventricular Work = Steady External Ventricular Work plus Pulsatile External Ventricular Work

Both steady and pulsatile components can be considered to have potential and kinetic subdivisions (Milnor et al 1966), but such divisions depend on the techniques of pressure and flow measurement, and particularly on the degree of narrowing caused by a cuff-type flow transducer. In what follows I will assume that pressure is measured end-on to the direction of flow, and that the velocity profile is flat, so that kinetic energy need not be calculated separately.

It has been shown (Morris and O'Rourke 1965, Porje 1967, Milnor et al 1966, O'Rourke 1968) that description of ascending aortic and pulmonary arterial pressure/flow relationships as vascular impedance permits one to calculate directly the steady and pulsatile components of ventricular work – steady work as mean pressure × mean flow, and pulsatile work from flow harmonics and vascular impedance as

$$\frac{1}{2} \sum_{n=1}^{N} (Q_n)^2 . Z_n . \cos \phi_n$$

where Q_n is modulus of the nth flow harmonic and Z_n and ϕ_n are modulus and phase respectively of impedance at this frequency. It has been shown that the two components of ventricular work have definite and different physiological significance (in sharp contrast to the concept of potential and kinetic components of ventricular work whose separation is a caprice of measurement). Steady external ventricular work represents energy lost in maintaining steady flow through small resistance vessels while pulsatile external work represents energy lost in the arterial system as a consequence of intermittent ventricular ejection. The ratio of pulsatile to total external left ventricular work is normally around 10 percent, but may increase markedly under abnormal circumstances (O'Rourke 1967). The ratio of pulsatile to total external right ventricular work is normally around 25 percent (Milnor et al 1966) but may be much higher in pulmonary vascular disease (Milnor et al 1968). The ratio of pulsatile to total external left or right ventricular work is an (inverse) index of arterial efficiency. This subject is explored further in Chapter 10.

TOTAL HEART WORK AND CARDIAC FUNCTION

The principal interest in external heart work is in separating the energy lost in maintaining steady flow – the heart's useful role – from that which is lost uselessly in arteries as a consequence of the heart's intermittency. It must be pointed out that external heart work – pulsatile and steady – account for a small and inconstant fraction of total energy generated by the heart. Most of this is lost within the heart itself (Braunwald 1969). When considering arterial function, external work is useful; when considering ventricular performance, external work is irrelevant. The subject of ventricular function and arterial properties is discussed further in Chapters 10 and 16.

REFERENCES

Alexander RS 1953 The genesis of the aortic standing wave. Circulation Research 1: 145–151
Anliker M, Steetler JC, Niederer P, Holenstein R 1978 Prediction of shape changes of propagating flow and pressure pulses in human arteries. In: Bauer RD, Busse R (eds) The arterial system Springer Verlag Berlin 15–34
Aperia A 1940 Haemodynamical studies. Scandinavian Archives of Physiology 83: Supplement 1, 1–230
Atabek HB, Lew HS 1966 Wave propagation through a viscous incompressible fluid contained in an initially elastic tube. Biophysical Journal 6: 481–503
Avolio AP 1976 Haemodynamic studies and modelling of the mammalian arterial system. PhD Thesis University of New South Wales Sydney

Avolio AP 1980 Multi-branched model of the human arterial system. Medical and Biological Engineering and Computing 18: 709–718

Avolio AP, O'Rourke MF, Mang K, Bason PT, Gow BS 1976 A comparative study of pulsatile arterial hemodynamics in rabbits and guinea pigs. American Journal of Physiology 230: 868–875

Bellhouse BT, Bellhouse FH 1969 Fluid mechanics of model normal and stenosed aortic valves. Circulation Research 25: 693–704

Bergel DH 1978 Mechanics of the arterial wall in health and disease. In: Bauer RD, Busse R (eds) The arterial system Springer Verlag Berlin 3–14

Bergel DH, Milnor WR 1965 Pulmonary vascular impedance in the dog. Circulation Research 16: 401–415

Bourgeois MJ, Gilbert BK, Donald DE, Wood EH 1974 Characteristics of aortic diastolic pressure decay with application to the continuous monitoring of changes in peripheral vascular resistance. Circulation Research 35: 56–66

Bourguignon MH, Wagner HN 1979 Non invasive measurement of ventricular pressure throughout systole. American Journal of Cardiology 44: 466–471

Bramwell JC, Hill AV 1922 Velocity of transmission of the pulse wave and elasticity of arteries. Lancet 1: 891–892

Braunwald E 1969 The determinants of myocardial oxygen consumption. Physiologist 12: 65–93

Brown BG, Bolson E, Frimmer M, Dodge HT 1977 Quantitative coronary arteriography. Estimation of dimensions, hemodynamic resistance and atheromatous mass of coronary artery lesions using the arteriogram and digital computation. Circulation 55: 329–337

Caro CG, Pedley TJ, Schroter RC, Seed WA 1978 The mechanics of the circulation. Oxford University Press New York

Cournand A, Ranges HA 1941 Catheterisation of the right atrium in man. Proceedings of the Society for Experimental Biology and Medicine 46: 462

Dick DE, Kendrick JE, Watson GL, Rideout VC 1968 Measurement of nonlinearity in the arterial system of the dog by a new method. Circulation Research 22: 101–111

Evans CL 1918 The velocity factor in cardiac work. Journal of Physiology (London) 52: 6–14

Evans CL, Matsuoka Y 1915 The effects of various mechanical conditions on the gaseous metabolism and efficiency of the mammalian heart. Journal of Physiology (London) 49: 378–405

Frank O 1899 Die Grundform des arteriellen Pulses. Erste Abhandlung Mathematische Analyse. Zeitschrift fur Biologie 37: 483–526

Frank O 1905 Der Puls in den Arterien. Zeitschrift fur Biologie 46: 441–553

Frank O 1930 Schatzung des Schlagvolumens des menschlichen Herzens auf Grund der Wellenund Windkesseltheorie. Zeitschrift fur Biologie 90: 405–409

Fry DL 1959 Measurement of pulsatile blood flow by the computed pressure gradient technique. Institute of Radioengineers Transactions on Medical Electronics M.E. 6: 259–264

Fry DL, Greenfield JC 1964 The mathematical approach to hemodynamics with particular reference to Womersley's theory. In: Attinger EO (ed) Pulsatile blood flow, McGraw New York p. 85–100

Gorlin R, Gorlin SG 1951 Hydraulic formula for calculation of the area of the stenotic mitral valve, other cardiac valves and central circulatory shunts 1. American Heart Journal 41: 1–29

Gould KL 1978 Pressure-flow characteristics of coronary stenoses in unsedated dogs at rest and during coronary vasodilation. Circulation Research 43: 242–253

Gould KL, Lee D, Lovgren K 1978 Techniques for arteriography and hydraulic analysis of coronary stenosis in unsedated dogs. American Journal of Physiology 235: 350–356

Green HD, Rapela CE 1964 Blood flow in passive vascular beds. Circulation Research 14 Supplement 1: 11–18

Greenfield JC JR, Fry DL 1965 Relationship between instantaneous aortic flow and the pressure gradient. Circulation Research 17: 340–348

Hamilton WF, Dow P 1939 An experimental study of the standing waves in the pulse propagated through aorta. American Journal of Physiology 125: 48–59

Hopkins RA, Hammon JW, Hale PA, Smith PK, Anderson RW 1979 Pulmonary vascular impedance analysis of adaption to chronically elevated blood flow in the awake dog. Circulation Research 45: 267–274

Katz LN 1927 Observations on the dynamics of ventricular ejection. American Journal of Physiology 80: 470–484

Katz LN 1931 Observations on the external work of the isolated turtle heart. American Journal of Physiology 99: 579–597

Kenner T 1978 Models of the arterial system. In: Bauer RD, Busse R (eds) The arterial system Springer Verlag Berlin p. 80–88

Kenner T 1979 Physical and mathematical modelling in cardiovascular studies. In: Hwang NH, Gross DR, Patel DJ (eds) Quantitative cardiovascular studies University Park Baltimore Ch. 2: 41–109

Laird JD 1980 Thomas Young, MD (1773-1829). American Heart Journal 100: 1–8

Levy MN 1979 The cardiac and vascular factors that determine systemic blood flow. Circulation Research 44: 739–746

Ling SC, Atabek HB 1966 Measurement of aortic blood flow in dogs by the hot film technique. Proceedings of the 19th annual conference on Engineering in Medicine and Biology San Francisco p. 113

McDonald DA 1960 Blood flow in arteries. 1st Edition Arnold London

McDonald DA 1968a Hemodynamics. Annual Review of Physiology 30: 525–556

McDonald DA 1968b Regional pulse wave velocity in the arterial tree. Journal of Applied Physiology 24: 73–78

McDonald DA 1974 Blood flow in arteries. 2nd Edition Arnold London

McDonald DA, Taylor MG 1956 An investigation of the arterial system using a hydraulic oscillator. Journal of Physiology (London) 133: 74–75

McDonald DA, Taylor MG 1959 The hydrodynamics of the arterial circulation. Progress in Biophysics and Biophysical Chemistry 9: 107–173

Milnor WR, Bergel DH, Bargainer JD 1966 Hydraulic power associated with pulmonary blood flow and its relation to heart rate. Circulation Research 19: 467–480

Milnor WR, Conti CR, Lewis KB, O'Rourke MF 1969 Pulmonary arterial pulse wave velocity and impedance in man. Circulation Research 25: 637–649

Morris MJ, O'Rourke MF 1965 Steady and pulsatile work of the left and right ventricles. Proceedings, Australian Physiological Society P. 35

Murgo JP, Westerhof N, Giolma JP, Altobelli SA 1980 Aortic

input impedance in normal man: relationship to pressure waveforms. Circulation 62: 105–116

Oddou C, Dantan P, Flaud P, Geiger D 1979 Aspects of hydrodynamics in cardiovascular research. In: Hwang NH, Gross DR, Patel DJ (eds) Quantitative Cardiovascular studies, University Park Baltimore Ch. 10, P. 457–492

O'Rourke MF 1967a Steady and pulsatile energy losses in the systemic circulation under normal conditions and in simulated arterial disease. Cardiovascular Research 1: 313–326

O'Rourke MF 1967b Pressure and flow waves in systemic arteries and the anatomical design of the arterial system. Journal of Applied Physiology 23: 139–149

O'Rourke MF 1968 Impact pressure, lateral pressure and impedance in the proximal aorta and pulmonary artery. Journal of Applied Physiology 25: 533–541

O'Rourke MF 1980 Vascular Impedance: a call for standardisation. In: Kenner T, Hinghoffer-Szalkay Berlin Pleum in press

O'Rourke MF 1980 Comments on pulmonary vascular impedance analysis of adaption to chronically elevated blood flow in the awake dog. Circulation Research 46: 731

O'Rourke MF 1981 Physiological Reviews, American Physiological Society. Vascular impedance in studies of arterial and cardiac function. (in press)

O'Rourke MF, Avolio AP 1980 Pulsatile flow and pressure in human systemic arteries; studies in man and in a multi-branched model of the human systemic arterial tree. Circulation Research 46: 3, 363–372

O'Rourke MF, Taylor MG 1966 Vascular impedance of the femoral bed. Circulation Research 18: 126–139

O'Rourke MF, Taylor MG 1967 Input impedance of the systemic circulation. Circulation Research 29: 365–380

O'Rourke MF, Blazek JV, Morreels CL, Krovetz LJ 1968 Pressure wave transmission along the human aorta; changes with age and in arterial degenerative disease. Circulation Research 23: 567–579

Poiseuille JLM 1840 Recherches expérimentales sur le mouvement des liquides dans les tubes de très petits diamètres. Comptes Rendus Hebdomadaires des seances de l'Academie des Sciences 11: 961–967, 1041–1048

Porjé IG 1967 The energy design of the human circulatory system. Proceedings, 7th International Conference on Medical and Biological Engineering Stockholm p 153

Prec O, Katz LN, Sennett L, Roseman RH, Fishman AP, Hwang W 1949 Kinetic energy of the heart in man. American Journal of Physiology 159: 483–491

Remington JW, Hamilton WF 1947 The evaluation of the work of the heart. American Journal of Physiology 150: 292–298

Remington JW 1963 The physiology of the aorta and major arteries, Handbook of Physiology American Physiological Society Washington D.C. Volume 2 Circulation 2: 799–838

Remington JW, Noback CR, Hamilton WF, Gold JJ 1948 Volume elasticity characteristics of the human aorta and prediction of the stroke volume from the pressure pulse. American Journal of Physiology 153: 298–308

Reuben SR, Swadling JP, de J Lee G 1970 Velocity Profiles in the main pulmonary artery of dogs and man, measured with a thin-film resistance anemometer. Circulation Research 27: 995–1001

Spencer MP, Johnson FR, Denison AB 1958 Dynamics of the normal aorta. 'Inertance' and 'Compliance' of the arterial

system which transforms the cardiac ejection pulse. Circulation Research 6: 491–500

Taylor MG 1957a An approach to an analysis of the arterial pulse wave. 1. Oscillations an attenuating line. Physics in Medicine and Biology 1: 258–269

Taylor MG 1957b An approach to an analysis of the arterial pulse wave. 2. Fluid oscillations in an elastic pipe. Physics in Medicine and Biology 1: 321–329

Taylor MG 1965 Wave travel in a non-uniform transmission line, in relation to pulses in arteries. Physics in Medicine and Biology 10: 539–550

Taylor MG 1959b An experimental determination of the propagation of fluid oscillations in a tube with a viscoelastic wall; together with an analysis of the characteristics required in an electrical analogue. Physics in Medicine and Biology 4: 63–82

Taylor MG 1964 Wave travel in arteries and the design of the cardiovascular system. In: Attinger EO (ed) Pulsatile blood flow, McGraw New York p 343–372

Taylor MG 1965b Wave travel in a non-uniform transmission line, in relation to pulses in arteries. Physics in Medicine and Biology 19: 539–550

Taylor MG 1966a The input impedance of an assembly of randomly branching elastic tubes. Biophysical Journal 6: 29–51

Taylor MG 1966b Wave transmission through an assembly of randomly branching elastic tubes. Biophysical Journal 6: 697–716

Taylor MG 1967 The elastic properties of arteries in relation to the physiological functions of the arterial system. Gastroenterology 52: 358–363

Taylor MG 1969 The optimum elastic properties of arteries. In: Wolstenholme GEW, Knight J (eds) Ciba Foundation Symposium on circulatory and respiratory mass transport, Churchill London p 136–147

Taylor MG 1973 Hemodynamics. Annual Review of Physiology 35: 87–116

Wemple RR, Mockros LF 1972 Pressure and flow in the systemic arterial system. Journal of Biomechanics 5: 629–641

Westerhof N, Sipkema P, Elzinga G, Murgo JP, Giolma JP 1979 Arterial impedance. In: Hwang HC, Gross DR, Patel DJ (eds) Quantitative Cardiovascular studies, University Park Baltimore 3: 111–150

Westerhof N, Bosman F, de Vries CJ, Noordergraaf A. 1969 Analog studies of the human systemic arterial tree. Journal of Biomechanics 2: 121–143

Womersley JR 1955 Method for the calculation of velocity, rate of flow and viscous drag in arteries when the pressure gradient is know. Journal of Physiology (London) 127: 553–563

Womersley JR 1957 oscillatory flow in arteries; the constrained elastic tube as a model of arterial flow and pulse transmission. Physics in Medicine and Biology 2: 178–187

Womersley JR 1957b The mathematical analysis of the arterial circulation in a state of oscillatory motion. Wright Air Development Center, Technical Report WADC-TR, 56–614

Womersley JR 1958 Oscillatory flow in arteries; the reflection of the pulse wave at junctions and rigid inserts in the arterial system. Physics in Medicine and Biology 2: 313–323

Young T 1808 Hydraulic investigations subservient to an intended Croonian lecture on the motion of the blood. Philosophical Transactions of the Royal Society (London) 98: 164–186

PART 2

The arteries as vascular conduits (steady flow factor)

5

Function of arteries as vascular conduits

NORMAL CONDUIT FUNCTION

The most important function of arteries is to deliver an adequate supply of blood to peripheral organs and tissues at all times and with all changes in their metabolic activity. Comment has been made (Ch. 1) on how effectively this is done, with an almost imperceptible mean pressure gradient between the ascending aorta and a peripheral artery more than one metre distant, and with the capacity for cardiac output to increase perhaps six fold, and muscle blood flow perhaps twelve fold without symptom or sign of arterial insufficiency. This efficiency of conduit function is a consequence of wide arterial calibre and correspondingly low resistance.

Values of resistance for different parts of a vascular bed have been calculated from detailed measurements of vascular geometry (Table 1.1). These data were used to construct Figure 1.6. From these data one can predict resistance changes in the whole vascular bed when a segment of artery is progressively narrowed (Figs. 5.2, 5.3, 5.6). Under normal circumstances resistance of a typical peripheral artery is about 1.3 percent of its whole vascular bed, while the resistance of the aorta upstream is of like magnitude. When the organ is active, resistance of aorta and artery remains constant, and so increased relative to that of the dilated vascular bed. One would not however expect to see mean pressure fall by more than 10–15 mm Hg between the ascending aorta and distal part of a major artery in the leg, even in strenuous exercise and with torrential flow along the artery.

CONDUIT FUNCTION IN DISEASE

Atherosclerosis is the most common disease in the western world and the most frequent cause of disability and death in our society. The clinically-apparent ill effects of atherosclerosis usually arise from narrowing and obstruction of arteries, with ischemia, fibrosis or infarction of the organ or tissue downstream.

Atherosclerosis does of course disorganise elastic components of the aortic and arterial wall, leading to impaired distensibility of these vessels, and altering 'cushioning' function of the arterial system. Such effects are often associated with dilation rather than stenosis, particularly in the aorta (Stehbens 1979). These effects on cushioning function, though important, (Chapter 13) are usually less important than the effects of atherosclerosis in limiting organ blood flow.

The problem of arterial narrowing is probably the most important and most frequent faced by clinicians today. Arterial narrowing is the most common cause of death in the western world. Arterial narrowing also can be attacked surgically, and in most hospitals vascular surgical procedures are being performed with increasing frequency, and better results. The crucial questions are:–
(i) What is a 'critical' stenosis?
(ii) At what stage in the process of narrowing is an organ's viability threatened?
(iii) When should a narrowed artery be bypassed? There are no simple answers to these questions, as evidenced by the range of values used in different studies and quoted by different authorities and in different textbooks (Table 5.1). In individual

Table 5.1 Assessment of altered conduit function with different degrees of reduction in arterial diameter

Degree of narrowing as decrease in diameter	Comment	Source
>50%	'Significant'	Abrams and Adams 1969
	'May produce a gradient and therefore a perfusion defect'	King and Douglas 1978
	Criterion for obstructive lesion, Veterans Administration controlled trial of stable angina	Murphy et al 1977
>70%	Criterion for obstructive lesion, N.H.L.B.I. controlled trial of unstable angina.	Scheidt 1977
	'Significant stenosis'	Sabiston 1979
>80%	'Reduction of blood flow in the basal state'	Julian 1979
	'Severe obstructive lesion'	Braunwald et al 1980

cases, note must be taken of other factors, including symptoms, degree of peripheral vasodilation, and presence or absence of collateral vessels. It is not the purpose of this book to give detailed advice on therapy, but rather to discuss mechanisms that may allow informed decisions to be made in particular cases. In addressing the above questions, one should also seek answers for other related questions which apply to arterial disease as it affects any vascular bed, but may as an example be directed to the coronary circulation:–

1. Concerning the appearance and progression of clinical features of coronary artery disease –
   a. Why is coronary artery disease silent for many years before symptoms arise?
   b. Why is coronary artery disease usually well advanced by the time that symptoms arise?
   c. Why do the ill effects of coronary artery disease often come on suddenly and progress rapidly?
2. Concerning the presence of obvious atherosclerosis without clinical manifestations –
   a. Why do some have no symptoms yet have severe and extensive coronary atherosclerosis?
   b. Why do some have no myocardial infarct despite total coronary artery obstruction?
3. Concerning myocardial infarction without complete obstruction of a coronary artery –
   a. Why do some suffer acute myocardial infarction without complete obstruction of an artery, and with no evidence of recent

thrombosis or spasm or recent progression of atherosclerosis?

In passing it might be noted that the questions set out here have been under study for over 80 years, well before Herricks's classical description of 'The symptoms of acute coronary obstruction' (Herrick 1912a). Herrick (1912b) referred carefully to previous studies, and stressed the importance of collateral vessels, considering these responsible for myocardial viability in patients with obstructive lesions who died without history of anginal pain, and to be important in those who survived a clinically–apparent episode. His advice on therapy even implied early ambulation and attempts to limit infarct size. 'If these cases are recognized, the importance of absolute rest in bed for several days is clear . . . . The hope for the damaged myocardium lies in the direction of securing a supply of blood through friendly neighbouring vessels so as to restore as far as possible its functional integrity'. Following other work (including that of Friedberg and Horn 1939) who described myocardial infarction in the absence of coronary occlusion, and of Blumgart et al (1941) who showed that only two thirds of patients with acute myocardial infarction had acute coronary occlusion*), the term 'Myocardial Infarction' came to be applied to the clinical syndrome that Herrick had described. These were dark days: emphasis

* In the most recent studies, De Wood et al (1980) have shown 87% of patients with complete obstruction within the first 4 hours of symptoms and 65% between 12–24 hours.

was placed on irreparable damage and need for prolonged bed rest while the infarct fibrosed, in contrast to Herrick's more optimistic advice. The modern approach to coronary care constitutes a return to Herrick in terms of short hospitalisation, and early aggressive attempts to improve collateral flow and limit infarct size (Sobel and Braunwald 1980). 'Myocardial Infarction' is an inappropriate diagnosis for a patient suffering thirty minutes of oppressive chest pain, and whose myocardium is still viable but starved of blood. The term 'Myocardial Infarction' seems to have been responsible for the fatalism and therapeutic nihilism of the last forty years.

A good case can be made for abandoning this term – at least as an initial diagnosis – and for substituting Herrick's "Acute Coronary Obstruction", Pantridge's "Acute Coronary Attack", or even the term "Myocardium Infarcting". All of these are more in keeping with the modern approach to coronary care than "Myocardial Infarction" – a term which implies that ischemic damage is irreversible or inevitable.

At this stage it is desirable to identify some sources of confusion in this area. These relate to the disease process itself, to techniques of investigation, and to theoretic analysis and interpretation. These will be directed at the coronary circulation, but the same principles apply *mutatis mutandis* to other vascular beds.

Atherosclerosis usually narrows an artery in an irregular fashion, resulting not in a small circular opening, but in an oval, slitlike or even crescentic orifice. The lumen of the affected section of artery is often irregular with variations in cross sectional shape. The affected segment of artery is usually compared to the vessel upstream or downstream, but this may either be narrowed above by the same disease, or dilated downstream in the mysterious process of post-stenotic dilation (Roach 1972, Stehbens 1979). These factors can make interpretation of absolute and relative narrowing quite imprecise.

Arterial narrowing is assessed in life by arteriography or after death by dissection, arteriography, or preparation of casts. The latter two techniques are rarely employed by pathologists on a regular basis. Dissection at autopsy is performed with the artery undistended; it will identify complete

obstruction but will not be able to quantify narrowing with any precision. Coronary arteriography is routinely performed in two or more projections so as to visualise the whole extent of all major arteries and to assess luminal assymetry. Technical quality of cine–angiograms vary considerably from institution to institution, and from operator to operator, but even for the one angiogram, different observers can give different interpretations for the degree of arterial narrowing (Brown et al 1977).

Practical clinical considerations

Different guidelines have been offered for documentation of coronary artery stenosis. Those of the American Heart Association are shown in Table 5.2. These are realistic in giving a range for a particular 'percent stenosis'. When one calculates the resistance of arterial segments from Poiseuille's formula, one gets some idea of how crude coronary arteriography can be. For '75 percent stenosis', lumenal diameter varies from 25–49 percent of upstream diameter, so that resistance (Ch. 4) varies 15 fold. For '90 percent stenosis', lumenal diameter ranges from 10–24 percent of upstream diameter, so that resistance varies 30 fold; for '99 percent stenosis', lumenal diameter ranges from 1–9 percent of that upstream so that resistance varies 10 000 fold. Assessment of lumenal obstruction in different publications is

Table 5.2 Recommended reporting system (American Heart Association 1975) for different degrees of measured reduction in diameter of a coronary artery

Reported degree of stenosis, percent	Measured reduction in lumen diameter, percent
'50'	26–50
'75'	51–75
'90'	76–90
'99'	>90

Table 5.3 Conversion table relating reduction in arterial diameter to reduction in cross-sectional area at a stenosis

Diameter Reduction percent	Area Reduction, percent
30	51
50	75
70	91
80	96
90	99

made difficult by its expression as reduction in lumenal diameter in some (including the American Heart Association report) and lumenal area in others. There is surprisingly no consensus on this matter and one has to be careful to ensure what is meant in each report. Table 5.3 compares reduction in diameter and in area.

A meticulous quantitative approach to angiographic documentation has been developed by Brown et al (1977). This entails laborious measurement of angiographic dimensions in two planes, correction of distortion, alignment, and construction of a three dimensional representation of the arterial segment in a digital computer. Though not perfect, this constitutes a refreshing attempt to provide precise quantification of the arteriogram.

Many clinical and other studies of coronary artery disease have compared different features of the disease to the coronary arteriogram with the tacit assumption that this is the absolute 'Gold' standard. Perhaps there is nothing better to use but one must appreciate that the gold standard is not 24 (or even 14) carat.

The last source of confusion is apparent in many articles on arterial obstruction. The literature on theoretical treatment of arterial stenosis includes many simplistic articles written by clinicians and some unrealistically complicated treatments by engineers who have no apparent contact with biological reality and the (relative) imprecision of physiological measurement. A consensus appears now to be emerging on the details of disturbed blood flow in arterial stenosis and how this can be explained from physical principles (Berguer and Hwang 1974, Young et al 1975, Logan 1975, Gould et al 1978, Gould 1980).

Physical principles in arterial stenoses

Factors which determine pressure drop across a stenosis have been investigated extensively in physical models (May et al 1963 ab, Young and Tsai 1973 ab, Berguer and Hwang 1974, Logan 1975) and in animal experiments (Young et al 1975, Gould 1978, 1980, Gould and Lipscomb 1974, Gould et al 1974, 1975, 1978). Formulae derived have been applied to calculate resistance across coronary artery stenoses in man (Brown et al 1977, 1979).

The pressure drop across an arterial stenosis depends on (1.) the viscous properties of blood within the stenosis and (2.) the effects of convergence into and divergence of flow out of the stenosis and the flow separation and turbulence in the vessel downstream (Fig. 5.1). This can be expressed by the formula:—

$$\triangle P = F.V + S.V^2 \text{ (Gould 1978)}$$

where P is pressure gradient across the stenosis, V is blood velocity in the artery upstream and F is the coefficient of pressure loss due to viscous friction within the stenosis (dependent on viscosity of blood, length of the stenosis and absolute diameter of the stenosis – according to Poiseuille's Law), and S is the coefficient of pressure loss due to flow separation (dependent on relative percent stenosis, divergence angle of the stenosis and blood density). F is equivalent to hydraulic resistance as derived from Poiseuille's law. The first term depends on velocity alone, while the second term depends on velocity squared and represents the non-linear term from Toricelli's formula for an orifice (p. 44).

Under normal circumstances, with an unobstructed artery, flow is laminar and the second term does not apply – there is no convergence, divergence or turbulence. As the artery is progressively narrowed, the second term emerges and becomes larger and larger as relative narrowing and angle of divergence increase.

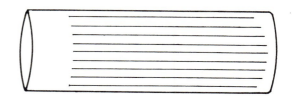

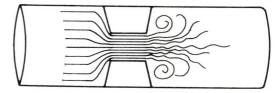

Fig. 5.1 Flow in a normal artery (above) and in a stenotic artery (below). Energy is lost within the stenosis (where if laminar flow is maintained, pressure drop can be calculated from Poiseiulle's formula), and beyond the stenosis where flow separation and turbulence occur.

In considering a stenosis it has been shown that the unsteady (pulsatile) components of flow are of little importance (Young et al 1974, Gould 1980) and that assymetry of the stenosis does not appreciably affect application of these formulae (Gould 1978).

In detailed consideration of the effects of arterial stenoses, all these different factors need to be considered. The non-linear terms are difficult to handle and introduce complexities that can distract attention from the major pathophysiological problems, and the questions raised previously. To a first approximation it is useful to consider only the viscous frictional loss within the stenosis itself. In doing so, one knows that one will be *underestimating* the effect of the stenosis to a degree that will depend among other things on the severity of the stenosis and the angle of divergence of the blood stream beyond. This type of simplified analysis assumes that flow into, through, and out of, the stenosis remains laminar. Such an analysis however provides the same answers as a more complicated treatment to the questions previously raised, and emphasises the importance of narrowing beyond 50 percent reduction in diameter, and of the resistance of the other components of the vascular bed. In applying it one just has to bear in mind that another (non-linear) factor will increase calculated resistance and decrease flow further at high degrees of obstruction.

Linearised approximation of an arterial stenosis

With respect to steady flow, the vascular bed can be regarded as a large number of hydraulic resistances (Fig. 5.2). The individual capillary resistances can be added in parallel to give total capillary resistance, and that of arterioles, small arteries, venules etc. likewise. With resistance of different segments of the vascular bed expressed in this way (Table 1.1), one can add each in series to determine the total resistance of the bed. From this single resistance, one can calculate flow for any given mean pressure.

Figure 5.3 shows resistance of different segments of a vascular bed calculated from data of Schleier (1918), together with the change in resistance of an arterial segment 0.5 cm long and of the whole bed when this segment is progressively narrowed. The calculations are applied as though Poiseuille's law was in effect, so that resistance increases inversely with the fourth power of arterial radius.

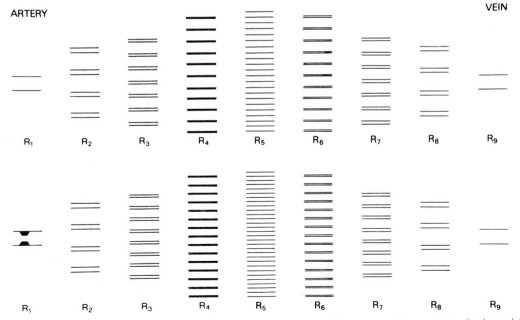

Fig. 5.2 The resistance of a vascular bed is the sum of all its component vessels. Under normal circumstances (top) arterial resistance R_1 is very low in comparison to total resistance ($R_1 + R_2 + R_3 + R_4 + \ldots . R_n$). Arterial obstruction (bottom) needs to be severe before arterial obstruction R_1 becomes appreciable in relation to the sum of other resistances

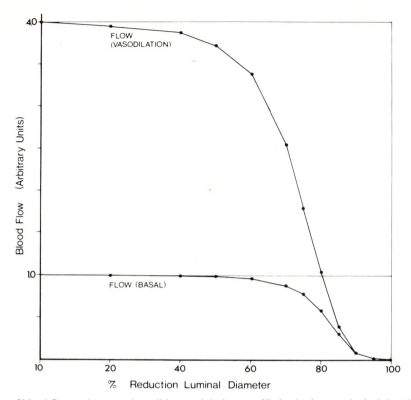

Fig. 5.3 Calculation of blood flow under control conditions and during vasodilation in the vascular bed described by Schleier, with progressive reduction in calibre of a 0.5 cm arterial segment. Change in resistance of this segment calculated from Poiseiulle's formula

With change in arterial radius from 1.5 to 0.15 mm (0 to 90 percent reduction in diameter), the resistance of the arterial segment increases 10 000 fold, while that of the whole vascular bed increases only 13 times. The reason for this disparity is that resistance of the arterial segment is initially very low – some 0.2 percent of the total. It is only when the lumen is reduced by more than 80 percent of the original diameter (from 3.0 to 0.6 mm) that its resistance exceeds that of the rest of the vascular bed, whereafter, with greater degrees of constriction, arterial resistance totally dominates that of all other components of the bed.

Figure 5.3 shows blood flow calculated from the hydraulic equivalent of Ohm's law (Flow Perfusion Pressure ÷ Total Resistance) for this vascular bed at different degrees of arterial constriction. It is clear that at 50 percent reduction in arterial calibre, flow is only slightly reduced (to 98.2 percent) and at 75 percent constriction to 77 percent

of original flow. Beyond this, small further constrictions cause marked reductions in flow:– a change from 0 to 75 percent constriction causes a 23 percent reduction in flow, but a further constriction from 75 to 80 percent causes a further 25 percent reduction. Below 70 percent constriction blood flow is little altered by changes in arterial calibre, but over 70 percent obstruction, the resistance of the narrowed arterial segment dominates the resistance of the whole vascular bed, so that tiny changes in calibre cause marked changes in blood flow.

These considerations apply to blood flow through a vascular bed under resting conditions. Also shown in Figure 5.3 is the effect of graded arterial constriction on blood flow during arteriolar vasodilation. This was calculated in the same way as before but with arteriolar resistance reduced so that initial total resistance was one quarter of that under resting conditions. It is obvious

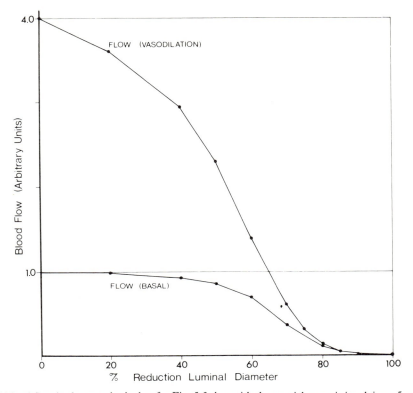

Fig. 5.4 Calculated blood flow in the vascular bed as for Fig. 5.3, but with the arterial stenosis involving a 5 cm length of artery

that the effect of constriction is more marked during hyperemia, and becomes apparent at lower degrees of arterial constriction. At 50 percent arterial obstruction, blood flow is reduced by less than 2 percent under resting circumstances but by 7 percent during vasodilation. At 80 percent obstruction, blood flow is reduced to 58 percent under resting circumstances, but to 26 percent during vasodilation. Another point becomes apparent from consideration of the effects of vasodilation in Figure 5.3. Under resting conditions, arteriolar vasodilation could completely offset the effects of arterial constriction and maintain flow up to 80 percent constriction. Beyond this compensation would quickly fail.

Figure 5.4 examines the effect of increasing the length of the arterial stenosis from 0.5 to 5.0 cm. Again, resistance of the arterial segment was calculated by assuming this to increase inversely with the fourth power of arterial radius. Again the effect was explored under control conditions and in simulated arteriolar vasodilation. In-

creasing length of the stenosis shifts both curves to the left so that reduction in blood flow occurs at a lesser degree of narrowing. Here 50 percent stenosis is much more important than before, with 15 percent reduction in basal flow and 43 percent reduction in hyperemic flow.

Figures 5.3 and 5.4 have been prepared from measured vascular parameters and resistance calculated from Poiseuille's law. Use of Poiseuille's law is an oversimplification under these circumstances and because of nonlinear terms related to velocity squared, one would expect that such a treatment would underestimate the effects of arterial stenosis. One would expect resistance to increase more with greater degrees of stenosis than shown here, and one would expect the changes with hyperemia to be even more marked. Even with this simplified treatment however, one sees the total dependence of blood flow on arterial calibre when degree of stenosis approaches and exceeds 70 percent.

Changes in blood flow shown in Figs 5.3 and 5.4 depend on the arbitrarily determined length of stenosis. When length of the stenosis is lengthened, decline in blood flow is more gradual with increasing stenosis, but with a shorter stenosis, blood flow is better maintained to a higher degree of constriction, but then plummets precipitously with further constriction.

Figure 5.5 shows the effects of graded coronary artery occlusion on experimentally measured flow through the coronary vascular bed under resting circumstances and during hyperemia induced by an arterial injection of hypaque. This figure (from Gould et al 1974) is typical of such studies and shows the same general features as Figures 5.3:– little fall in resting blood flow until arterial diameter is reduced by more than 70 percent, and marked fall thereafter, but greater relative reduction of blood flow by arterial constriction during vasodilation. The effects of lengthening the narrowed arterial segment as shown in Figure 5.4 agree well with the experimental results of Feldman et al (1978) and show that increasing the length of an arterial stenosis even at only 50 per-

cent reduction in lumenal diameter can appreciably reduce hyperemic flow.

Functional effects of stenosis

What is a 'critical' stenosis?

The above considerations permit an enlightened approach to the question of 'critical' stenosis, if not a definite answer. One would not expect an arterial stenosis to be hemodynamically significant, even if elongated, up to 50 percent reduction in lumenal diameter. Beyond 50 percent stenosis, capacity for increased blood flow during activity would be progressively impaired, but arteriolar vasodilation should compensate for arterial constriction up to 75–80 percent obstruction. Beyond 80 percent occlusion, one would expect reduction in basal flow, inability to increase blood flow during activity, and marked reduction in flow accompanying any further encroachment on lumenal diameter. These comments are in general

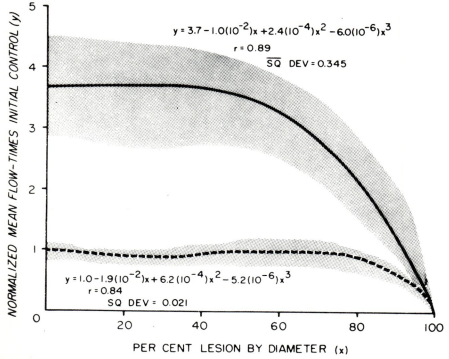

Fig. 5.5 Experimentally determined relationship between coronary artery constriction (abscissa), and basal flow (dotted line) and hyperemic response (unbroken line) on the ordinate. From Gould et al (1974)

agreement with clinical interpretation of 'critical', 'significant', and 'high grade' arterial stenosis.

In individual cases it would be desirable to measure pressure gradient across a stenosis at rest and during activity in order to assess its importance. This can readily be done for assessing the severity of femoro-popliteal arterial obstruction, where pressure can be measured simultaneously in the arm and affected leg before and immediately after treadmill exercise. Direct measurement of pressure gradient in a coronary artery can only be done at surgery, and under basal conditions. Measurement of pressure gradient across a carotid obstruction is a simple and frequently-performed procedure in diagnosis and at operation.

Pressure gradient across an arterial stenosis depends on blood flow through the stenosis. If collateral vessels are well developed, blood flow will be low and the gradient, small. In the presence of adequate collateral flow, even a 95 percent stenosis may not be 'critical' and so may not warrant surgery. In assessment of 'critical' or 'significant' stenosis, the pressure gradient (and the symptoms of ischemia) are probably much more sensitive than the arteriogram.

What is responsible for appearance and progression of clinical features of coronary artery disease?

These can readily be answered from consideration of Figure 5.3–5.6. Symptoms do not arise until arterial resistance becomes an appreciable fraction of total resistance and so is sufficient to limit blood flow. At this stage the disease itself will be obvious on angiography or at autopsy, with lumenal diameter reduced to <50 percent of original, and lumenal area to <25 percent of original at least. Symptoms are likely to arise first when the organ is active when, with peripheral vasodilation, arterial resistance is a relatively higher proportion of total resistance. Because of compensatory vasodilation (Gould et al 1974), a localised stenosis is unlikely to alter blood flow appreciably until calibre is reduced by 70 percent, and cross sectional area by 91 percent. Thereafter, progression of disease even by small amounts will cause marked reduction in blood flow, and appearance or progression of symptoms.

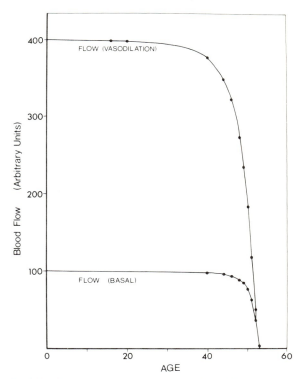

Fig 5.6   Change in resting and hyperemic blood flow in the vascular bed, as calculated in Fig. 5.3, but with reduction in cross sectional area progressing at a steady rate such as to reduce cross sectional diameter to 50% of original after 40 years. For explanation, see text

Figure 5.6 illustrates the effects of steadily progressive disease on blood flow into a vascular bed. This shows changes in basal and hyperemic flow to an organ (assuming this to be four times basal) over a period of 53.3 years. Resistance of the arterial segment is calculated assuming Poiseuille's law to apply as in Figures 5.3–5.4. It is assumed that the obstructive disease progresses at a steady rate, sufficient to narrow the lumen to 50 percent of its original diameter over 40 years, and to progress thereafter at the same rate. At forty years, resting flow is hardly altered and capacity for maximal (assumed to be fourfold) blood flow only slightly reduced. Further decrease in resting flow is relatively minor for a further eight years, but after this, resting and hyperemic flow fall precipitously.

As with the other figures, this is an oversimplification. Atherosclerosis does not progress at a constant rate; the lumen does not remain circular; thrombosis may completely occlude the lumen at any time. The analysis does not include the non-linear terms that are known to apply. But inclusion of these would accentuate the steep fall in flow when stenosis is severe. What one sees in life is precisely what one would predict from physical principles pertaining to blood flow through a tube whose calibre is progressively narrowing in one or more short segments:– a long period without compromised flow and without symptoms, anatomically severe stenosis at the time that symptoms are first apparent, and rapid progression of clinical features thereafter.

Why may severe and obvious coronary atherosclerosis be asymptomatic?

Absence of symptoms in the presence of gross antherosclerosis is often attributed to development of collateral vessels, and to effort insufficient to require additional blood flow. Such may be the case, but this apparent discrepancy can be explained along the same lines as before when one considers the insensitivity of diagnostic and autopsy procedures in distinguishing small differences in arterial narrowing. One certainly is often surprised that patients with what is shown to be severe atherosclerosis and arterial narrowing have no symptoms whereas others with an apparently similar degree of disease are severly symptomatic. The problem appears to be in distinguishing subtle differences within severe atherosclerosis. A difference between 70 and 80 percent arterial narrowing (Fig. 1.3) may be quite inapparent in a coronary arteriogram and would probably not be distinguished at autopsy, but such a difference is sufficient to almost halve resting blood flow, more than halve blood flow during vasodilation, and eliminate vasodilatory compensation for impaired basal flow. A further five percent reduction in calibre may be sufficient to reduce basal flow below the level required for organ viability. The difference in arterial calibre required to maintain adequate flow, cause ischemia on activity, or lead to infarction at rest is very narrow, and too narrow to be always perceived and identified with current techniques.

Why may myocardial infarction occur in the absence of coronary artery obstruction?

This subject has been much explored in recent years since the early systematic studies of Friedberg and Horn (1939) and Blumgart et al (1941). From the physical principles discussed here, one can readily appreciate that arterial stenosis may be sufficiently severe to reduce blood flow below that required to maintain tissue viability. Total arterial occlusion is not required. In Figure 5.3 a 90 percent arterial obstruction reduced blood flow to 10 percent of the basal and 3 percent of the hyperemic level – surely a trickle only and quite inadequate to maintain life. In their autopsy series, which has been confirmed by many since, Blumgart et al (1941) found that almost one third of their patients with apparently transmural infarction did not have complete coronary artery occlusion. Virtually all of these patients however had severe atherosclerotic arterial narrowing, and probably of sufficient degree to cause infarction, according to the arguments presented here.

These points must I believe be considered when attempting to understand the onset and progression of symptomatic arterial disease. Other factors of course must be considered as well, including formation and dissolution of platelet thrombi, spasm (particularly in the coronary system), and the role of increased organ activity in causing ischemia and necrosis (particularly subendocardial ischemia and subendocardial infarction). The physical principles however apply to anything that narrows an arterial lumen, be it atheroma, spasm, platelet thrombi, or a combination of these.

REFERENCES

Abrams HL, Adams DF 1969 The coronary arteriogram. 2. Structural and functional aspects. New England Journal of Medicine 281: 1336–1342
American Heart Association Committee Report Austen WG chairman 1975 A reporting system on patients evaluated for coronary artery disease. Circulation 51: 7–34
Beurguer R, Hwang NHC 1974 Critical arterial stenosis: a theoretical and experimental solution. Annals of Surgery 180: 39–50
Blumgart HL, Schlesinger MJ, Zoll PM 1941 Angina pectoris,

coronary failure and acute myocardial infarction. Journal of the American Medical Association 116: 91–97

Braunwald E 1974 Reduction of myocardial infarct size. New England Journal of Medicine 291: 525–526

Braunwald E, Cohn PF, Ross RS 1980 Ischemic heart disease. In: Isselbacher KJ, Adams RD, Braunwald E, Petersdorf RG, Wilson JD (eds) Harrison: Principles of internal medicine, McGraw Hill New York p. 1116–1124

Brice JG, Dowsett DJ, Lowe RD, 1964 Hemodynamic effects of carotid artery stenosis. British Medical Journal 2: 1363–1366

Brown BG, Bolson E, Frimmer M, Dodge HT 1977 Quantitative coronary arteriography. Estimation of dimensions, hemodynamic resistance and atheroma mass of coronary artery lesions using the arteriogram and digital computation. Circulation 55: 329–337

Brown BG 1979 Letter to the editor. Circulation 60: 1196

Brown BG, Pierce CD, Peterson RB, Bolson EL, Dodge HT 1979 A new approach to clinical investigation of progressive coronary atherosclerosis. Circulation 60: Supplement 2: 66

Byar D, Fiddian RV, Quereau M, Hobbs JT, Edwards EA 1965 The fallacy of applying the Poiseuille equation to segmented arterial stenosis. Americal Heart Journal 70: 216–24.

De Wood MA, Spores J, Notske R, Mouser LT, Burroughs R, Golden MS, Lang HT 1980 Prevalence of total coronary occlusion during the early hours of transmural myocardial infarction. New England Journal of Medicine 303: 897–902

Feldman RL, Nichols WW, Pepine CJ, Conti CR 1978 Hemodynamic significance of the length of a coronary arterial narrowing. American Journal of Cardiology 41: 865–871

Friedberg CK, Horn H 1939 Acute myocardial infarction not due to coronary artery occlusion. Journal of the American Medical Association 112: 1675–1679

Fronek A, Coel M, Bernstein EF 1978 The importance of combined multisegmental pressure and Doppler flow velocity studies in the diagnosis of peripheral arterial occlusive disease. Surgery 84: 840–847

Gensini GG 1975 Coronary Arteriography. Futura Mt. Kisco New York p. 260–271

Gould KL 1978 Pressure-flow characteristics of coronary stenosis in unsedated dogs at rest and during coronary vasodilation. Circulation Research 43: 242–253

Gould KL 1980 Dynamic coronary stenosis. American Journal of Cardiology 45: 286–292

Gould KL 1981 New technology for coronary heart disease. Journal of the American Medical Association 245: 689–694

Gould KL, Lipscomb K, Hamilton GW 1974 Physiologic basis for assessing critical coronary stenosis. American Journal of Cardiology 33: 87–94

Gould KL, Lipscomb K 1974 Effects of coronary stenosis on coronary flow reserve and resistance. American Journal of Cardiology 33: 48–55

Gould KL, Lipscomb K, Calvert C 1975 Compensatory changes of the distal coronary vascular bed during progressive coronary constriction. Circulation 51: 1085–1094

Gould KL, Lee D, Lovgren K 1978 Techniques for arteriography and hydraulic analysis of coronary stenosis in unsedated dogs. American Journal of Physiology 235: H350–H356

Herrick JB 1912 a The symptoms of acute coronary obstruction. Society Proceedings; Association of American Physicians p. 1971–1972

Herrick JB 1912b Clinical features of sudden obstruction of the coronary arteries. Journal of the American Medical Association 59: 2015–2020

Humphries J, Juller L, Ross RS 1974 Natural history of ischemic heart disease in relation to arteriographic findings: a twelve year study of 224 patients. Circulation 49: 489–497

Hurst JW, Logue RB, Walter PF 1978 Coronary atherosclerotic heart disease. IN: The heart Hurst JW ed McGraw New York p. 1156–1290

Julian DG 1979 Diseases of the coronary arteries. In: Cecil: Textbook of Medicine Beeson PB, McDermott W, Wyngaarden JB (eds) Saunders Philadelphia p. 1223–1238

King SB, Douglas JS 1978 Interpretation of the coronary arteriogram. In: The Heart Hurst JW (ed) McGraw New York p. 403–412

Laing SP, Greenhalgh RM 1980 Standard exercise test to assess peripheral arterial disease. British Medical Journal 1: 13–16

Lawrie DJ, Levinsky RA, Lewis RM 1975 A mathematical model describing the effects of coronary artery stenosis on coronary blood flow in resting and stressed dogs. Cardiovascular Research Centre Bulletin 13: 52–60

Levy MN 1979 The cardiac and vascular factors that determine systemic blood flow. Circulation Research 44: 739–746

Logan SE 1975 On the fluid mechanics of human coronary artery stenosis. IEEE Transactions on Biomedical Engineering B.M.E. 22: 327–334

McMahon MM, Brown BG, Cukingnan R, Rolett EL, Bolson E, Frimmer M, Dodge HT 1979 Quantitative coronary angiography: measurements of the 'critical' stenosis in patients with unstable angina and single vessel disease without collaterals. Circulation 60: 106–113

Mann FC, Herrick JF, Essex HE, Baldes EJ 1938 The effect on the blood flow of decreasing the lumen of a blood vessel. Surgery 4: 249–252

May AG, Van De Berg L, De Weese JA, Rob CG 1963 Critical arterial stenosis. Surgery 54: 250–259

Murphy ML, Hultgren HN, Detre K, Thomsen J, Takaro T 1977 Treatment of chronic stable angina. A preliminary report of survival data of the randomised Veterans Administration Cooperative Study. New England Journal of Medicine 297: 621–627

Oliva PB, Breckenridge JC 1977 Arteriographic evidence of coronary arterial spasm in acute myocardial infarction. Circulation 56: 366–374

Poiseuille JLM 1840 Recherches experimentales sur le mouvement des liquides dans les tubes de tres petits diamétres. Comptes Rendus Hebdomadaires des seance de l'Academie des Sciences 11: 961–967, 1041–1048

Proudfit WL 1980 Methods used to compare the medical management of coronary atherosclerotic heart disease with coronary bypass surgery. In The Heart Hurst JW (ed) Update 2 Bypass surgery for obstructive coronary disease McGraw New York p. 3–11

Roach MR 1972 Post-stenotic dilatation in arteries In Bergel DH ed. Cardiovascular fluid dynamics. London Arnold p. 111–140

Sabiston DC 1979 Surgical treatment of coronary artery disease. In: Beeson Pb, McDermott W, Wyngaarden JB (eds) Cecil: Textbook of Medicine Saunders Philadelphia p. 1238–1242

Santamore WP, Walinsky P 1980 Altered coronary flow responses to vasoactive drugs due to coronary stenoses in the dog. American Journal of Cardiology 45: 276–285

Scheidt S 1977 Unstable angina: medical management — or surgery. Cardiovascular Medicine 2: 541–543

Schleier J 1918 Der Energieverbrauch in der Blutbahn. Pflugers Archiv Fur Die Gesamte Physiologie 173: 172–223

Shipley RE, Gregg DE 1944 The effect of external constriction of a blood vessel on blood flow. American Journal of Physiology 141: 289–296

Sobel BE, Braunwald E 1980 Management of acute myocardial infarction. In: Braunwald E (ed) Heart disease, Saunders Philadelphia 1353–1386

Stehbens WE 1979 Hemodynamics and the blood vessel wall. Thomas Springfield

Vlodover Z, Frech R, Von Tassel R, Edwards JE 1973 Correlation of the antemortem coronary arteriogram and the postmortem specimen. Circulation 47: 162–169

Weale FE 1964 Hemodynamics of incomplete arterial obstruction. British Journal of Surgery 51: 689–693

Young DF, Tsai FY 1973 Flow characteristics in models of arterial stenosis 1. Steady flow. Journal of Biomechanics 6: 395–410

Young DF, Tsai FY 1973 Flow characteristics in models of arterial stenosis 2. Unsteady flow. Journal of Biomechanics 6: 547–559

Young DF, Cholvin NR, Roth AC 1975 Pressure drop across artificially induced stenosis in the femoral arteries of dogs. Circulation Research 36: 735–743

PART 3

The arteries as vascular cushions (pulsatile flow factors)

6

Analysis of arterial waves

THE PULSE IN THE TIME DOMAIN

It is current conventional clinical practice (Hurst and Schlant, 1978, Wallace 1979, Braunwald 1980) to describe the recorded intra-arterial pressure pulse in terms of its peak and nadir (systolic and diastolic pressures) and in terms of the presence or absence of inflections and secondary oscillations on the systolic and diastolic part of the wave. A critique of this has been given (O'Rourke 1971) and will be expanded in Chapter 17. One can go beyond such simple descriptions and obtain important physiological information from the time delay between various inflections on the pulse – i.e. pulse wave velocity over a known length of artery from the delay in the foot of the wave between proximal and distal recording sites, and the duration of ventricular ejection from the interval between the foot of the wave and incisura in the proximal aorta. (In measuring ejection duration, it is important to distinguish between the incisura and the foot of the diastolic wave; the first is caused by aortic valve closure, the second by wave reflection from peripheral arterioles. The two do not always coincide).

One can also measure time delay between different inflections and wavelets in the pulse in order to gauge the return of echos from peripheral reflecting sites and the period of arterial 'resonance'. This approach was utilised at length and exclusively by Frank, Hamilton, Remington, Alexander, Spencer and others over a period of more than fifty years (Frank, 1905, Hamilton and Dow 1939, Alexander 1953, Remington 1963, Remington and O'Brien 1970) and more recently in association with harmonic analysis by O'Rourke (1967, 1971), Wetterer and Kenner (1968), Wes-

terhof et al (1979), Sipkema et al (1980) and Murgo et al (1980). The major problem with this approach is in identification and interpretation of inflections and wavelets and in exclusion of artifact. Use of catheter tip manometers by Murgo and colleagues has been a major advance in this area.

Analysis of the pulse in the time domain has been the standard approach not only of clinicians, but also of the vast majority of physiologists up until 20 years ago when Donald McDonald established the value of harmonic analysis of arterial pulses and the concept of the arterial system in steady-state oscillation. Up till then, the only accredited approach to the study of the pulse was in its analog form – as pressure varying with time, and in terms which were at best semi-quantitative, and at worst, almost pure whimsy.

THE PULSE IN THE FREQUENCY DOMAIN

McDonald introduced an alternative concept – description of pressure as varying with frequency:– the arterial pulse as comprising a mean value and a series of harmonic sine waves occurring at multiples of heart rate frequency (Fig. 6.1).

McDonald's work was described in his review with Michael Taylor (McDonald and Taylor, 1959) and in his monograph (McDonald, 1960). Both reveal the restrained excitement of a careful scientist who has uncovered new information which previously lay buried in the undulations of the pulse. McDonald's approach to study of arterial phenomena was based almost totally on harmonic analysis of arterial pulses. He and his colleagues John Womersley, and later Michael

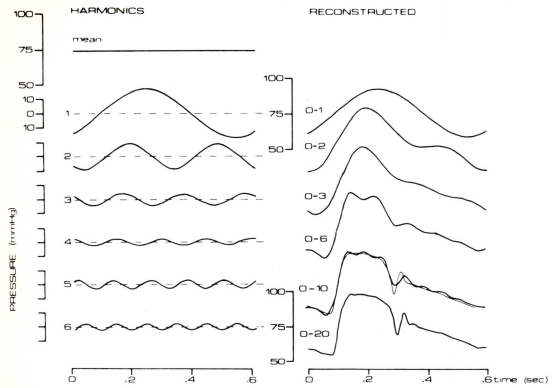

Fig. 6.1 Example of a Fourier series. *Left*: The mean term and first six harmonics of a pressure wave from the ascending aorta of a dog.
Right: Individual harmonics added to reproduce the original wave. Agreement is close with the first six harmonics added (0–6), better with the first 10 harmonics (0–10), while the resynthesised wave is almost identical to the original wave (the thin line in the second bottom trace) with addition of the first 20 harmonics (0–20). From Westerhof et al (1979)

Taylor, freely admitted that they were not the first to utilise this analysis, quoting its earlier application by Broemser, Aperia and Porjé, among others (Broemser. 1930, Aperia 1940, Porjé 1946). It must be said however that McDonald and his colleagues were responsible for establishing the validity of this approach, and so popularising its use. One single factor was responsible for this:– the theoretic studies by McDonald's mathematical colleague, John Womersley. Womersley (1957) showed that non-linearities in the equations of motion which relate pressure gradient and flow in an artery are quite small, and can, to a first approximation, be neglected. This supposition has been repeatedly confirmed. The foundation is solid. It is one thing to describe a pressure pulse as a series of harmonic sine waves, as McDonald's predecessors had done, but quite another to assume linearity and so regard each harmonic component as un-

iquely related to the corresponding harmonic of flow at the same point or pressure at another point. With linearity demonstrated – to a first approximation – this became possible, so that a technique used for describing a pulse wave became the basis for comparing pulsatile phenomena throughout the arterial system.

Lack of competence in the German language prevents me from giving a proper appreciation of German and Austrian scientists, principally Drs. Wetterer, Kenner and colleagues in Munich, Erlangen and Graz (see Wetterer and Kenner 1968). Their work, much performed quite independently, supported and extended that of the British group.

McDonald's concept of the arterial system in steady-state oscillation was fiercely resisted by physiologists of the classical school as evidenced by authoritative reviews by Remington (1963) and by Spencer and Denison (1963) in the First Hand-book of Physiology of the American Physiological Society. It is now generally accepted by physiologists, as evidenced by the prominent place it is accorded in recent textbooks (Milnor 1974, Little 1977, Berne and Levy 1979) and in the most recent edition of the Handbook (Gow 1980). From this point in time it appears hardly to warrant the type of controversy that it initially generated. McDonald (1960) pointed out that 'the most obvious feature of blood flow in arteries is that it is pulsatile', and (McDonald and Taylor 1959) that 'the most striking feature of the pulse is its regularity'. What was more logical than applying a standard practice in the physical sciences for regularly-repeated fluctuations in stress, strain, heat, electricity and sound to regularly-repeated pulsations in arteries?

We are quite familiar with this concept as it applies to music and description of musical waves. A series of musical waves takes the same form as the arterial pulse (Fig. 6.2). Both are described as oscillations against time, one of sound intensity, the other of pressure, flow or diameter. The only difference is in the time scale. The musical wave is

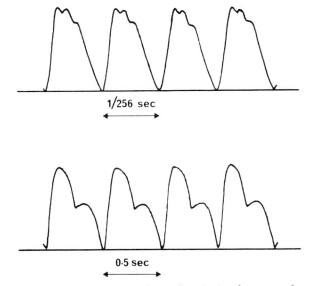

Fig. 6.2 The musical notes from a flute (top) at frequency of middle C (256/sec) and the arterial pressure waves in a dog (bottom) at heart rate frequency of 120 minute^{-1}. In both cases, waves are regularly repeated with the same contour, and can be described in terms of secondary fluctuations and inflexions, or as Fourier series

repeated perhaps 256 times per second (for middle C) and the pulse perhaps two per second (at heart rate 120 min^{-1}). We never refer to inflections or secondary oscillations of sound waves, but rather to their harmonic content – the amplitude of the first, second, third, fourth etc. harmonics at (for middle C) 256, 512, 1024, 2048 etc. cycle sec^{-1} (Hertz). Obviously, with the wave regularly repeated, the higher harmonics must occur at multiples of the basic frequency; if they did not, there would be a different carry-over from one wave to the next, so that successive waves would not be identical. What distinguishes the tone and character of a musical wave at a given pitch (frequency) is its content of higher harmonics. An arterial pulse wave can be described in precisely the same way. Both musical wave and pulse wave have (in theory) an infinite number of harmonic components. Limitations of recording systems and (for sound) of the human ear restrict amplitude of higher frequencies. This has been discussed on page 19 in relation to dynamic accuracy of manometers and flowmeters. In practice, most of the energy of the arterial pulse — pressure, flow, or diameter — is contained in the first five harmonics with amplitude decreasing progressively after the first harmonic (Figs. 6.1, 6.3). The sharp inflections of a pulse are dependent on registration of higher harmonics. The technique of breaking down a wave such as a pressure of flow pulse into its component harmonics was first described by Fourier (a comptemporary of Napoleon (McDonald 1974)) in studies of heat. The technique of Fourier Analysis is described in Appendix 2; this is usually performed in a digital computer, but can be done with the aid of a small sophisticated pocket calculator. Figure 6.1 shows an arterial pressure wave together with its first six harmonics, and its progressive resynthesis from 1, 2, 5, 10 and 20 harmonics. While most energy of the arterial pressure wave is contained in its first five harmonics, below 10 hertz, venous waves with sharper inflections and secondary waves have relatively more energy in higher harmonics (Patel et al 1965). Implications of this with respect to dynamic accuracy of recording systems has been discussed on page 19.

One of the original concerns in applying harmonic analysis to pulse waves was the presence of slight variations in heart rate. The heart does not beat with the same precise regularity that a tuning fork vibrates. McDonald and colleagues were well aware of this, but expressed surprise that this was one of the principal complaints of conventional physiologists. These, in considering the pulse wave as a transient in analog form, assumed that each pulse was damped to extinction before the next arrived. McDonald predicted that this same damping would lead to each pulse behaving as though it were part of a steady state oscillation, repeated with precisely the same contour and frequency, even in the presence of small alterations in heart rate. Subsequent analyses, performed while the heart rate was varying quite markedly (O'Rourke and Taylor 1966) confirmed this to be the case.

Figure 6.3 shows pressure and flow waves recorded at the same site in the femoral artery, and their breakdown into mean values and component harmonics. It is clear that the mean value for pressure is relatively high in comparison to mean flow, while the harmonics – expressed in mm Hg and ml sec^{-1} – are of similar amplitude. The relationship between pressure and flow at this point can be described as input impedance by relating mean values and corresponding harmonics of pressure and flow waves – the first harmonic of pressure to the first harmonic of flow, the second to the second, and so on. The impedance graph that results takes the same form as electrical or hydraulic impedance – a graph of modulus (amplitude of pressure/amplitude of flow) and phase (delay of flow after pressure) plotted against frequency. This shows the response that would be seen – the pressure that would be generated – for steady and pure sinusoidal flow at these frequencies at this point. Caro and McDonald (1961) actually determined impedance in the pulmonary artery with sinusoidal flow generated by a hydraulic oscillator. The results were similar to those obtained by comparing corresponding harmonics of simultaneously – recorded pressure and flow waves (Patel et al 1963). Use of a hydraulic oscillator is technically difficult, and virtually impossible to apply without altering mean flow and so physiological function of tissues downstream. It is far simpler, and more realistic to utilise the heart as flow source and de-

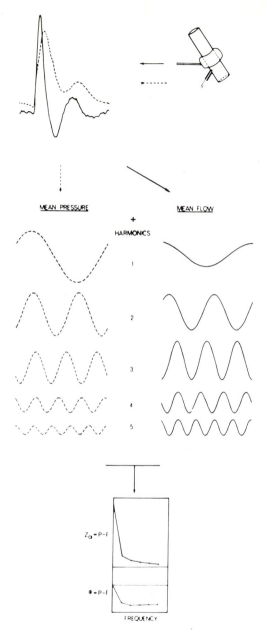

Fig. 6.3 Pressure (broken line) and flow (solid line) waves in the femoral artery of a dog, broken down into mean terms and Fourier series, the first 5 components of which are shown. From mean values and corresponding harmonics, impedance modulus (Z_0) and phase ø may be determined as a function of frequency (bottom) – modulus as the amplitude of pressure harmonic divided by amplitude of corresponding flow harmonic, and phase as the delay between corresponding harmonics. From O'Rourke and Taylor (1966), with permission American Heart Association Inc.

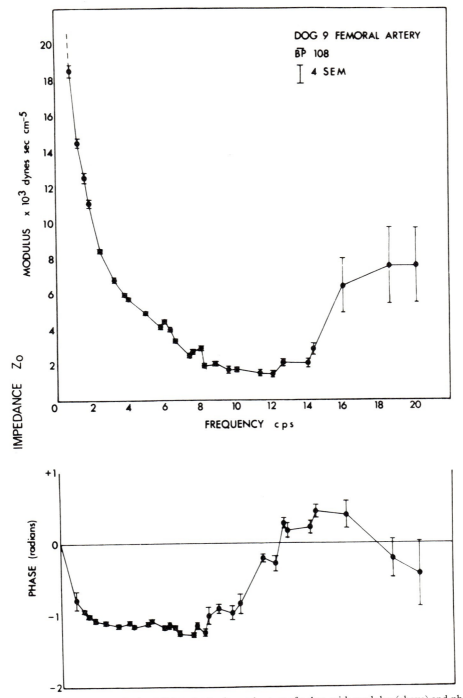

Fig. 6.4 Vascular impedance under control conditions in the femoral artery of a dog, with modulus (above) and phase (below) plotted against frequency. Impedance was determined from Fourier analysis of a series of 57 waves recorded in a dog with heart block, whose heart was paced at different frequencies. Abscissa cycle sec^{-1} or Hertz. From O'Rourke and Taylor (1966) with permission American Heart Association Inc.

termine the frequency–dependent behaviour of
the vascular bed (input impedance) by relating
harmonic components of the compound pressure
wave to corresponding harmonics of the input
flow wave.

One of the restrictions of harmonic analysis is
evident in Figure 6.3. With the heart beating at 1
sec^{-1}., impedance data points are obtained at 1, 2,
3, 4 ... Hertz. No information is obtained at intermediate frequencies. With a hydraulic oscillator, one can of course obtain impedance results

over a continuous range of frequencies by slowly
increasing speed of the driving motor. Input impedance can however be obtained over a wide frequency range by inducing heart block and pacing
the heart at different rates. Figure 6.4 shows the
results of such an experiment. Evidence of linearity is apparent from the impedance plots which
show near superposition of modulus and phase
values irrespective of what harmonic pair they
were calculated from.

Figure 6.5 shows flow wave and pressure *gradient* waves in the femoral artery, their component
harmonics, and the relationship of harmonics as
longitudinal impedance. As discussed in Chapter 4,
longitudinal impedance is determined by the regional properties of the aorta alone, not as with
input impedance, properties of the whole vascular
bed. It should be noted that while flow contour
and harmonic content are similar to that in the
ascending aorta, pressure gradient and longitudinal impedance are vastly different to aortic pressure wave and input impedance respectively. Amplitude of the differential pressure wave is very

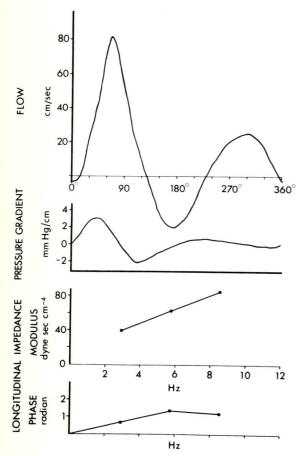

Fig. 6.5 *Longitudinal impedance* is the relationship between
differential pressure (pressure gradient/cm along an artery) and
flow in the artery. *Top*: Recorded flow (solid line) and pressure
gradient in the femoral artery of a dog, as published by
McDonald (1960).
Bottom: Modulus (above) and phase (below) of longitudinal
impedance calculated from Fourier analysis of these waves. In
contrast to imput impedance, longitudinal impedance modulus
increases progressively with frequency, while phase is always
positive, and approaches 90° with increasing frequency.

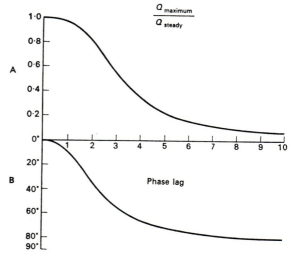

Fig. 6.6 Womersley's theroretic determination of the
relationship between pulsatile flow and pressure gradient in an
artery.
Top: Amplitude of oscillatory flow harmonic as a fraction of
amplitude of steady flow component. 1.0 corresponds to
Poiseuille's value of 1/8.
Bottom: Phase lag of flow after pressure
Abscissa is Womersley's non dimensional parameter α
(α = radius $\times \sqrt{\text{angular frequency} \div \text{kinematic viscosity}}$)
which determines kinematic similarity of flow. The flow ratio,
can be displayed in terms of longitudinal impedance, with
features similar to that in Fig. 6.5. From Womersley (1955.)

low, and its mean value is small in comparison to component harmonics. The modulus of longitudinal impedance is low at zero frequency (mean value) and increases with increasing frequency. Longitudinal impedance is of mainly historical interest. It is of little practical value (in contrast to the great usefulness of input impedance) and is shown again here for the sake of completeness, and to stress the difference between arteriovenous pressure difference (from which input impedance is calculated) and pressure gradient along a segment of artery. The theoretic longitudinal impedance of a vascular segment has been determined by Womersley (1957), and is usually displayed in a different form, as a graph of normalised modulus (compared to Poiseuille resistance expressed as 1.0), and phase lag (delay of flow after pressure – Figure 6.6). This subject is discussed in detail by McDonald (1960 and 1974). Longitudinal impedance will not be mentioned again, but input impedance will be discussed repeatedly.

Figure 6.7 shows results obtained from a comparison of corresponding harmonic components of pressure waves at different sites between the aortic arch and iliac artery (the waves in Figure 9.3). The progressive rise in the first two harmonics, and the early dip and later rise of the third, fourth and fifth was one of the first features noted by McDonald and Taylor, and attributed by them to peripheral wave reflection and non-uniform arterial elasticity (McDonald 1960, Taylor 1965). This data may also be displayed as a graph of amplification against frequency in comparing corresponding harmonics of pressure waves in the aortic arch to those in the iliac artery (Fig. 9.15).

Frequency spectrum analysis

The technique of frequency spectrum analysis was first applied to arterial pressure/flow relationships by Randall (1958). Its full potential was exploited by Taylor (1966) who stressed that the mathematical technique ought to be applied only when the heart is made to beat irregularly. In frequency spectrum analysis, a long train of simultaneously-recorded pressure and flow waves (or differential

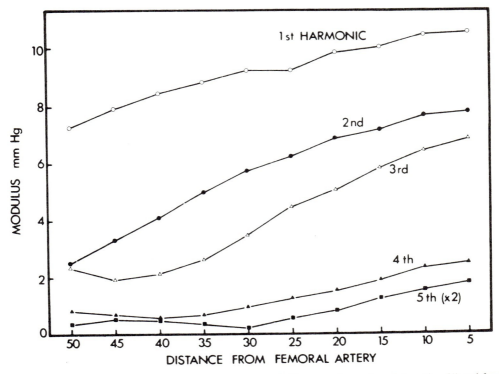

Fig. 6.7 Amplitude of the first five harmonics of pressure waves recorded between the aortic arch (position 50) and femoral artery of a wombat. Individual waves are shown in Fig. 9.3. From O'Rourke 1967

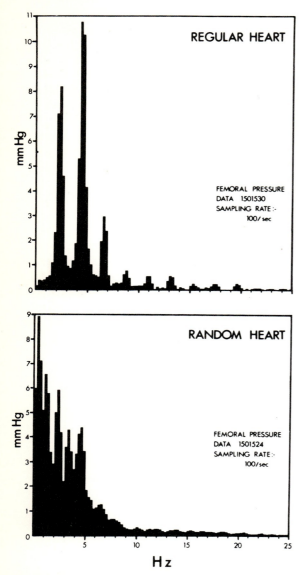

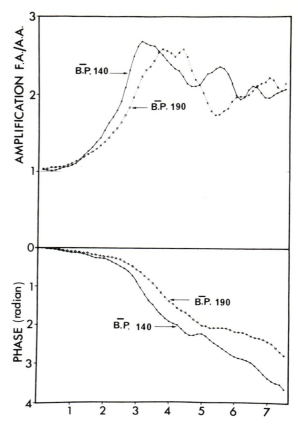

Fig. 6.9 Amplification (above) and phase difference (below) of pressure in the aortic arch and femoral artery of a dog under control conditions (closed circles) and with increased mean arterial pressure (open circles). Pulse wave velocity approximately 7.8 m sec^{-1} under control conditions and approximately 10.4 m sec^{-1} at the higher pressure. From O'Rourke (1970), with permission American Heart Association Inc.

Fig. 6.8 Amplitude of frequency components of femoral artery pressure waves with the heart beating regularly (above) and with cardiac irregularity induced by random electrical stimulation (below). From Taylor (1966) with permission American Heart Association Inc.

pressure and flow, or pressure and pressure) are recorded, digitised, and the frequency spectrum is obtained by auto- and cross-correlation techniques or by Fast Fourier transform algorithms. One obtains from this, graphs of spectral energy of the waves, input impedance, longitudinal impedance, or pressure wave amplification respectively. With the heart beating regularly, energy is confined to the harmonics of the waves, but when the heart is beating irregularly, energy is spread more evenly (Fig. 6.8). In the latter case, one can obtain pressure amplification (Fig. 6.9) or input impedance (Fig. 6.10) over a wide and evenly spaced band of frequencies such as can only otherwise be obtained with heart block and artificial pacing, as in Fig. 6.4.

The mathematical technique of frequency spectrum analysis is more complicated than Fourier analysis and a digital computer is required. This type of analysis is widely used in the physical sciences, and appropriate computer software is easily available. It is surprising that it is not utilised more frequently, particularly in analysis of data from patients with atrial fibrillation.

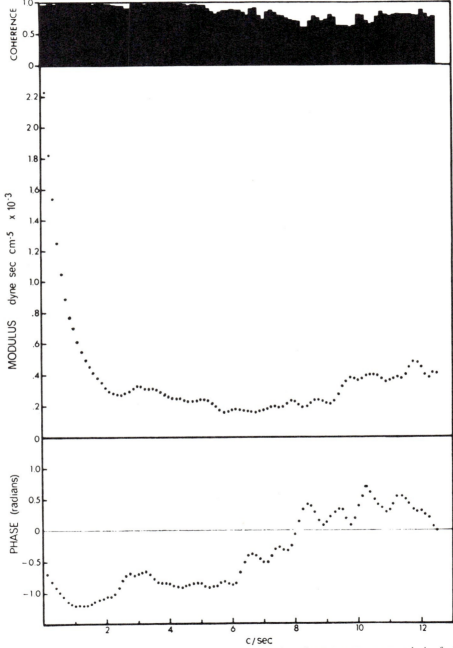

Fig. 6.10 Vascular impedance in the ascending aorta of a dog, determined from frequency spectrum analysis of a long series of pressure and flow waves recorded during random electrical stimulation of the heart Abscissa: cycle sec^{-1}. From Taylor 1966 with permission American Heart Association Inc.

REFERENCES

Alexander RS 1953 The genesis of the aortic standing wave. Circulation Research 1: 145–151

Aperia A 1940 Haemodynamical studies. Scandinavian Archives of Physiology 83: Supplement 1 1–230

Berne RM, Levy MN 1977 Cardiovascular Physiology 3rd ed. Mosby St Louis.

Braunwald E 1980 Heart Disease. Saunders Philadelphia p. 22–24

Caro CG, McDonald DA 1961 The relation of pulsatile pressure and flow in the pulmonary vascular bed. Journal of Physiology (London) 157: 426–453

Gow BS 1980 The Handbook of Physiology, Section 2. The Cardiovascular System Volume II Vascular smooth muscle. Bohr DF, Somloy O, Sparks HV Jr, Geiger SR (eds). The American Physiological Society Bethesda Marylands Circulatory Correlates: Vascular impedance resistance and capacity: 14: 353–408

Hamilton WF, Dow P 1939 An experimental study of the standing waves in the pulse porpagated through aorta. American Journal of Physiology 125: 48–59

Hurst JW, Schlant RC 1978 Examination of the arteries and their pulsations. In: Hurst JW (ed) The Heart McGraw New York p. 183–192

Little RC 1977 Physiology of the heart circulation. Year Book Medical Publishers Chicago

McDonald DA 1960 Blood flow in arteries. 1st Edition Arnold London

McDonald DA 1974 Blood flow in arteries. 2nd Edition Arnold London

McDonald DA, Taylor MG 1959 the hydrodynamics of the arterial circulation. Progress in Biophysics and Biophysical Chemistry 9: 107–173

Milnor WR 1974 The Circulation. In: Mountcastle VB (ed) Medical Physiology Mosby St. Louis p. 839–1026

Murgo JP, Westerhof N, Giolma JP, Altobelli SA, 1980 Aortic input impedance in normal man: relationship to pressure wave forms. Circulation 62, 1: 105–116

O'Rourke MF 1967 Pressure and flow waves in systemic arteries and the anatomical design of the arterial system. Journal of applied Physiology 23: 139–149

O'Rourke MF 1970 Arterial hemodynamics in hypertension. Circulation Research 26 Suppl. 2: 123–133

O'Rourke MF 1971 The arterial pulse in health and disease. American Heart Journal 82: 687–802

O'Rourke MF, Taylor MG 1966 Vascular impedance of the femoral bed. Circulation Research 18: 126–139

O'Rourke MF, Taylor MG 1967 Input impedance of the systemic circulation. Circulation Research 20: 365–380

Patel GJ, De Freitas FM, Fry DL 1963 Hydraulic input impedance to aorta and pulmonary artery in dogs. Journal of Applied Physiology 18: 134–140

Patel DJ, Mason DT, Ross J Jr., Braunwald E 1965 Harmonic analysis of pressure pulses obtained from the heart and great vessels of man. American Heart Journal 69: 785–794

Porjé IG 1946 Studies of the arterial pulse waves particularly in the aorta. Acta Physiologica Scandinavia 13: (Suppl. 42) 7–68

Randall JE 1958 Statistical properties of pulsatile pressure and flow in the femoral artery of the dog. Circulation Research 6: 689–698

Remington JW 1963 The physiology of the aorta and major arteries. Handbook of Physiology, American Physiological Society Washington DC Volume 2 Circulation 2: 799–838

Remington JW, O'Brien LJ 1970 Construction of aortic flow pulse from pressure pulse. American Journal of Physiology 218: 437–447

Sipkema P, Westerhof N, Randall OS 1980 The arterial system characterised in the time domain. Cardiovascular Research 14: 270–290

Spencer MP, Denison AB 1963 Pulsatile blood flow in the vascular system. Handbook of Physiology, American Physiological Society Washington DC Volume 2 Circulation 2: 839–864

Taylor MG 1964 Wave travel in arteries and the design of the cardiovascular system. In: Attinger EO (ed.) Pulsatile Blood Flow McGraw New York p. 343–372

Taylor MG 1966 Use of random excitation and spectral analysis in the study of frequency – dependent parameters of the cardiovascular system. Circulation Research 18: 585–595

Wallace AG 1979 Arterial pressure and pulses. In: Beeson PB, McDermott W, Wyngaarden JB (eds) Cecil Textbook of Medicine Saunders Philadelphia p. 1074

Westerhof N, Sipkema P, Elzinga G, Murgo JP, Giolma JP 1979 Arterial impedance. In: Hwang HC, Gross DR, Patel DJ (eds.) Quantitative cardiovascular studies, Univeristy park Baltimore Ch 3 p. 111–150

Wetterer E 1954 Flow and pressure in the arterial system, their hemodynamic relationship and the principles of the measurement. Minnesota Medicine 37: 77–86

Wetterer E, Kenner T 1968 Grundlagen der dynamik des arterienpulses. Springer Verlag, Berlin

Womersley JR 1955 Method for the calculation of velocity, rate of flow and viscous drag in arteries when the pressure gradient is known. Journal of Physiology 127: 553–563

Womersley JR 1957 The mathematical analysis of the arterial circulation in a state of oscillatory motion. Wright Air Development Center Technical Report W.A.D.C.–T.R. 56–614

7

Wave reflection

Over the years there has been, and there continues now, considerable controversy about wave reflection in arteries – whether it occurs at all under normal circumstances, and if so, how much wave reflection occurs, whence it arises, and whether re-reflection of reflected waves is possible. The argument presented here is that wave reflection does occur, and is usually intense, that it arises predominantly from normally constricted arterioles and that re-reflection is a definite and important determinant of pulse wave contour. Most differences in opinion among different workers in this field as to intensity of reflection can be explained on the basis of timing of reflected waves and on the basis of interaction of reflected waves from different sites with each other and with the incident wave generated by the heart.

The first known reference to wave reflection in the arterial system was by Galen who described the effects of occluding an artery with a ligature. This was referred to again by Harvey (1649) in his letters to Jean Riolan, when defending his concept of the blood's circulation – and in unequivocal terms '. . *unde et fluxus inhibitur et impetus refringitur . . . eo quod supra ligaturam reverberatur*'.

It is obvious that the pressure impulse generated by the heart moves away from the heart at a finite speed. This pulse wave velocity can be calculated from the time taken for the foot of the wave to travel a measured distance, say from the ascending aorta to the femoral artery. Wave velocity averages some 7 metres sec^{-1} over this interval (Ch. 4). It is obvious that between heart beats the wave has sufficient time to travel over a far greater length than any arterial network in the mammalian body. What happens to the wave? Is it damped to extinction in the small peripheral vessels or is it reflected *i.e.* turned back upon itself, at arterioles, branching points, or other points of discontinuity in the vascular tree? If the wave were damped out completely, and so there were no reflection of any form at the heart, one would expect that the pressure wave in the ascending aorta would have the same contour as the ascending aortic flow wave. This is precisely what one sees at the mouth of a uniform elastic tube of great length when it is filled with a liquid and a flow impulse is generated at its origin (Wetterer 1954, McDonald and Taylor 1959, McDonald 1974, Kouchoukos et al 1970). But the ascending aortic pressure wave is quite different to the ascending aortic flow wave (Fig. 7.1). This is the first evidence of wave reflec-

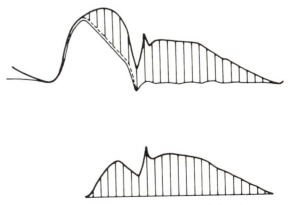

Fig. 7.1 *Top*: Pressure and flow waves recorded in the ascending aorta of a dog. In the absence of wave reflection, and if the heart were a pure flow source, the pressure wave would be expected to be almost identical to the flow wave. This is shown as the dotted line. The shaded area is the difference between actual pressure and this predicted pressure wave. After Kouchoukos et al 1970.
Bottom: The shaded area between recorded pressure and predicted pressure in the absence of wave reflection. This appears to be biphasic, suggesting the presence of two peripheral reflecting sites at different distances from the heart

tion. The next point is that pressure waves (and flow waves) in the aorta and other arteries often show very obvious secondary fluctuations in diastole. If the ventricle beats but once per cardiac cycle, and if the arteries themselves do not contract actively (a hypothesis that was first refuted by Harvey in 1628) the only possible explanation for this secondary wave is some type of wave reflection. This was discussed at length by Otto Frank (1899, 1905, 1926, 1930) in relation to the first accurate recordings of intra-arterial pressure.

That wave reflection exists must, I believe, be accepted as a matter of fact. One must then seek the mechanism and answer the questions – How much? From where? How often? A satisfactory explanation will have to account for the contour of pressure waves in different arteries under different conditions, and the contour of flow waves as well, together with the relationships of different harmonic components of these waves to each other. The explanation will also have to reconcile the views of those who consider wave reflection to be absent or inapparent under some conditions (Peterson 1954, Morkin 1967, Murgo et al 1977, Westerhof et al 1979, Bourguignon and Wagner 1979, Wagner

1980) and will have to account too for disappearance of the diastolic pressure fluctuations under some circumstances in experimental animals (as when arterial pressure is markedly increased, Wetterer 1954 (Fig. 7.2) or the aorta is occluded (O'Rourke 1970, O'Rourke and Cartmill 1971) and their appearance after apparent absence in other cases, as in an adult human on development of cardiogenic or hypovolemic shock or during the Valsalva manouver (O'Rourke 1971). Such explanations can, I believe, be given for all conditions and for all animals, and for man, on the basis of different degrees of interaction between incident and reflected waves, and between different reflected waves from more than one peripheral site.

EVIDENCE AGAINST WAVE REFLECTION EXPLAINED

Before proceeding, it would be desirable to consider and explain some of the evidence quoted against the view that wave reflection is a major factor in determining pulse wave contour.

It is often pointed out that arterial pressure

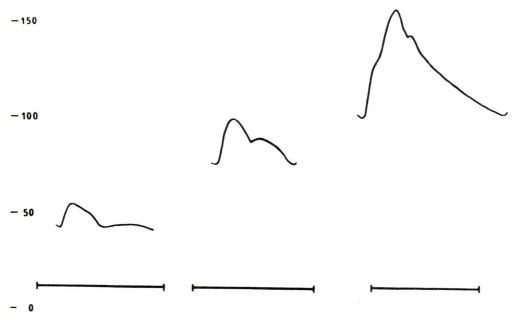

Fig. 7.2 Effect of increasing pressure on contour of pressure waves in the ascending aorta of a rabbit. Diastolic waves are apparent at lower pressures but absent when arterial pressure is abnormally high. With hypertension the diastolic wave is replaced by a late systolic pressure peak. From O'Rourke 1970, after data rearranged from Wetterer (1954), with permission American Heart Association Inc.

waves sometimes have no diastolic wave at all, and that pressure during diastole appears to fall in an exponential fashion after aortic valve closure, just as it might in an elastic chamber or *Windkessel* in which pulse wave velocity was infinite. Absence of diastolic pressure fluctuations in waves showing such contour permits change in peripheral resistance or arterial compliance to be determined on the basis of the simple *Windkessel* model (Warner et al 1953, Bourgeois et al 1974, Simon et al 1979). This finding is not at variance with the concept of travelling and reflected waves. Pressure

pulse contour in older human subjects characteristically shows such exponential decline without secondary waves during diastole (Freis et al 1966, O'Rourke et al 1968, Fig. 7.3). This is explained on the basis of arterial degeneration with age causing increased pulse wave velocity (Ch. 12) so that reflected waves from all peripheral sites return early, during systole, and interact with the incident waves so that all fuse; as a result there is no discretely identifiable wave reflection during diastole, and so no obvious diastolic wave, but just a gradual smooth exponential decline in pressure

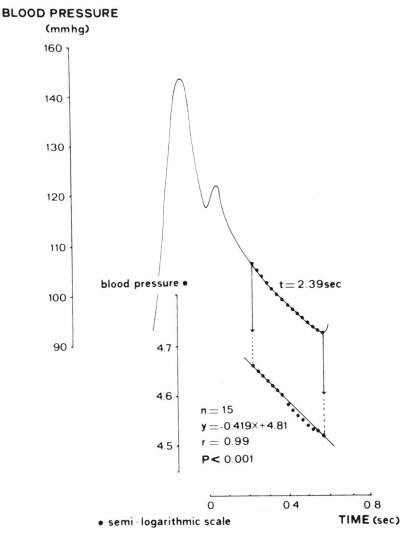

Fig. 7.3 Pressure recorded under control conditions from the brachial artery of an adult human subject. In this case diastolic pressure decline is utilised for determination of arterial compliance. (From Simon et al 1979)

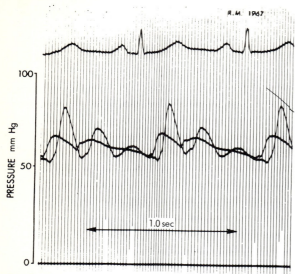

Fig. 7.4 Pressure waves recorded simultaneously in the aortic arch and brachial artery of an adult patient with hypotension and clinical features of peripheral vasoconstriction. Damped natural frequency of both manometer systems exceeded 20 Hz. From O'Rourke (1970) with permission American Heart Association Inc.

(O'Rourke 1971). This explanation uncovers an important problem in the clinical application of the techniques described by Bourgeois and Simon. These techniques are not applicable if systole shortens or if wave velocity falls (as it does in cardiac failure and shock) when the diastolic wave reappears and can become very prominent indeed (Fig. 7.4). This matter draws attention to the two simple models of the arterial system (Ch. 4) – on the one hand, the Windkessel, in which pressure changes instantaneously throughout, there is no reflection, and pressure falls exponentially during diastole, and on the other hand the tube of finite length with finite wave velocity and definite wave reflection. This is discussed again in Chapter 9. Under some circumstances, as when pulse wave velocity is high, the whole arterial system behaves like a Windkessel while under other circumstances it behaves like an elastic tube with obvious wave reflection. Otto Frank effected an uneasy compromise between these two concepts over 50 years ago (see McDonald and Taylor (1959) for further discussion), referring to the *Grundform* or basic exponential decline or the pressure pulse and the *Grundschwingung* or superimposed oscillation due to wave reflection. The

conflict is readily resolved by the obvious explanation:– if a tubular model is short enough, and wave velocity fast enough, and if excitation is long enough, all incident and reflected waves will fuse and the tubular model will behave like a Windkessel (Wetterer 1954, Wetterer et all 1977).

The anatomical design of the arterial system is not conducive to discrete wave reflection. McDonald quoted his colleague John Womersley as saying 'if you wanted to design a perfect sound absorber you could hardly do better than a set of tapering and branching tubes with considerable internal damping such as the arterial tree'. To which one could add that with the enormous variation in length to peripheral arterial terminations, one would expect that any wave reflections would return at different times, and so cancel each other completely. And yet one does see diastolic oscillations of pressure and flow which are sometimes up to half the amplitude of the original wave (Fig. 7.4). The most logical explanation for this is that in the mammalian body, peripheral reflecting sites are so grouped at the extremities of the body as to produce a single functionally-disctete reflecting site. As shown by Taylor (1966) and as discussed later (Ch. 9), reflected waves in mammals do cancel each other out at high frequencies, but at low frequencies – less than approximately 8 Hz. in the dog and man at normal pulse wave velocity – appear to be arising from one functionally discrete site at each end of the body (O'Rourke and Taylor 1967, O'Rourke 1967). This is the single most surprising aspect of arterial function – that reflected waves appear to arise from one functionally discrete site despite the fact that the major individual reflecting sites, the arterioles, (see p. 88) are distributed spatially over a great distance. In our studies of reflection in man and experimental animals, the only animal in which reflection did not appear under any circumstances was the snake (Avolio et al 1980). In the snake, spatial dispersion of individual reflecting sites is apparently sufficient to cause full cancellation of individual reflected waves so that no single functionally-discrete site is apparent; in the snake, arterial pressure falls exponentially after even the sharpest and briefest perturbation.

In his earlier studies McDonald (1960) calculated peripheral reflection coefficient in systemic arteries as approximately 0.35. On the basis of this and of his work with Womersley on wave attenuation in travel, he considered that the effects of wave reflection on arterial phenomena would be relatively small, and argued strongly against the idea of high wave reflection leading to 'standing waves' in the arterial system. Hamilton and Dow had introduced this concept in 1939 to explain the presence of diastolic pressure waves and their reciprocity in upper and lower body arteries. In the second edition (1974) of his monograph, McDonald admitted that his estimation of wave reflection was too low but on the basis of high viscous damping still would not concede that reflected waves could traverse, then retraverse the arterial system with sufficient amplitude to retain a discrete identity. McDonald's writing on this subject is somewhat contradictory in that while he showed evidence of strong wave reflection in data analysed in the frequency domain, he would not acknowledge the same evidence of discrete reflection in pressure displayed in the time domain – in pulse wave contour. McDonald accepted the presence of secondary diastolic waves in the arterial pulse but would not concede that these were due to reflection and rereflection of the original wave. This is the single issue in McDonald's classic monograph on which his views and my own are at odds.

Other studies, often still quoted to refute the concept of strong wave reflection are those of Peterson and Shepard (1955) and of Starr (1957). Peterson and Shepard generated a pressure wave in the femoral artery of a dog by a rapid injection of blood and found that the resulting impulse, travelling retrogradely along the aorta was barely detectable in the ascending aorta. This is not a good argument against wave reflection. Reflected waves return from many arteries, the femoral artery being just one of these. A more realistic test would have been simultaneous generation of pressure waves in a dozen or more peripheral arteries. The femoral artery is the most obvious artery to the body's most distant point, but it appears to have no more importance in peripheral reflection than a dozen or so arteries of similar calibre. Interventions in one artery cause trivial changes at a distance. Occlusion of both femoral arteries causes little change in ascending aortic pressure wave contour or in aortic wave transmission (McDonald 1960,

O'Rourke 1969) – a fact that can be interpreted to indicate normally high reflection coefficient in the femoral bed (p. 100). The findings of Peterson and Shepard are not supported in any case by the common finding of a pressure fluctuation of 5–20 mm Hg in the brachial artery of patients on cardiopulmonary bypass who are being perfused through the femoral artery.

Starr's experiments were performed on human cadavers. After artificially generating a pressure wave in the aorta, he measured only a small retrograde reflected wave and found no evidence of secondary reflection at the aortic valve or in the upper part of the body. Starr's experiments were done under circumstances of apparent gross peripheral arteriolar relaxation (death). In living patients, when blood pressure is low and peripheral resistance is high, a short, sharp ventricular ejection produces an extremely prominent diastolic wave. So prominent is this diastolic wave in patients with cardiogenic shock, in whom hypotension, vasoconstriction, and short ventricular ejection are combined, (Fig. 7.4), that it can interfere with identification of the cardiac incisura, and so cause problems in timing of arterial counterpulsation (Ch. 13).

REFLECTION OF A TRANSIENT PULSE

In explaining pulse transmission and reflection, it is useful to consider a simple elastic tube, and the pressure waves that result in this when a flow wave is generated at its origin (McDonald and Taylor 1959). Figure 7.5 shows pressure waves in such a tube with the tube clamped at different distances from its origin. The effects of wave reflection are seen as echos after the initial wave, occurring at shorter and shorter intervals when the tube is clamped closer and closer to its mouth. After the wave is generated in this case, both origin and end of the tube behave as closed end reflecting sites. The wave is seen to bounce back and forth between origin and termination of the tube until damped to extinction as a result of the (necessarily) incomplete reflection at each end and attenuation cause by viscosity of the tubular wall and contained fluid. With successive reflections, the mean pressure rises as a result of the tube's further dis-

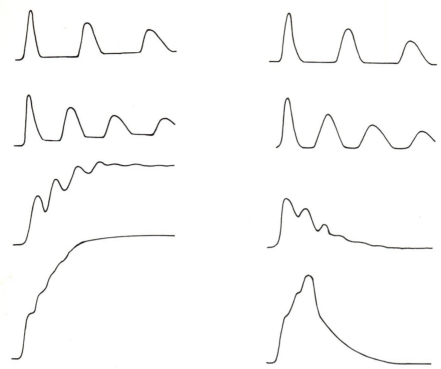

Fig. 7.5 Diagrammatic representation of pressure waves in the proximal part of a long distensible tube following a brief injection of fluid. The first pulse in each case is the result of fluid input. Subsequent pulses are echos from the distal closed end of the tube. From above down, the tube is occluded closer and closer to its mouth. Figures on the left side relate to a totally occluded tube. Figures on the right relate to a tube whose distal obstruction is subtotal. Data rearranged from that published by McDonald and Taylor (1959)

tension by the volume of fluid injected.

The waves a, b, and c in Figure 7.5 are taken from McDonald and Taylor (1959). The wave (d) is added to illustrate the effect that might be expected if the tube were occluded even closer to its origin. The mean level of pressure will increase even higher than in cases a, b, and c (which is what one would expect with the same flow pulse injected into a tube of smaller capacity) but the reflected waves summate with the incident wave so that wave reflection is far less apparent than when the tube is occluded at a greater distance. Indeed cases b, c, and d are the only ones relevant to the mammalian arterial system, where reflected waves from peripheral sites return just after, at the end of, or during ventricular ejection.

The simple tubular model used to obtain data for Figure 7.5 differs in a number of respects from the systemic arterial tree. For a start, both ends are completely closed so that mean pressure rises by a certain level as the result of fluid injection. The

terminations of the arterial tree (the arterioles) permit slow and steady blood flow so that mean pressure falls to its original value before the next cardiac cycle. In the model experiments, allowance can be made for this by assuming an exponential fall in pressure from the peak of ejection, and drawing pressure oscillations around this line. The results (Fig. 7.5, right), show pressure waves similar to those recorded in arteries under different conditions. The similarity (Fig. 7.2) to those recorded during hypotension, (case b), control conditions (case c) and hypertension (case d) is apparent.

The waves synthesised from experimental data in Figure 7.5 show obvious reflection in cases b and c, but not in case d. Yet these three waves would be recorded at the mouth of a tube with the same degree of peripheral reflection. Were the duration of injection shorter in case (d) the reflected wave would be just as apparent as in case (c). Were the duration of injection in case (c) lengthened, the reflected wave would be as inapparent as in case (d). This illustrates the important point of reflected wave summation. Wave reflection may be apparent only as a deviation of the contour of pressure wave from the contour of flow input. Only when the period of ejection is short, or when the reflected wave returns late, can the reflected wave be identified as a distinct discrete entity.

Figure 7.1 shows pressure and flow waves recorded in the ascending aorta by Kouchoukos et al (1970) together (dotted line) with the pressure one would predict in the absence of wave reflection. The shaded area represents the pressure difference which is attributable to wave reflection. This appears to be biphasic, as shown in the lower part of Figure 7.1., with a smaller systolic and larger diastolic component. Evidence to be presented later suggests that there are two functionally discrete reflecting sites in the systemic circulation, one representing the resultant of all individual reflecting sites in the upper part of the body, and the other, further away, representing the resultant of all individual reflecting sites in the lower part of the body. In Figure 7.1, the late systolic peak may be due predominantly to wave reflection from the upper body and the diastolic wave, predominantly to wave reflection from the lower part of the body.

Harvey's description of Galen's experiment has been noted. Occlusion of an artery by a ligature causes reflection of the pressure wave at the liga-

ture. Yet also as noted, under normal circumstances arterial occlusion causes little change in the pressure wave upstream, even immediately above the ligature (p. 81). Only if the artery is severed downstream, or when the arterial bed downstream is dilated, does occlusion of an artery cause a substantial change in pressure pulse contour upstream. An extension of Harvey's logic would lead one to conclude that wave reflection in a vascular bed under normal circumstances is already quite high.

ANALYSIS OF WAVE REFLECTION IN STEADY-STATE OSCILLATION

When considering the arterial pulse in the frequency domain, and when interpreting pressure/pressure, and pressure/flow relationships in terms of wave reflection, it is important to know what behaviour one would expect of sinusoidal waves travelling to and fro in tubular models of the arterial system.

Pressure waves

Figure 7.6 shows a simple tubular model of the arterial system, excited at its origin by a pump which generates sinusoidal flow. The amplitude of

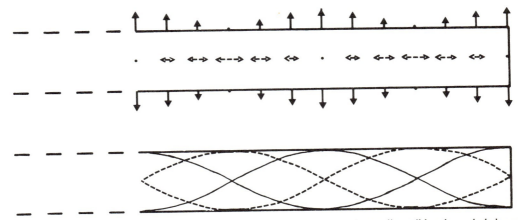

Fig. 7.6 *Top*: Pressure (solid lines with arrows) and flow (dashed lines with arrows) along a distensible tube occluded completely at its right end and activated by a sinusoidal oscillation. At the closed end pressure fluctuations are maximal and flow oscillations, zero. Back along the tube maxima and minima of pressure alternate with corresponding minima and maxima respectively of flow. The position of these antinodes and nodes are determined by pulse wave velocity of the tube and the frequency of the sinusoidal oscillation.
Bottom: Pressure and flow oscillations at different points along this tube can be represented by the solid line (for pressure) and the broken line (for flow)

pressure waves generated in this tube will be determined by the tube ending. If the tube is completely occluded, then the patterns of pressure back along the tube can be determined from this end, when one knows wave velocity of the tube and the frequency of the pump.

Figure 7.7 (a) shows pressure wave distribution along this tube at that one instant in time when amplitude of the incident wave is greatest at the tube ending. There will be at this time a sinusoidal distribution of pressure along this tube with successive maximal and minimal values whose position will depend on wave velocity of the tube (c) and pump frequency (n). The position of the second maximum of pressure back along the tube will represent one full wavelength (one complete sine wave will be inscribed between this point and the closed end) and this wavelength λ from the tube end is given by the elementary formula $\lambda = \dfrac{c}{n}$ If

wave velocity in the tube were 8 metre sec^{-1}, and if frequency were 4 Hz, the wavelength would be two metres. If frequency were increased to 8 Hz, or wave velocity were reduced to 4 metre sec^{-1}, wavelength would fall to 1 metre, so that the maximum of pressure would be seen 1 metre from the closed tubular end. The second smaller wave in Figure 7.7(a) represents the reflected wave returning from the closed end with amplitude 80 percent of the incident wave and with the same phase (*i.e.* the same timing). This will travel back along the tube and add to the incident wave so that the resultant wave will be 1.8 times the amplitude of the initial wave. The peak of the reflected wave, and of the resultant wave will be seen 1 wavelength back from the closed end.

Figure 7.7(a) shows pressure distribution along the tube at that instant in time when pressure amplitude is greatest at its closed end. With sinusoidal input into the tube, pressure amplitude at this point will vary with time, first falling to zero, then to a minimal value equal in amplitude but opposite in sign at one half pump cycle, then will pass through zero to its maximal positive value again at the end of one full pump cycle. In other words pressure amplitude at the tube end varies sinusoidally with time, while pressure amplitude along the tube varies sinusoidally with distance. One quarter wavelength back from the closed end (*i.e.* 50 cms back if wave velocity were 8 metre sec^{-1} and frequency 4 Hz), pressure oscillation would be zero, and would remain zero through the whole cycle while on each side of this point, pressure would vary sinusoidally with time but with a much smaller amplitude than at the closed end. At sites a short distance away on either side of this point, amplitude of oscillation will be equal but of opposite sign *i.e.* one will be positive by a given amount while the other will be negative by the same amount; they are 180° out of phase. Along the tube, amplitude varies sinusoidally with distance, but phase changes abruptly from 180° positive to 180° negative at one quarter and three quarter wavelength back from the closed end. One half wavelength back from the end, (100 cm back with wave velocity 8 metre sec^{-1} and frequency 4 Hz), pressure oscillation would be the same as that both at the closed end and one wavelength back, but of opposite sign (180° phase difference).

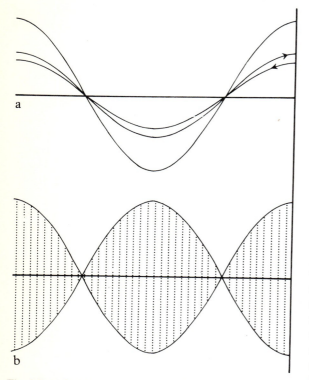

Fig. 7.7 (a) Incident wave (arrow pointing right), reflected wave (arrow pointing left), and resultant wave (top) of sinusoidal pressure when pressure is highest at the end of an elastic tube.
(b) The pressure wave envelope in this tube. For explanation, see text.

The pressure oscillation along this tube can be displayed in the form of an envelope (Fig. 7.7(b)) which shows a maximal amplitude at the tubular end, and at one half wavelength, and again at one wavelength, and with minimal values at one quarter and three quarter wavelength. At any one point along the tube, pressure will vary in sinusoidal fashion with a modulus or maximal amplitude as shown by the wave envelope at that point. The wave envelope shows modulus or maximal amplitude of the sine wave at any point while giving no indication of phase.

The patterns shown in Figure 7.7 are determined by wave travel and reflection so that their position can be predicted from the reflecting site when one knows wave velocity of the tube and frequency of the pump. The patterns are not determined by the position of the pump along the tube. If this tubular model (Fig. 7.6) is excited not by a simple sine wave, but by a compound wave

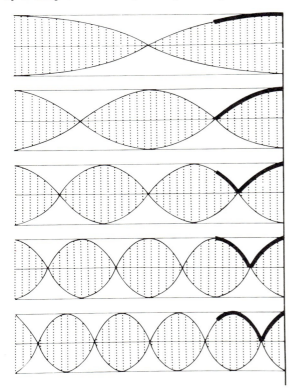

Fig. 7.8 The pressure wave envelope over the last 50 cms of an elastic tube, completely occluded at its end, for the first 5 harmonics of a compound pressure wave. Wave velocity 8 metre sec⁻¹; frequency of compound wave, 2 sec⁻¹. For explanation, see text. (Compare with Fig. 6.7.)

containing different harmonics – like an arterial pulse wave – the same principles will apply, with the position of different maxima and minima of pressure modulus along the tube depending on the frequency of the different harmonics. If the pump frequency were 2 sec⁻¹, and wave velocity were 8 metre sec⁻¹, one wavelength would be 4 metres for the first harmonic, 2 metres for the second harmonic, 4/3 metres for the third harmonic, 1 metre for the fourth, and 0.8 for the fifth. Figure 7.8 shows the wave envelopes for the first five harmonics of a compound wave (assuming these to be of equal amplitude) in the last metre of a tube, with wave velocity 8 metre sec⁻¹ and frequency 2 Hz. Highlighted are the changes in modulus one would expect over the last 50 cms of this tube for the first five harmonics of the compound pressure wave. These changes in pressure modulus are very similar to those of pressure waves recorded along the aorta to the femoral artery of dogs (McDonald 1974) and other mammals (Fig. 6.7) and represent good evidence of a strong reflecting site in the vascular bed just beyond the last reflecting site.

In Figure 6.7, the fluctuation in modulus of pressure wave harmonics along the aorta is superimposed on a general increase in amplitude between the aortic arch and iliac artery. This is not seen in the simple tubular model, but has been a consistent finding in dogs and other mammals. This has been investigated in detail by Taylor (1964, 1965, 1967) who has shown that this general increase in modulus of all pressure wave harmonics along the aorta to peripheral arteries is explained by the progressive increase in stiffness of the aorta and other arteries away from the heart – the non-uniform elasticity of arteries. Taylor (1964) calculated the change in amplitude of pressure wave harmonics in a simple tubular model such as Figure 7.6 but in which arterial distensibility was reduced by a factor of three between the most proximal and most distal point. Figure 7.9 shows the relative amplitude of pressure oscillations as a function of frequency between the origin and end of such a tube, when this was scaled to represent the distance between the ascending aorta and femoral artery. The general increase of all frequencies is attributable to decreasing arterial distensibility, and the oscillation, to peripheral wave

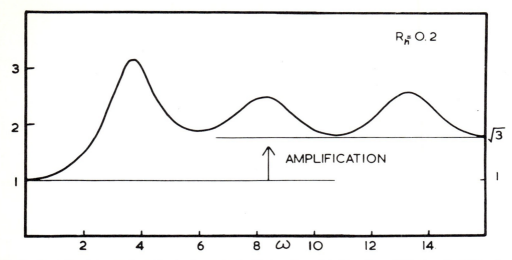

Fig. 7.9 Ratio of peripheral to central amplitude of pressure oscillations in a tube whose distensibility is reduced by a factor of 3 between its origin and distal end. Abscissa – circular frequency ω (ω = frequency × 2π). (Compare with Fig. 6.10) from Taylor 1965. In: Attinger ED (ed) Pulsatile Blood Flow McGraw-Hill, New York. With permission.

reflection. The greatest increase in pressure amplitude occurs at that frequency where the distance from inlet to tubular termination represents one quarter wavelength. Figure 6.9 shows pressure amplification between the aortic arch and femoral artery of a dog, obtained from frequency spectrum analysis of pressure waves recorded simultaneously at both sites. These results correspond well with Taylor's predictions of pressure transmission in a model showing non-uniform distensibility. Figure 6.9 shows also the effects on pressure amplification of raising mean arterial pressure. As one would predict, the amplification curve is shifted to the right with peak amplification now occuring at a higher frequency. This is attributable to the increase in pulse wave velocity at the higher mean pressure. At the higher pulse wave velocity, wavelength is increased; the distance from aortic arch to femoral artery represents one quarter wavelength at a higher frequency. (In Figure 6.9 the increase in pulse wave velocity is apparent in a lower phase angle of the amplification plot; this represents a decreased delay of femoral pressure oscillations after aortic arch oscillations.)

In attempting to simplify a subject which is difficult conceptually to grasp, I have omitted consideration of changes in phase of pressure waves along the aorta and in its branches. From the sim-

ple modelling studies, one would expect such changes in phase to occur, and indeed they do. Evidence of such change is the fluctuation in relative phase of aortic and femoral pressure waves at low frequencies as seen in the lower part of Figure 6.9. These fluctuations become less apparent at higher frequencies as a result of reflected wave interaction; they are usually inapparent above 8 Hz in dogs and man. Further details on changes in phase and in apparent phase velocity along the aorta may be found in McDonald (1960, 1974) and O'Rourke (1967).

Pressure flow relationships: hydraulic or vascular impedance

In the tubular model it was noted that pressure amplitude was least at one quarter and three quarter wavelengths from the closed end, and greatest at the end, and at one half and one wavelength back. These pressure oscillations in a tube with closed end are associated with corresponding flow oscillations which are one quarter pump cycle or 90° out of phase, both in time and place (Fig. 7.6). At the end of the tube, flow oscillation is (necessarily) zero, while pressure oscillation is maximal. At one quarter wavelength back, pressure oscillation is minimal while flow oscillation is maximal. (One can look at this as minimal particle displacement in the lateral direction (pressure) and maximal displacement in the horizontal direction (flow)).

Impedance is a standard and well accepted term in physics for describing the relationship between alternating voltage and current (electrical impedance), and the sinusoidal components of pressure and gas flow (acoustic impedance) or of pressure and liquid flow (hydraulic impedance). The term hydraulic impedance is usefully applied to the simple tubular model to describe the relationship between sinusoidal pressure and associated sinusoidal flow. Since the relationship is pressure ÷ flow, and since pressure in the tube is maximal where flow is minimal, and *vice versa*, one would expect to find the same maxima and minima at the same positions along the tube as one sees for pressure. This indeed is the case. Taylor (1957 a,b) studied impedance in theoretic models of an elastic tube, and also in a real tube. Results are shown in Figure 7.10. As for pressure there are maxima and minima of impedance modulus along the tube, with minima at one quarter and three quarter wavelength, and with maxima at the tube end and at one half and one wavelength back. Just as for pressure, the precise positions of maxima and minima along the tube are determined by the position of the tubular end (not by its origin) and by wave velocity of the tube, and the frequency of an oscillation travelling in the tube.

Taylor's (1957) impedance patterns in tubular models of the arterial system are similar to those determined subsequently in experimental animals, and in man. The concept of vascular impedance gives important insight into vascular properties and arterial function, and is discussed in detail in chapters 8–10. Figure 6.4 shows typical results obtained from pressure and flow waves recorded in the femoral artery of a dog. Impedance modulus is seen to fall from a very high value (the peripheral resistance) to a minimal value at around 10 Hz, then to rise to a maximal value at 20 Hz. One could interpret these results to indicate that the peripheral reflecting site was located at one wavelength from the recording site at 40 Hz (assuming 10 Hz to represent one quarter, and 20 Hz one half wavelength). Assuming wave velocity to average 10 metre sec^{-1} in the arteries downstream, the reflecting site would be calculated as

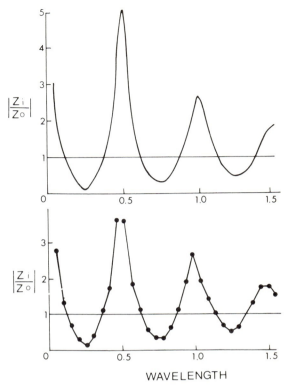

Fig. 7.10 Modulus of input impedance (as a function of characteristic impedance)
Top: calculated for a uniform transmission line
Bottom: measured in a rubber tube
Abscissa: wavelength. (From Taylor 1957, as reproduced by McDonald 1974) (Compare with Fig. 6.4), with permission of the Institute of Physics, Bristol

being 25 cms away. This distance corresponded to a point just below the knee, and appeared to be a credible distance to a functional reflecting site in the vascular bed.

The results of impedance determination in Figure 6.4 are typical of those determined in experimental animals and in man. The results differ from impedance patterns in the simple tubular model in showing no large maximal value of impedance modulus after the initial minimum. When these results became available, Taylor resumed his modelling studies, and showed that the experimentally determined patterns were attributable to the effects of branching, and different lengths to individual reflecting sites in the vascular bed (Taylor 1966, 1967). Effects of blood and arterial wall viscosity, and of non-uniform arterial elasticity played a subsidiary role.

The phase difference between pressure and flow in a tubular model and in arteries is more readily understood and is more important than phase differences of pressure oscillations. It is apparent from Fig. 7.6 that pressure and flow oscillations in a simple tube are one quarter pump cycle or 90° out of phase. But this phase (graphed below in Fig. 4.3) would be expected in an inviscid system to change abruptly from −90° (flow leading pressure) between zero and one quarter wavelength to +90° (pressure leading flow) at one quarter wavelength, then back to −90° at one half wavelength. In Taylor's multibranched model, the same general pattern was seen (Ch. 8) but the fluctuations in impedance phase (the phase difference between pressure and flow) were more gradual and disappeared at higher frequencies where phase settled close to zero. This pattern of impedance phase is precisely what one sees in experimental studies (e.g., Fig. 6.4), and as with the fluctuations in modulus, can readily be attributed to wave reflection in the vascular bed downstream.

PERIPHERAL REFLECTION COEFFICIENT

Taylor (1957a) has shown that reflection coefficient in a tubular model can be calculated as:–

$$R = \frac{Z_t - Z_o}{Z_t + Z_o}$$

where Z_t is terminal impedance of a tube and Z_o its characteristic impedance. Characteristic impedance is the impedance of the tube in the absence of wave reflections. In experimental studies it is estimated as the value of impedance modulus about which oscillations occur (O'Rourke and Taylor, 1966, 1967, McDonald 1974). When Z_t is infinite (an elastic tube with a completely closed end), and characteristic impedance finite, R will approximate to +1 i.e. there will be 100 percent reflection. When accurate experimental determinations of vascular impedance became available, Taylor (Taylor 1966, O'Rourke and Taylor 1966) showed that this same calculation revealed a peripheral reflection coefficient of approximately 0.8 (i.e. 80 percent reflection) for the femoral vascular bed. (In Fig. 6.4, if one takes Z_t as 57 00 dyne sec cm^{-5} and Z_o as 6 000 dyne sec cm^{-5},

R is calculated as 51/63 or 0.81.) This reflection coefficient was higher than previously estimated by McDonald (1960), and indeed close to the near 100 percent suggested by Hamilton and Dow (1939). McDonald subsequently (1974) conceded that his low estimation of reflection coefficient was based on an erroneous value of Z_t and accepted the higher value as being closer to the truth. Bergel and Milnor (1965) made the same error as McDonald in calculating reflection coefficient for the pulmonary vascular bed; their estimate of 0.32 should be 0.52 (Morris 1966).

In his studies of randomly – branching networks of tubes, Taylor (1966, 1967) showed that while 80 percent reflection was a reasonable estimate for individual vascular terminations, it was a maximal value for the whole vascular bed under basal conditions. The effects of wave reflection from different sites led to cancellation of reflection at higher frequencies, so that reflection coefficient fell to zero from its value of 0.8 at lower frequencies. The actual behaviour of reflection coefficient as a function of frequency is difficult to predict precisely; it will depend on the path length to individual peripheral reflecting sites and degree of dispersion of these individual sites. In proximal arteries of dogs and man, little wave reflection is apparent at frequencies greater than 8 Hz. In peripheral arteries, little wave reflection is usually apparent over 16 Hz.

SITES OF WAVE REFLECTION

One would expect that wave reflection could arise from any discontinuity in calibre or distensibility along the arterial tree where there is a change in vascular impedance. Possible reflecting sites are branching points, areas of alteration in arterial distensibility, and high resistance arterioles.

The present consensus is that the arterioles are the major sites of wave reflection in the systemic circulation. As blood flows through the systemic circulation, blood pressure falls but little over long distances in the arteries, then falls precipitously over a short distance in the arterioles. This fact, together with the observed effects of vasodilator drugs on arterial pressure waves, was the main argument advanced by Hamilton (1944),

Porjé (1946) and McDonald (1960) in coming to this conclusion. Later evidence has reinforced these views, especially the calculations of peripheral reflection coefficient from impedance determinations, as just discussed, and the findings that intra-arterial injection of a vasodilator agent can virtually abolish all evidence of wave reflection in a peripheral vascular bed (O'Rourke and Taylor,

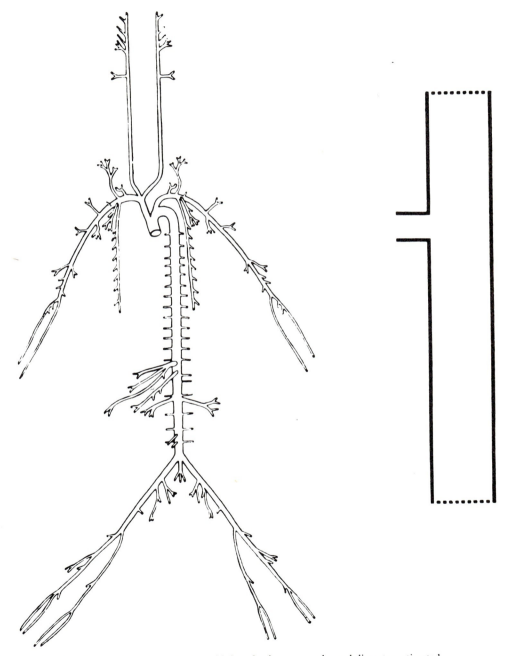

Fig. 7.11 *Left*: The systemic arterial system of a dog with lengths drawn to scale, and diameter estimated.
Right: The arterial system of a dog represented by a single tube, incompletely occluded at both ends, and which receives blood from the heart one third of the way along its length. (From O'Rourke, 1967)

1966, (p. 101)). Vasodilator agents do not alter arterial branching; their known effects on large arteries are quite incapable of explaining the marked fall in peripheral reflection that accompanies their intra-arterial injection.

The effects of changing arterial distensibility along the arterial tree is one of the known causes of wave reflection. The effects of this are usually analysed differently (as in Fig. 7.9) but they amount to the same thing – generation of small retrograde reflected waves as the anterograde wave travels from the heart down the progressively stiffening aorta, and into the even less extensible peripheral arteries. Though an important factor to consider, these effects are still minor in comparison to the influence of peripheral arteriolar tone.

In the past, and even in some recent studies, emphasis has been placed on branching points in major arteries as important sites of wave reflection (Remington 1963, Wetterer et al 1977, Westerhof et al 1978, 1979, Murgo et al 1980). Early evidence of pressure wave transmission suggested that wave reflection arose from the region of the aortic bifurcation or pelvic branches of the iliac artery (Hamilton and Dow 1939, Alexander 1953, Remington 1963). This work drew attention to the distal aorta and initiated a search for some anatomical, histological or physiological change in the aorta or iliac arteries in this region. There was much speculation on this which came to nothing. As seen from the ascending aorta, this site appears to behave as a functionally discrete reflecting site, but so does the upper thigh when impedance measurements are taken in the descending aorta, and the knee area when measurements are made in a femoral artery. In all cases the distal site appears to represent nothing more than the resultant of all individual reflecting sites in the vascular bed downstream. Studies of the aorta and its branches have failed to disclose any particular characteristic of the aortic bifurcation; it appears to behave like any other arterial bifurcation.

The effects of arterial branching on wave reflection were studied from the theoretic aspect by Womersley (1958). This work is discussed in detail in McDonald (1974). In life, the measured increase in cross sectional area of arteries at branching points is between 1.15 and 1.25. This is precisely the range of values calculated for minimal impedance change and minimal wave reflection. Womersley calculated that the wave reflection from a large arterial junction like the aortic bifurcation would be very low – perhaps two per cent or so. His calculations suggested that reflection from branching sites in smaller arteries may be greater than this. Nonetheless, the weight of all evidence suggests that the effects of arterial branching on wave reflection are trivial. Indeed one could readily argue that nature's design of arterial branching appears to be such as to minimise wave reflection.

SECONDARY REFLECTION OF REFLECTED WAVES

The presence of prominent diastolic fluctuations in the earliest recorded accurate pressure waves led Otto Frank (1899, 1905) and his followers to

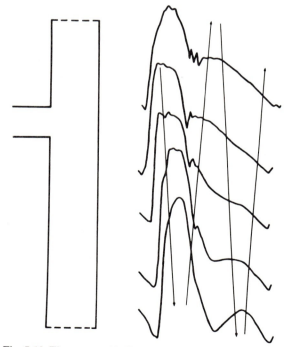

Fig. 7.12 The asymmetric T model of the arterial system (left), and at right, pressure waves recorded between the aortic arch (top), iliac artery (bottom) and intermediate sites in a dog. A line is drawn parallel to the foot of the wave to indicate travel of the initial impulse generated by ventricular ejection. Reflection and re-reflection of this impulse can explain wave contour at different sites. (From O'Rourke 1970) with permission of the American Heart Association Inc.

refer to arterial resonance and even to calculate (from pulse wave velocity and the time or *Grundschwingung* between peaks of the pressure pulse in a peripheral artery) the length of the arterial resonating system. In dogs, when pulse wave velocity averages 6 metre sec^{-1} between proximal aorta and femoral artery and period of the 'resonant' wave is 0.2 seconds, this is calculated as 60 cm. Frank believed that this resonance was superimposed on the basic shape or *Grundform* of the arterial pressure pulse, which he considered to decay exponentially from the time of aortic valve closure, as in a *Windkessel*. This concept was carried further by Hamilton and Dow (1939) who introduced the concept of aortic 'standing waves' to explain apparently simultaneous peaks of pressure waves in lower body arteries, the diastolic pressure wave and the reciprocal fluctuations of pressure in upper and lower body about a 'node' in the descending thoracic aorta.

These concepts of Frank and followers, and of Hamilton and colleagues assume not only in-tense reflection of pressure waves generated by the heart, but also reflection again and again within the arterial tree. McDonald quite properly criticised the concept of resonance and of standing waves as being physically impossible when wave reflection is considerably less than 100 percent and when in addition the wave is being damped during travel between reflecting sites. As discussed (p. 81) McDonald in 1974 accepted the higher value of wave reflection but would never concede that appreciable rereflection of waves was possible. There must be some prospect of compromise between the views of these distinguished physiologists. I would like to think that they were all right, in different ways:– that McDonald was correct in criticising ideas that were based on physical impossibility (and in Frank's case use of two incompatible models of the arterial system at the same time), but that he was unrealistic in expecting precise and complete application of physical principles to a biological system when others were referring to their partial application. 'Resonance'

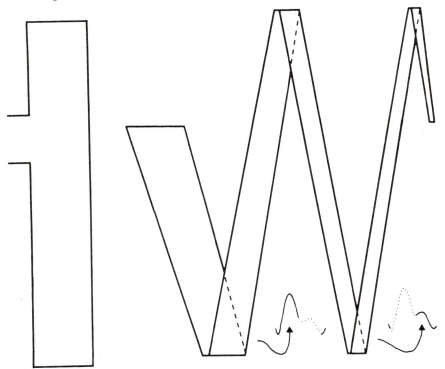

Fig. 7.13 Wave travel and reflection in a tubular model of the arterial system (bottom) 60 cms long, assuming attenuation 0.05 neper/cm and reflection coefficient 0.75. The primary peak of the femoral pressure wave is attributable to summation of incident and reflected waves after the first reflection, while the diastolic wave is attributable to summation of incident and reflected waves at the second reflection in the lower part of the body

certainly cannot occur in a biological system with incomplete reflection and strong attenuation, but neither from the purists point of view can 'anemia' if this is truly regarded as complete lack of blood. The concepts of resonance, standing waves and nodes are, I believe, of some value provided one does not take these terms literally as meaning what they would in a physical system.

The compromise suggested (O'Rourke 1967, 1971, Ch. 8) is similar to that advanced by Wetterer (1954) and Wetterer and Kenner (1968) that rereflection of reflected waves does occur, and that a form of damped resonance does develop between reflecting sites in the upper and lower parts of the body. This concept, with wave reflection occurring between lumped arteriolar terminations in the upper and lower parts of the body (Figs. 7.11, 7.12) will be advanced to explain the major features of pressure waves, flow waves and impe-

dance patterns in different arteries of different animals under different conditions (Chs. 8, 9).

This compromise was considered, and rejected by McDonald (1974) on the basis of heavy attenuation of the pulse over long lengths of artery. McDonald considered the pulse as travelling to the feet and back, rather than to a lumped reflecting site in the region of the pelvis, some 40 cms (not 100 cms) distant. When the pulse is considered to travel over some 60 cm in the asymmetric T model of the arterial system suggested by impedance studies (Chs. 8, 9), and when experimentally-determined values of reflection coefficient and attenuation are used (Fig. 7.13), the compromise appears to be quite reasonable.

In explaining arterial function and pulse wave shape, many things are important, but the most important of all appears to be reflection and rereflection of the arterial pulse.

REFERENCES

Alexander RS 1953 The genesis of the aortic standing wave. Circulation Research 1: 145–151

Apéria A 1940 Haemodynamical studies. Scandinavian Archives of Physiology 83 Suppl 1: 1–230

Avolio AP, O'Rourke MF, Webster M 1980 Pulsatile hemodynamics in the arterial system of the snake. Proceedings, Twenty eighth International Congress of Physiological Sciences

Bergel DH, Milnor WR 1965 Pulmonary vascular impedance in the dog. Circulation Research 16: 401–415

Bourgeois MJ, Gilbert BK, Donald DE, Wood EH 1974 Characteristics of aortic diastolic pressure decay with application to the continuous monitoring of changes in peripheral vascular resistance. Circulation Research 35: 56–66

Bourguignon MH, Wagner HN 1979 Non-invasive measurement of ventricular pressure throughout systole. American Journal of Cardiology 44: 466–471

Frank O. 1899 Die Grundform des arteriellen Pulses. Erste Abhandlung. Mathematische Analyse. Zeitschrift Für Biologie 37: 483–526

Frank O 1905 Der Puls in den Arterien. Zeitschrift für Biologie 46: 441–553

Frank O 1930 Schatzung des Schlagvolumens des menschlichen Herzens auf Grund der Wellenund Windkessel theorie. Zeitschrift für Biologie 90: 405–409

Freis ED, Heath WC, Luchsinger PC, Snell RE 1966 Changes in the carotid pulse which occur with age and in hypertension. American Heart Journal 71: 757–765

Hamilton WF 1944 The patterns of the arterial pressure pulse. American Journal of Physiology 141: 235–241

Hamilton WF, Dow P 1939 An experimental study of the standing waves in the pulse propagated through aorta. American Journal of Physiology 125: 48–59

Harvey W 1628 De motu cordis et sanguinis in animalibus. William Fitzer Frankfurt Translated by Franklin KJ 1957 Blackwell Oxford

Harvey W. 1649 De circulatione sanguinis. Translated by Franklin KJ 1957 Blackwell Oxford

Kouchoukos NT, Sheppard LC, McDonald DA 1970 Estimation of stroke volume in the dog by a pulse contour method. Circulation Research 26: 611–623

McDonald DA 1960 Blood flow in arteries. 1st edition Arnold London

McDonald DA 1974 Blood flow in arteries. 2nd edition Arnold London

McDonald DA, Taylor MG 1956 An investigation of the arterial system using a hydraulic oscillator. Journal of Physiology (London) 133: 74–75

Morkin E 1967 Analysis of pulsatile blood flow and its clinical implications. New England Journal of Medicine 277: 139–146

Morris MJ 1955 Pressure and flow in the pulmonary vasculature of the dog. Thesis for BSc Med. University of Sydney

Murgo JP, Westerhof N, Giolma JP, Altobelli SA 1981 Manipulation of ascending aortic pressure and flow wave reflections with the Valsalva Manouver: relationship to input impedance. Circulation 63: 122–132

Murgo JP, Westerhof N, Giolma JP, Altobelli SA 1980 Aortic input impedance in normal man; relationship to pressure waveforms. Circulation 62: 105–116

Newman DL, Greenwald SE, Bowden NLR 1979 An in-vivo study of the total occlusion method for the analysis of forward and backward pressure waves. Cardiovascular Research 13: 595–600

O'Rourke MF 1967 Pressure and flow waves in systemic arteries and the anatomical design of the arterial system.

Journal of Applied Physiology 23: 139–149

O'Rourke MF 1969 Effects of major artery occlusion on pressure wave transmission along the human aorta. Proceedings of the Australian Physiological and Pharmacological Society p. 24

O'Rourke MF 1970 Arterial hemodynamics in hypertension. Circulation Research 26: Supplement 2 123–133

O'Rourke MF 1971 The arterial pulse in health and disease. American Heart Journal 82: 687–802

O'Rourke MF, Blazek JV, Morreels CL, Krovetz LJ 1968 Pressure wave transmission along the human aorta; changes with age and in arterial degenerative disease. Circulation Research 23: 567–579

O'Rourke MF, Cartmill TB 1971 Influence of aortic coarctation on pulsatile hemodynamics in the proximal aorta. Circulation 44: 281–292

O'Rourke MF, Taylor MG 1966 Vascular impedance of the femoral bed. Circulation Research 18: 126–139

O'Rourke MF, Taylor MG 1967 Input impedance of the systemic circulation. Circulation Research 20: 365–380

Pepine CJ, Nichols WW, Curry RC Jr., Conti CR 1979 Aortic input impedance during nitroprusside infusion. A reconsideration of afterload reduction and beneficial action. Journal of Clinical Investigation 64: 643–654

Peterson LH 1954 The dynamics of pulsatile blood flow. Circulation Research 2: 127–139

Peterson LH, Shepard RB 1955 Some relationships of blood pressure to cardiovascular system. Surgical Clinics of North America 35: 1613–1628

Porje IG 1946 Studies of the arterial pulse wave particularly in the aorta. Acta Physiologica Scandinavica 13 Supplement 42: 7–68

Simon AC, Safar ME, Levinson JA, London GM, Levy BI, Chau NP 1979 An evaluation of large arteries compliance in man. American Journal of Physiology 237: H 550–H 554

Sipkema P, Westerhof N, Randall OS 1980 The arterial system characterised in the time domain. Cardiovascular Research 14: 270–279

Sperling W, Bauer RD, Busse R, Korner H, Pasch TH 1975 The resolution of arterial pulses into forward and backward waves as an approach to the determination of characteristic impedance. Pflugers Archives 355: 217–227

Starr A 1955 Studies made by simulating systole at necropsy. State of peripheral circulation in cadavers. Journal of Applied Physiology 11: 174–180

Taylor MG 1957a An approach to an analysis of the arterial pulse wave. 1. Oscillations in an attenuating line. Physics in Medicine and Biology 1: 258–269

Taylor MG 1957b An approach to an analysis of the arterial pulse wave. 2. Fluid oscillations in an elastic pipe. Physics in Medicine and Biology 1: 321–329

Taylor MG 1964 Wave travel in arteries and the design of the cardiovascular system. In: Attinger EO (ed) Pulsatile blood flow McGraw New York p. 343–372

Taylor MG 1965a Wave travel in a non-uniform transmission line, in relation to pulses in arteries. Physics in Medicine and Biology 10: 539–550

Taylor MG 1966a The input impedance of an assembly of randomly branching elastic tubes. Biophysical Journal 6: 29–51

Taylor MG 1966b Use of random excitation and spectral analysis in the study of frequency-dependent parameters of the cardiovascular system. Circulation Research 18: 585–595

Van Den Bos GC, Westerhof N, Elzinga G, Sipkema P 1976 Reflection in the systemic arterial system: effects of aortic and carotid occlusion. Cardiovascular Research 19: 565–573

Warner HR, Swan HJC, Connolly DC, Tompkins RG, Wood EH 1953 Quantitation of beat to beat changes in stroke volume from the aortic pulse contour in man. Journal of Applied Physiology 5: 495–507

Westerhof N, Sipkema P, van den Bos GC, Elzinga G 1972 Forward and backward waves in the arterial system. Cardiovascular Research 6: 648–656

Westerhof N, Van den Bos GC, Laxminarayan S 1978 Arterial reflection, In: Bauer RD, Busse R (eds) The Arterial System Springer Berlin p. 48–62

Wetterer E 1954 Flow and pressure in the arterial system, their hemodynamic relationship and the principles of their measurement. Minnesota Medicine 37: 77–86

Wetterer E, Bauer RD, Busse R 1977 Arterial dynamics. INSERM Eurotech 92 Cardiovascular and Pulmonary Dynamics 71: 17–42

Wetterer E, Bauer RD, Busse R 1978 New ways of determining the propagation coefficient and the viscoelastic behaviour of arteries in situ. In: Bauer RD, Busse R (eds) The Arterial System Springer Berlin p. 35–47

Wetterer E, Kenner TH 1968 Grundlagen der Dynamik des Arterienpulses. Springer Berlin

8

Vascular impedance: the relationship between pressure and flow

'We are apt to think of mathematical definitions as too strict and rigid for common use, but ... (using them) we discover identities which were not obvious before and which our definitions obscured rather than revealed ... we pass quickly and easily from the mathematical concept of form in its static aspect to form in its dynamic relations; we rise from a conception of form to an understanding of the forces which give rise to it.'
(*D'Arcy W. Thompson* 'On Growth and Form' 1917)

The relationship between pressure and flow is not apparent from inspection of wave contour. It is possible of course to compare the amplitude of pressure and flow waves and to measure the delay between peaks and secondary oscillations of pressure and flow waves. Little more is possible from analysis carried out in the time domain, i.e. from pressure and flow displayed as waves, unless one perturbs the arteries artificially with discrete identifiable impulses, as done by Anliker et al (1968) and Sipkema et al (1980). Fresh insight however is gained by expressing pressure/flow relationships as vascular impedance, through analysis of pressure and flow in the frequency domain.

The term 'Impedance' is often used loosely by clinicians to describe the opposition to blood flow into a vascular bed, especially in relation to the effects of vasodilator drugs on peripheral arterioles. This is inappropriate since vascular impedance has a particular and specific meaning and is strictly analogous with electrical, mechanical and acoustic impedance in the physical sciences. Like these, vascular impedance is displayed as a graph of modulus (amplitude of pressure harmonic divided by amplitude of corresponding flow harmonic) and phase (delay of flow harmonic after corresponding pressure harmonic) plotted against frequency (Figs. 6.3, 6.4, 8.1).

Application of the concept of impedance to cardiovascular studies appears to have been first suggested by the British mathematician John Womersley in 1955 (McDonald, 1974), and its value is dependent on the near linearity of pressure/flow relationships that he was first to explore and evaluate. Taylor, in McDonald's laboratory, subsequently laid the foundation to the interpretation of vascular impedance through his studies of impedance in theoretic, electrical and hydraulic models of the circulation during the 1950s (Taylor 1957a,b, 1959; McDonald and Taylor, 1959) but it was Randall and Stacy (1956) from Missouri who published the first data from an experimental animal. Numerous studies have since been reported, and vascular impedance is now firmly established in the scientific literature, (see McDonald, 1974; Noble 1979, Westerhof et al 1979, O'Rourke 1981) and in textbooks (Milnor 1974, Little 1977) as the appropriate description of pulsatile pressure/flow relationships.

IMPEDANCE IN A TYPICAL PERIPHERAL VASCULAR BED

With the exception of the ascending aorta and pulmonary artery, vascular impedance has been studied more intensively in the femoral artery than in any other vessel (Randall and Stacy, 1956; Randall 1958, McDonald 1974, O'Rourke and Taylor, 1966; Taylor, 1966a). This artery can be considered to supply a typical peripheral vascular bed, and is an ideal site for determining impedance under a variety of conditions, since pressure and flow can be measured with minimal operative trauma, and with an animal very lightly anesthetised, and the effects of vasodilation and vasoconstriction can be examined without causing large alterations in mean arterial pressure. The patterns of impedance in other peripheral arteries, though differing in detail (*vide infra*) show the same general features and the same changes under different conditions as those in the femoral artery.

Impedance under basal conditions

Figure 6.4 shows femoral vascular impedance determined in a dog with surgically-induced heart block, and whose heart could be paced at different frequencies. Pacing was induced in order to obtain values of impedance modulus and phase between the harmonic frequencies at the regular heart rate. Impedance modulus is seen to fall smoothly from its value at zero frequency (the resistive term calculated from mean pressure ÷ mean flow) to a minimum at 11–12 Hertz and subsequently to rise again at higher frequencies. Impedance phase is zero for the resistive term at zero frequency, then becomes negative (flow leading pressure) and stays negative up to 11–12 hertz when phase crosses zero to become positive. Figure 6.4 is a typical plot of vascular impedance for the femoral vascular bed. The data in this figure give powerful support for the contention that non-linearities in pulsatile pressure-flow relationships are very small. Although the heart was paced at different rates, so that data plotted at any one frequency had been calculated from different harmonics of pressure and flow waves at different heart rates, all values of modulus and phase fell along the smooth curve. The relatively large standard errors at high frequencies were not unexpected since these were derived from the eighth, ninth and tenth harmonics which were of very low amplitude and so subject to considerable experimental error. Linearity appeared to be preserved even under extreme circumstances. Figure 8.1 shows femoral vascular impedance determined from a series of pressure and flow waves recorded during sinus arrhythmia. Although heart rate was varying greatly, values of impedance calculated for each wave fell along the same smooth curve with very little scatter except at high frequencies (above 12 Hz). At 3 Hz, the first harmonic of a short pressure or flow wave corresponded to the third harmonic of a long wave at one Hz, yet the values of modulus and phase of impedance calculated from each were almost exactly the same. It was surprising to find such consistent results under conditions which theoretically invalidated the use of steady-state analysis. In applying harmonic analysis to pressure and flow waves, one assumes that they are part of a series of identical waves repeated with precise regularity. Results shown in Figure 8.1 imply that even with variations in heart rate, each wave appears to behave as though it were regularly repeated, even though it is not. As for the impedance results in Figure 6.4, the data displayed in Figure 8.1 give impressive support for the concept that non linearities in pressure-flow relationships can, to a first approximation, be ignored. Similar evidence of linearity has been found for pulsatile pressure/flow relationships in other vascular beds by us and by others (Noble et al, 1967; Bergel and Milnor, 1965).

Effects of alteration in mean arterial pressure

When mean arterial pressure is increased, no matter how, the curves of modulus and phase are shifted to the right, so that the minimum of modulus and phase cross-over occur at a higher frequency; when mean pressure is reduced, impedance curves shift to the left (Fig. 8.2). These changes in modulus and phase are quite independent of any concurrent alteration in peripheral resistance. They are seen whether peripheral resistance increases, decreases, or remains constant, and with alterations in mean pressure brought about by alterations of arteriolar tone or by changes in cardiac output. These same findings are seen in all vascular beds, and are attributable to changes in wave velocity between recording and peripheral reflecting sites, with consequent differences in timing of reflected waves from peripheral sites.

Effects of vasoconstriction and vasodilation

In a peripheral vascular bed, the effects of change in arteriolar tone can be examined independently of changes in mean pressure by injecting a vasoactive drug into the artery of supply, and taking records before the drug has been redistributed to the rest of the body. This technique was used to obtain data for Figures 8.3–8.6.

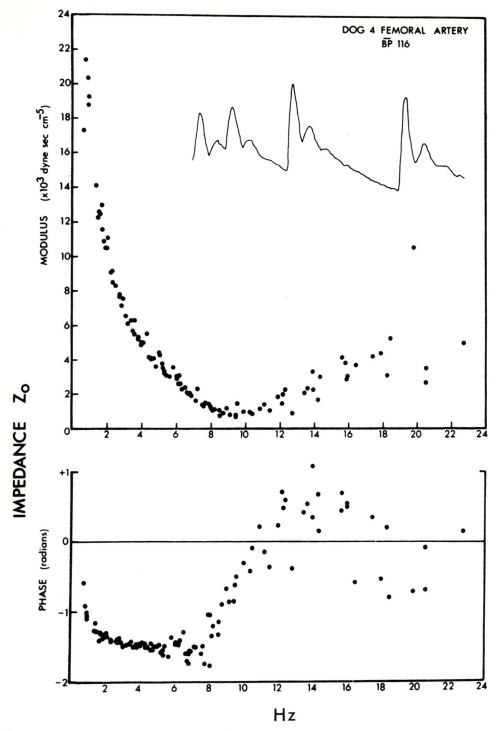

Fig. 8.1 Vascular impedance under control conditions in the femoral artery of a dog. Impedance was determined from a series of 11 waves recorded during marked sinus arrhythmia. (From O'Rourke and Taylor 1966) with permission American Heart Association Inc.

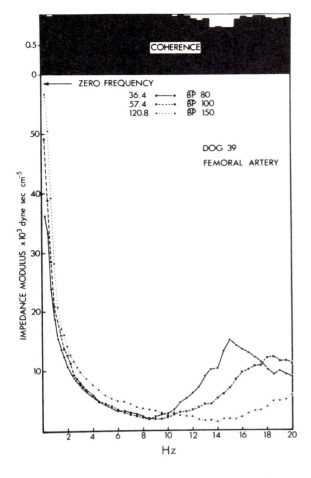

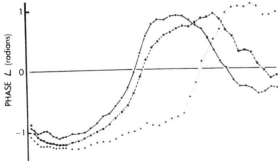

Fig. 8.2 Vascular impedance in the femoral artery of a dog under control conditions with mean arterial pressure 80 mmHg, and during infusion of norepinephrine at mean arterial pressure 100 mmHg and 150 mm Hg. Peripheral resistance, initially 36.4 dyne sec cm⁻⁵ rose to 57.4 then 121 dyne sec cm⁻⁵. Shift of impedance curves to the right is attributable to increase in mean pressure, and in pulse wave velocity (From O'Rourke 1970) with permission American Heart Association Inc.

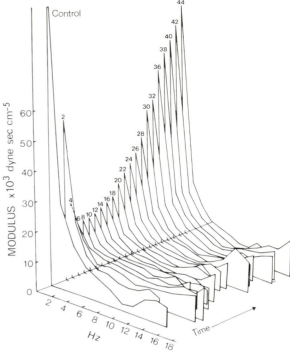

Fig. 8.3 Effects of vasodilation on the modulus of vascular impedance in the femoral artery of a dog. Time course of impedance modulus is shown following intra-arterial injection of acetylcholine (100 μg in 1 ml) Each curve represents modulus determined from one pair of pressure and flow waves. Time in seconds following injection is shown above each curve (From O'Rourke and Taylor 1966) with permission American Heart Association Inc.

The effects of vasodilation on the modulus of femoral vascular impedance is shown in Figure 8.3. This shows impedance modulus determined from corresponding pairs of pressure and flow waves at two second intervals after intra-arterial injection of 100 μg acetyl choline chloride. With vasodilation, there was a fall of peripheral resistance to less than one seventh of its original value; this was associated with a fall in modulus calculated from the first, second, and third harmonics to one half or less of their original value, but with an increase in modulus of impedance derived from the fifth and higher harmonics. The net effect was a flattening of impedance modulus with loss of the distinct minimum at around 10 Hz. Peak effect was seen at eight seconds, and the drug had all but worn off at 44 seconds. Figure 8.4 shows the peak effect of arteriolar vasodilation of impedance

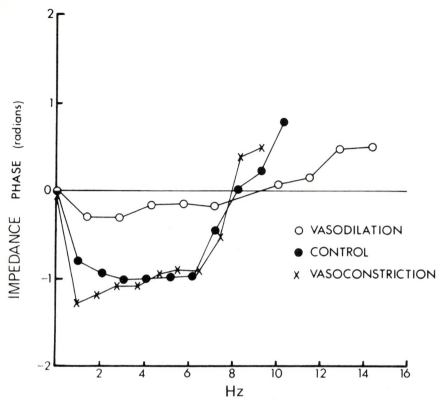

Fig. 8.4 Effects of vasodilation and vasoconstriction on the phase of vascular impedance in the femoral artery of a dog (From O'Rourke and Taylor 1966) with permission American Heart Association Inc.

phase. This showed less fluctuation than under normal conditions being far less negative up to eight Hz, and less positive above eight Hz. As with the change in modulus, this came on gradually, was most marked eight seconds after injection of acetyl choline and had all but worn off 44 seconds later. Figure 8.5 shows pressure and flow waves in the femoral artery under control conditions and during peak vasodilation. Under control conditions pressure and flow waves were quite dissimilar in contour, but with intense vasodilation, the waves were virtually identical. The effects of vasodilation on impedance and wave contour are precisely what one would predict from decrease in peripheral reflection coefficient, as explained later.

The effects of vasoconstriction on femoral vascular impedance (Figs. 8.4, 8.6) were less dramatic than those caused by vasodilation. Figure 8.6 was determined from harmonic analysis of wave pairs at four second intervals after intra-

arterial injection of noradrenaline 6 μg. The drug was injected with the artery occluded downstream so that the first two plots show the effects of reactive hyperemia. The maximal effect of vasoconstriction on impedance modulus and phase was seen between 15–30 seconds after injection, and comprised an increase in zero frequency component of impedance (peripheral resistance), more marked minimum of impedance at 8–10 Hz and more negative impedance phase below 3 Hz. These changes are explicable on the basis of increase in peripheral reflection coefficient.

EXPLANATION OF IMPEDANCE PATTERNS WITH MODELS OF THE PERIPHERAL VASCULAR BED

Impedance patterns under control conditions and the changes with alterations in mean arterial pres-

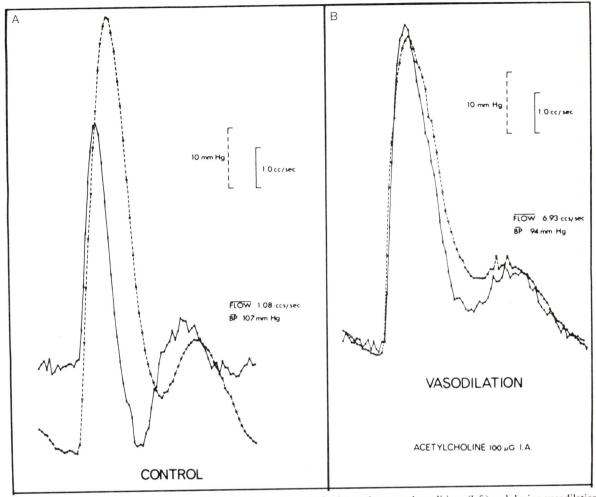

Fig. 8.5 Pressure and flow waves recorded from the femoral artery of a dog under control conditions (left) and during vasodilation induced by intra-arterial injection of acetylcholine (right). The waves have been drawn from the digital voltmeter output with pressure represented by a broken line, flow by an unbroken line. (From O'Rourke and Taylor 1966) with permission American Heart Association Inc.

sure and arteriolar tone in vessels downstream can be explained readily on the basis of wave travel in arteries downstream with reflection at peripheral arterioles.

The patterns of impedance modulus and phase under control conditions resemble those seen in a tube with a completely closed end (Ch. 7, Taylor 1957a,b, McDonald and Taylor 1959, McDonald 1974). In such a tube, (Fig. 7.10), impedance modulus and phase vary with frequency, having successive minima of modulus at frequencies where the distance to the closed end represents one quarter and three quarters of a wavelength, and an intervening maximum at one half wavelength; impedance phase fluctuates from near 90° negative to near 90° positive, with zero intercept at one quarter, one half, and three quarter wavelength. From Figure 8.1, one may interpret the first minimum of modulus and phase crossover to identify the frequency at which reflecting sites are one quarter wavelength away. Subsequent maxima and minima were not seen because impedance was not determined above 24 Hz, amplitude of pressure and flow components in the waves at

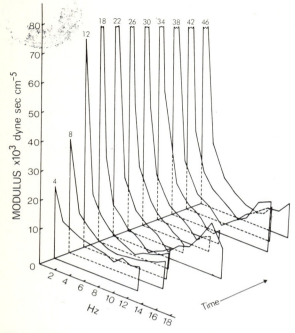

Fig. 8.6 Effects of vasodilation and vasoconstriction on the modulus of vascular impedance in the femoral artery of a dog. Time course of impedance modulus is shown following intra-arterial injection of norepinephrine (6 μg in 1 ml). Reactive hypermia is responsible for the shape of the first three curves. The control curve resembled that seen 18 seconds after injection of the drug. Time in seconds after injection appears above each curve (From O'Rourke and Taylor, 1966) with permission American Heart Association Inc.

these frequencies being very low, and within the noise level of recording instruments. Assuming pulse wave velocity to be 10 metre sec^{-1}., one can calculate wavelength at 10 Hz to be 10 ÷ 10 (Ch. 7) or 1.0 metre, so that distance to effective closed end reflecting site is 0.25 metre. This distance in the dogs studied corresponded to a point just below the knee. The results can be interpreted on the basis of such a point representing the resultant of all individual arterial terminations in the vascular bed downstream. This appeared to be a reasonable and realistic interpretation.

In the femoral and other vascular beds, impedance modulus never fluctuates to the same degree with frequency as it does in simple tubular models of the arterial system. Investigating this, Taylor (1965, 1966b) showed that such behaviour can be accounted for by the effects of blood and wall viscosity, non-uniform elasticity in central arteries,

and most importantly, the effects of spatial dispersion of peripheral terminations – the fact that arterial terminations in the paw are at a far greater distance from the recording site than those in the thigh. Figure 8.7 shows Taylor's (1966) model of a peripheral vascular bed. When realistic dimensions for vascular lengths and widths were used in this model, together with measured values of blood density and viscosity, and of arterial elasticity, and when a reflection coefficient of 0.8 was assumed, values of modulus and phase of impedance at its input were virtually identical to those recorded in the femoral artery of experimental animals under control conditions (Fig. 8.8).

Taylor's randomly-branched model was used to explain impedance changes brought about by vasodilation and vasoconstriction. Identical changes to those seen in the dog during vasodilation were brought about by reducing reflection coefficient at all individual terminations to zero, while identical changes to those seen during vasoconstriction were brought about by increasing reflection coefficient to 0.95 (Fig. 8.8).

These modelling studies provide simple, unifying explanations for impedance patterns under different conditions and for the vascular mechanisms responsible for these.

Patterns of modulus and phase of impedance under control conditions are explicable on the basis of a high (around 80 percent) reflection coefficient at peripheral arterioles in the vascular bed downstream. The frequency of impedance minimum and phase cross-over is determined by pulse wave velocity in the femoral artery and its radicles between measuring site and reflecting sites and on the average distance between recording and reflecting sites.

Changes in the frequency of impedance minimum and phase cross-over with changes in mean arterial pressure are attributable to alterations in pulse wave velocity and so in the time taken for return of reflected waves. As mean pressure rises, the arterial wall becomes stiffer, and pulse wave velocity rises (Schimmler 1965, O'Rourke 1970, Kenner 1972, McDonald 1974, Ch. 4). With rise in pulse wave velocity, and earlier return of wave reflection, the frequency increases at which the distance to reflecting sites represents one quarter wavelength (Ch. 7). Thus one can readily explain

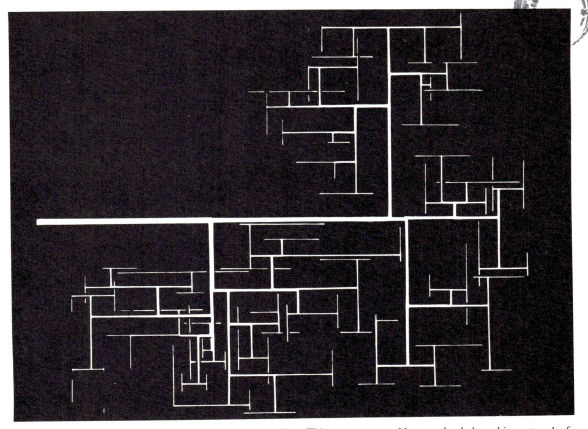

Fig. 8.7 Taylor's mathematical model of a peripheral vascular bed. This was represented by a randomly branching network of elastic tubes. From Taylor (1966b)

how increased mean pressure shifts impedance curves to the right, while decreased mean pressure shifts impedance curves to the left.

The large changes in femoral vascular impedance with vasodilation are attributable to decrease in reflection coefficient from around 80 percent to near zero. The relatively small changes in impedance with vasoconstriction are attributable to the already high resting arteriolar tone and the relatively small further increase in reflection possible with further increase in arteriolar tone.

Impedance data on the effects of vasodilator agents, and their interpretation provides further support for the concept (Hamilton 1944, McDonald 1974) that peripheral arterioles are the major sites of wave reflection, that reflection coefficient is normally high because of high resting arteriolar tone, and that branching sites in major arteries are relatively unimportant in generating

wave reflection. In the past, (Remington 1963) and even in some recent studies (Westerhof et al 1979), the importance of branching points in major arteries appears to have been overemphasised. The fact that wave reflection in a vascular bed can be virtually abolished with vasodilation alone argues strongly against branching points in large arteries playing any major role in wave reflection, and supports the evidence from other sources (Ch. 7, McDonald 1974).

IMPEDANCE IN REGIONAL VASCULAR BEDS

Impedance patterns in the subclavian artery of experimental animals are similar to those in the femoral artery (O'Rourke 1965, Attinger et al 1966, Cox and Pace 1975). The carotid artery

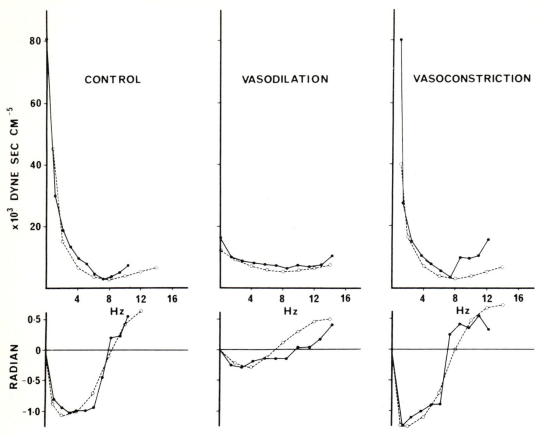

Fig. 8.8 Solid lines: Experimentally determined values of impedance modulus and phase in the femoral artery of a dog under control conditions and during intra-arterial injection of acetylcholine (centre) and norepinephrine (right). Dashed lines: Impedance at the input of Taylor's model of the femoral vascular bed with reflection coefficient 0.8 (left), zero (centre), 0.95 (right)

(Fig. 8.9) shows less evidence of wave reflection than the femoral and subclavian artery – with a less well marked minimum of impedance modulus and smaller variation in impedance phase. This is attributable to the lower peripheral resistance of this bed, doubtless due to relatively low arteriolar tone in cerebral arterioles.

In the renal artery, blood flow is high, arteriolar tone low, and distance to arteriolar terminations is short. Patterns of vascular impedance in this vessel under control conditions resemble those in the femoral artery of a small dog during vasodilation, as would be expected (Fig. 8.10).

IMPEDANCE CHANGES BETWEEN THE HEART AND PERIPHERAL ARTERIES

Figure 8.9 shows impedance determined from a series of pressure and flow waves in different arteries of the same animal under control conditions and at approximately the same mean arterial pressure. Similar data to these have been published by Attinger et al (1966) and Cox and Pace (1975). So as to make comparisons in arteries of differing calibre, flow was expressed in linear velocity (cm sec^{-1}) instead of volume flow (cm^3 sec^{-1}) and so impedance modulus in dyne.sec. cm^{-3} instead of dyne.sec.cm^{-5}. These impedance patterns are explicable on the same basis as those in the femoral artery. As would be expected, the frequency of the minimum of modulus and crossover of phase becomes progressively lower in arteries further from the periphery and closer to the heart. This is attributable in part to the longer distance to peripheral reflecting sites in arteries close to the heart, and in part to the lower wave velocity in the proximal aorta (Taylor 1965, McDonald 1974).

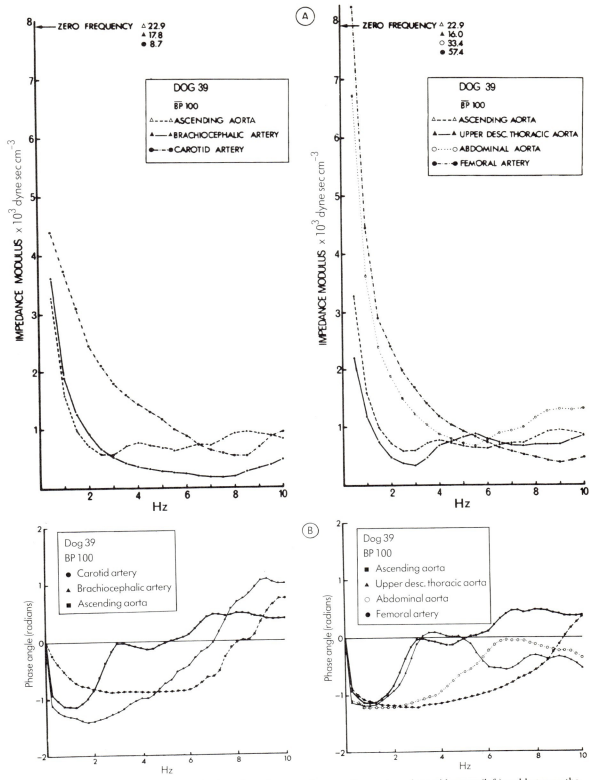

Fig. 8.9 A: Changes in modulus of vascular impedance between the ascending aorta and carotid artery (left) and between the ascending aorta and femoral artery (right) of a 21 kg dog. Modulus expressed in terms of linear flow velocity. Peripheral resistance shown above. B: Changes in impedance phase angle between the ascending aorta and carotid artery (left) and between the ascending aorta and femoral artery of the same dog. From O'Rourke (1967)

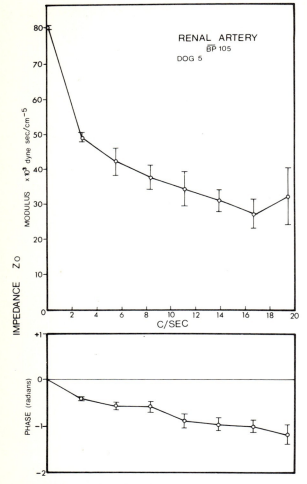

Fig. 8.10 Vascular impedance from the renal artery of a dog

The apparent or functionally discrete site of wave reflection has been calculated from impedance patterns in the aortic arch, abdominal aorta, and femoral artery – for the lower part of the body, and in the brachio-cephalic, left subclavian and carotid artery in the upper part of the body. Seen from the origin of the brachiocephalic or left subclavian origin, the peripheral reflecting site in a dog appears to be at a distance which corresponds to a region just above the axilla. Seen from the origin of the descending aorta however, the peripheral reflecting site appears to be further away, and to be located in the region of the pelvis. These findings in dogs are also apparent in other experimental animals (O'Rourke 1965, Avolio

1976, Avolio et al 1976) and in man (Mills et al 1970, O'Rourke and Avolio 1980). Consequences of this will be discussed in Chapters 9 and 10. Despite differences in size and shape, the upper body reflecting site in all mammals studied appears from the aortic arch to be located in the region of the mid upper arm, while the lower body reflecting site, seen from the same region behaves as though it were in the pelvic region. In all cases the reflecting site appears to be at a distance which reasonably approximates the average distance to all individual arterial terminations in the vascular bed downstream.

Ascending aortic impedance: Input impedance to the systemic circulation

Vascular impedance in the ascending aorta is of particular significance. Not only does this describe the relationship between pressure and flow at the root of the aorta, and so characterise the properties of the whole systemic circulation, but it also represents the hydraulic load presented by the systemic circulation to the left ventricle of the heart.

The original, and most subsequent experimental studies of ascending aortic impedance have been performed on dogs (Patel et al 1963, Attinger et al 1965, O'Rourke and Taylor 1967, Noble et al 1967, Cox and Pace 1975); there is now general agreement on the patterns observed, and the mechanisms responsible for these (McDonald 1974, O'Rourke 1981).

The principal features of ascending aortic impedance curves in dogs are seen in Fig. 8.11. From its value at zero frequency (the peripheral resistance), impedance modulus falls steeply to a minimal value which occurs at a lower frequency than in any other artery; from this first minimum, modulus rises slightly then falls again to a second minimum after which it rises to settle about a constant value above 12–15 Hz. Impedance modulus at frequencies greater than 1.5 Hz is usually less than one twentieth of the modulus at zero frequency. Phase angle is negative at low frequencies and shows two fluctuations which correspond to the two minima of modulus; phase approaches or crosses zero at the frequency of the second minimum of modulus. Such patterns of impedance are

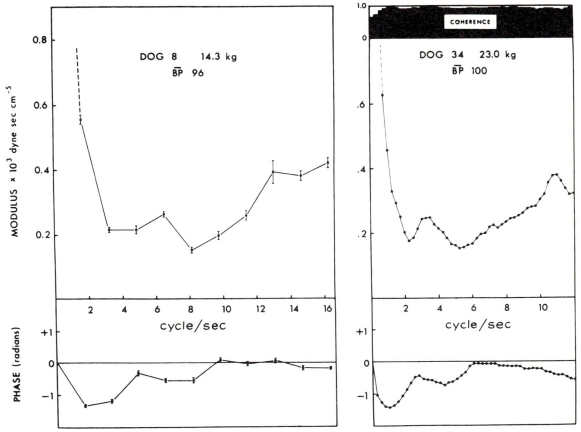

Fig. 8.11 Vascular impedance in the ascending aorta of a small 14.3 kg dog (left), and of a large 23 kg dog (right). (From O'Rourke and Taylor 1967) with permission American Heart Association Inc.

usually seen when impedance values are obtained over a wide range of frequencies as with the technique of frequency spectrum analysis (Taylor 1966a); sometimes however only one broad minimum of impedance modulus is observed (Fig. 8.12).

The fluctuations of impedance modulus and phase may be attributed as in other arteries to wave reflection in the vascular bed downstream. As expected from consideration of wave transmission and reflection, these fluctuations occur at lower frequencies in large dogs, and at higher frequencies in small dogs, but the patterns cannot be explained on the basis of a single functionally-discrete reflecting site in the vascular bed, since the second minimum of modulus does not occur at three times the frequency of the first minimum, and the intervening maximum does not occur at

twice this frequency, while impedance phase does not cross zero at close to these frequencies. As previously noted, impedance patterns in other arteries including the brachiocephalic and left subclavian arteries and descending thoracic aorta are readily explained on the basis of a single functionally-discrete reflecting site in the vascular bed downstream. However when impedance patterns in the ascending aorta are compared to those in the descending aorta (supplying the lower part of the body) and the brachiocephalic and subclavian arteries (supplying the upper part of the body), they appear to be a composite of those in these vessels (Fig. 8.13). This finding suggested (O'Rourke 1965, O'Rourke and Taylor 1967) that the patterns of impedance in the ascending aorta result from this vessel supplying two separate vascular beds – that in the upper part of the body

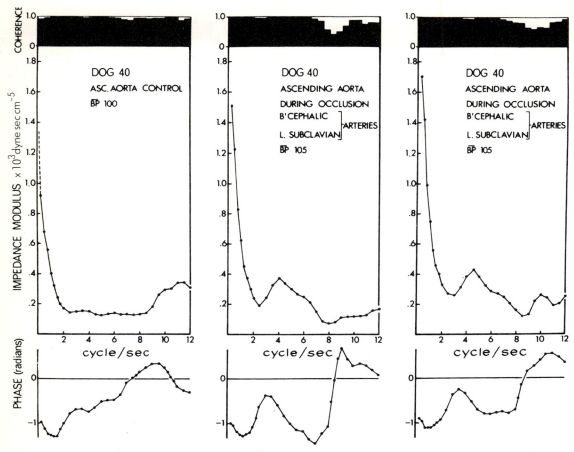

Fig. 8.12 Vascular impedance in the ascending aorta of a dog under control conditions (left) and on two occasions during occlusion of both the brachiocephalic and left subclavian arteries (From O'Rourke and Taylor 1967) with permission American Heart Association Inc.

where average pathlengths to reflecting sites are relatively short, and that in the lower part of the body where average pathlengths to reflecting sites are relatively long. The first minimum of impedance modulus in the ascending aorta was attributed to the presence of the lower body reflecting site, and the second minimum was attributed to the upper body reflecting site, while the absence of a definite intervening maximum was attributed to the interaction of reflections from these two sites. This interpretation was supported by the modelling studies of Taylor (1966b) and also by experimental determinations of ascending aortic impedance when arteries to the upper and lower parts of the body were occluded. When the brachiocephalic and left subclavian arteries are

occluded, ascending aortic impedance comes to resemble that in the descending thoracic aorta, with successive maxima and minima of modulus and fluctuations of impedance phase (Fig. 8.12), while occlusion of the descending thoracic aorta causes loss of the first minimum of impedance and phase fluctuation, so that the pattern comes to resemble that seen in the brachiocephalic and left subclavian arteries (Fig. 8.14).

In dogs, the position of upper and lower body reflecting sites was calculated from minima of impedance modulus in the ascending aorta, together with measured or assumed values of pulse wave velocity (O'Rourke 1965, 1967, O'Rourke and Taylor 1967). That in the upper body appeared as though it were located in the mid part of the up-

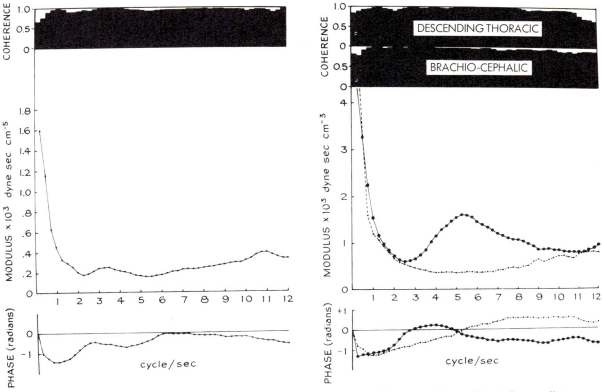

Fig. 8.13 Vascular impedance at three sites in a 23 kg dog at the same mean arterial pressure (100 mmHg). Left, ascending aorta; Right, upper descending thoracic aorta (solid line) and proximal brachiocephalic artery (broken line). From O'Rourke and Taylor, 1967) with permission American Heart Association Inc.

per limb, while that in the lower part of the body appeared as though it were located in the pelvic area, approximately twice as far distant as that in the upper body. The reflecting site in each case was considered to represent the resultant of all individual arterial terminations in the respective vascular bed. The presence of minima at lower frequencies in larger dogs than in smaller was attributed to the greater distance to reflecting sites in the larger than in smaller dogs while the similarity of impedance patterns in other respects was attributed to the similarity of body shape (O'Rourke and Taylor 1967, McDonald 1974, O'Rourke 1981). Figure 7.11 shows the simple model of the whole systemic arterial tree that was used to explain these impedance patterns. The ascending aorta supplies two vascular beds in parallel. The shorter arm of the asymmetric T represents arteries to the upper part of the body, and its end, the resultant of all individual arterial ter-

minations; the longer arm represents all arteries to the lower part of the body and its end, the resultant of all arterial terminations in the lower part. Minor modifications of this model can be used to explain impedance patterns in the ascending aorta of other experimental animals, and of man; the model can also be utilised to explain contour of pressure and flow waves in upper and lower body arteries (Chs. 9,11).

The effects of altering mean arterial pressure on ascending aortic impedance appear to be the same as in peripheral vascular beds (p. 97), with a shift of impedance curves to the right (higher frequencies) with increasing pressure and to the left (lower frequencies) when pressure is decreased (Fig. 8.15). Two other points have been noted with increasing arterial pressure. The first is that the first minimum shifts further than the second, as though increasing mean pressure increases pulse wave velocity more in lower body arteries than in

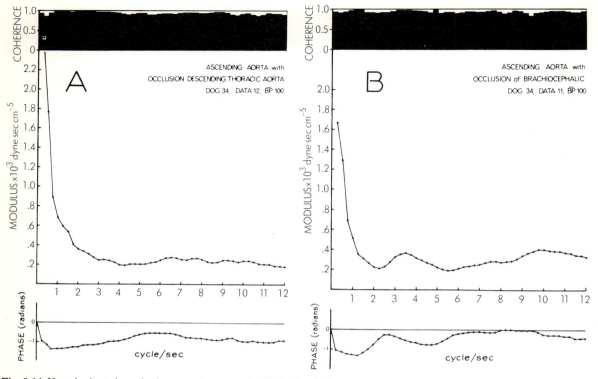

Fig. 8.14 Vascular impedance in the ascending aorta of a 23 Kg dog during occlusion of the descending thoracic aorta (left) and during occlusion of the brachiocephalic artery (right) (From O'Rourke and Taylor 1967) with permission American Heart Association Inc.

upper body arteries. The second is that the general level of impedance modulus may appear to fall. This has been attributed to flow measurements being taken with a cuff – type transducer which prevents arterial expansion at a higher distending pressure, so that flow velocity is overestimated and so, derived impedance modulus (expressed as dyne sec cm^{-5}) underestimated at the higher pressure. When flow is measured with a catheter tip transducer (and so arterial expansion is not restricted) and impedance modulus is expressed in terms of velocity flow (as dyne sec cm^{-3}) impedance modulus increases with increasing pressure to the same degree as does pulse wave velocity (Merillon et al 1980, Murgo et al 1980).

Some reports of ascending aortic impedance have found no obvious change in modulus or phase with alteration in mean distending pressure (Patel et al 1963, Abel 1971, Cox and Pace 1975). In these studies, mean pressure variations were relatively modest and the analytical technique

(Fourier analysis of wave pairs with the heart beating regularly) less sensitive than the technique of frequency spectrum analysis that we have been able to apply (Taylor 1966; O'Rourke and Taylor 1967).

Vasodilator and vasoconstrictor agents appear to have the same type of effect on ascending aortic impedance as on other beds (Fig. 8.15), with vasoconstriction causing little alteration in fluctuations of modulus and phase, and with vasodilation decreasing these fluctuations. However, since these agents have their effect through altering peripheral reflection, and since the effects of wave reflection in the ascending aorta are less marked than elsewhere (because of the partial cancellation of reflected waves from upper and lower body), these changes are less marked than in peripheral beds. Some (Patel et al 1963, Cox 1974) have been unable to demonstrate any change in frequency-dependent components of impedance with alterations in vasomotor tone. In Figure 8.16, effects on

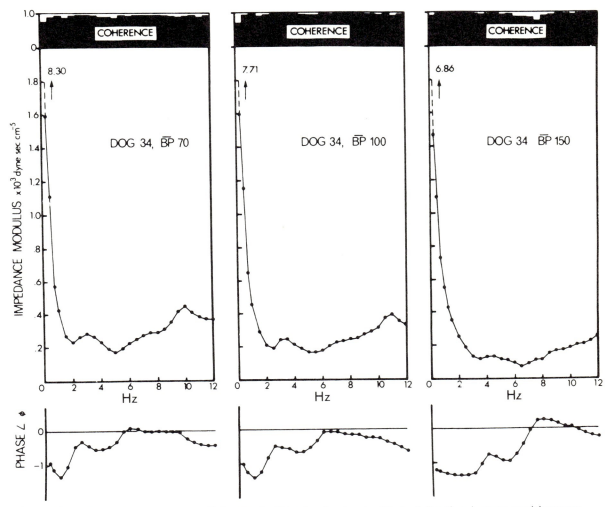

Fig. 8.15 Vascular impedance in the ascending aorta of a 23 kg dog showing the effects of alterations in mean arterial pressure unaccompanied by large changes in peripheral resistance. Peripheral resistance is shown inset at upper left (From O'Rourke 1970) with permission American Heart Association Inc.

arteriolar tone are combined with effects of altered mean arterial pressure. It was not possible to separate these different effects under experimental circumstances as it was in a peripheral vascular bed (p. 97); changes in mean pressure always accompanied alterations in arteriolar tone.

Ascending aortic impedance has been determined in a variety of experimental animals including sheep (O'Rourke 1965, Avolio 1976), rabbits and guinea pigs (Avolio et al 1976). Patterns are basically similar to those in dogs with minor differences which can readily be explained on the basis of differences in body size and shape, and

with the same asymmetric T conceptual model of the systemic arterial tree.

In sheep, rabbits and guinea pigs, impedance modulus falls steeply from its resistive value at zero frequency to a minimal value at a frequency somewhat higher than the resting heart rate, and with impedance phase, initially negative, approaching or crossing zero at the same frequency (Figs. 8.17, 8.18). As in dogs, the position of this functional reflection site appears to be in the region of the pelvis and to represent the resultant of all arterial terminations in the lower part of the body (Avolio et al 1976, Avolio 1976). The differ-

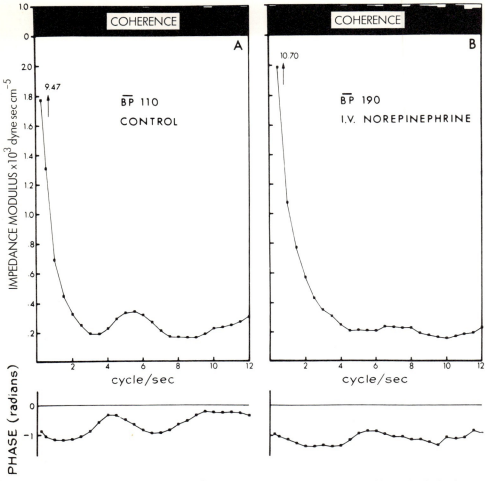

Fig. 8.16 Vascular impedance in the ascending aorta of a 25.5 kg dog (A) under control conditions, (B) during intravenous infusion of norepinephrine (approximately 5 μg min^{-1}), (C) during intravenous infusion of acetylcholine (approximately 100 μg min^{-1}) and (D) during infusion of isoproterenol (approximately 2 μg min^{-1}). Values of peripheral resistance are given in the upper left part of each panel (From O'Rourke and Taylor 1967) with permission American Heart Association Inc.

ences in frequency of the first minimum of impedance (approximately 2 Hz in sheep, 5 Hz in rabbits, 12 Hz in guinea pigs) are thus readily explained on the basis of differences in body length.

After the first impedance minimum, the patterns of ascending aortic impedance in rabbits and sheep are somewhat different to those seen in dogs, in that a second minimum of modulus often occurs at three times the frequency of the first, with an intervening maximum at twice this frequency. (Interpretations are impossible in guinea pigs because fluctuations occur at high frequencies where signal/noise ratio of instruments is low).

These findings suggest that the ascending aorta 'sees' only the one peripheral reflecting site in the lower part of the body. However when impedance is determined in the ascending aorta, descending aorta, and brachiocephalic artery of the same animal under similar circumstances (Fig. 8.19), one obtains the same information as in dogs:— evidence of upper and lower body reflecting sites, and ascending aortic impedance patterns which appear as a composite of those in the major vessels supplying the upper and lower parts of the body. The essential difference between rabbits and sheep on the one hand, and dogs on the other, is that the

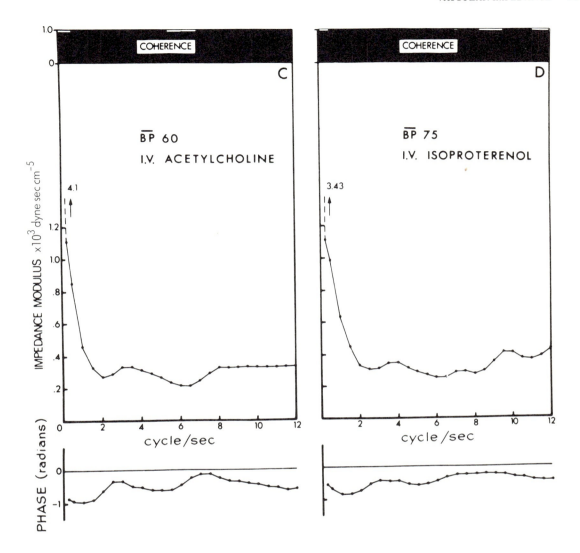

minimum of modulus and phase cross-over in the brachiocephalic artery occurs at three times (not twice as in dogs) the equivalent frequency in the mouth of the descending thoracic aorta. This suggests that in rabbits and sheep, the lower body reflection sites is relatively further away than the upper body reflection site as compared to dogs. When the apparent position of upper and lower body reflection sites is calculated from impedance minima and pulse wave velocity, however they appear to have the same relative position in sheep and rabbits as in dogs – in the region of the pelvis for the lower site and the mid upper arm for the

upper. Thus the difference in impedance patterns can be explained on the basis of differences in body shape. In rabbits and sheep the trunk is longer in comparison to the upper limbs than in dogs, so that the lower body reflecting site appears to be three times further away than the upper instead of twice as far away as in dogs. Thus the arterial system in rabbits and sheep is represented by the same basic asymmetric T model as used for dogs, only with a relatively shorter upper than lower branch (Fig. 9.17).

Differences in patterns of ascending aortic impedance in animals of different size and shape are

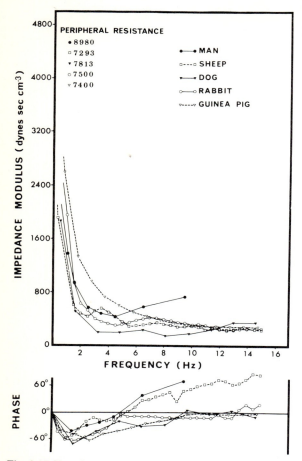

Fig. 8.17 Vascular impedance in the ascending aorta of five different mammals. Modulus expressed as dyne sec cm⁻³, as determined from linear flow velocity (From Avolio 1976)

thus readily explained on the basis of anatomical differences, with body length determining the frequencies at which impedance minima occur, and body shape determining the degree of interaction of reflection from upper and lower body sites. This subject will be pursued again in relation to impedance patterns in man and in relation to pressure and flow contour (Ch. 9 and 11).

Ascending aortic impedance and arterial models

Different models have been proposed to explain impedance patterns and pulse contour in systemic arteries (Ch. 4). The most realistic of these is that of Avolio (1976, 1980) which uses the same computational techniques as that of Taylor (1966b) which was previously used (p. 101) to explain impedance patterns in a peripheral vascular bed. Unlike Taylor's model, that of Avolio allows for different dimensions of arteries and different patterns of branching so that the geometrical pattern of a vascular bed or of the whole systemic arterial tree can be simulated.

Avolio applied this model to the systemic vascular bed of humans, sheep, rabbits and guinea pigs. Dimensions of major arteries were determined by dissection or post mortem angiography and values of arterial distensibility were calculated from measurements of pulse wave velocity prior to death. Using these values together with known values of blood viscosity and density, Avolio calculated impedance modulus and phase for the ascending aorta, upper descending aorta and brachiocephalic artery of sheep, rabbits and guinea pigs. Results (Fig. 8.20) were virtually identical to those determined experimentally. The position of apparent reflecting sites in the models corresponded to the position of sites determined experimentally. In all cases it was shown that the distributed arterial geometry could be approximated by an asymmetrical T tube with realistic dimensions (Fig. 9.17).

This model will be referred to in more detail in Chapter 9 where it will be used to explain impedance patterns and pulse contour in human systemic arteries.

PULMONARY VASCULAR IMPEDANCE

Pulmonary vascular impedance was first determined by Caro and McDonald (1961) in rabbits using a sinusoidal pump of variable frequency superimposed on steady flow, and measuring sinusoidal pressure fluctuation with Taylor's harmonic resolver. This technically difficult experiment has not to my knowledge been repeated and subsequent determinations have been made in the conventional manner by relating corresponding harmonics or frequency components of compound pressure and flow waves generated by the heart. It is important however to note that the results obtained with the sinusoidal pump are similar to those obtained from Fourier or frequency spectrum analysis of compound waves. Further studies

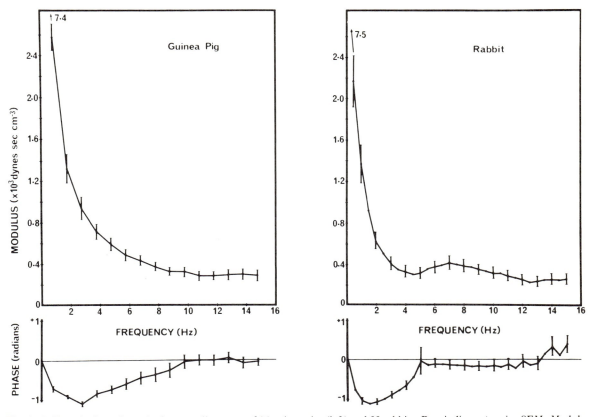

Fig. 8.18 Vascular impedance in the ascending aorta of 16 guinea pigs (left) and 22 rabbits. Bars indicate ± twice SEM. Modulus expressed in terms of linear flow velocity (From Avolio et al 1976)

of pulmonary vascular impedance have been performed in dogs (Patel et al 1963, Morris 1965, Bergel and Milnor 1965, Milnor et al 1967, Reuben et al 1971). There is now general agreement as to patterns observed and underlying mechanisms.

Pulmonary vascular impedance (Fig. 8.21) is basically similar to ascending aortic impedance, with four principal differences. The first difference is that pulmonary vascular resistance is much lower – about one tenth – the value of systemic vascular resistance, so that impedance modulus at zero frequency is far less than that in the ascending aorta, and the subsequent fall of modulus with frequency is less steep than in the ascending aorta. The second principal difference is that the pulmonary artery is more distensible at physiological pressures than the ascending aorta. As a result of this, pulse wave velocity is approximately half that in the ascending aorta, and the characteristic im-

pedance – the value of modulus about which fluctuations occur – is also approximately half that in the ascending aorta. The third difference is a consequence of the first two. With resistance one tenth that in the systemic circulation, and arterial distensibility one half that of the aorta, the ratio $\dfrac{Z_T - Z_O}{Z_T + Z_O}$ which determines reflection coefficient is far lower than that in the systemic circulation. Bergel and Milnor (1965) calculated this as 0.32, but the value would have been closer to 0.5 had they used pulmonary vascular resistance as Z_T, as now considered proper (McDonald 1974, p. 88). As a result of the relatively low reflection coefficient, fluctuations in impedance phase are less marked than in the ascending aorta. The last difference is that there is no apparent difference in wave reflection from both lungs, so that there appears to be one single functionally-discrete reflecting site in the pulmonary vascular bed. This is

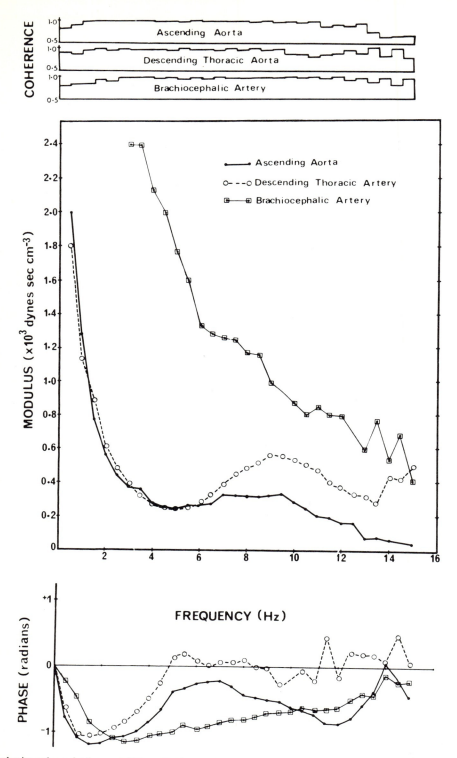

Fig. 8.19 Vascular impedance in the ascending aorta, descending thoracic aorta and brachiocephalic artery of a rabbit, at similar mean arterial pressure (From Avolio et al 1976)

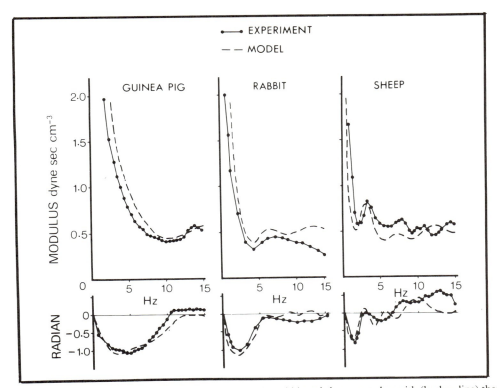

Fig. 8.20 Vascular impedance in the ascending aorta of a guinea pig, rabbit and sheep, together with (broken line) theoretically determined impedance in the ascending aorta of these three animals using Avolio's multi-branched model of the systemic circulation and measured arterial dimensions and vascular properties

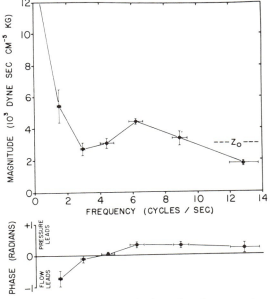

Fig. 8.21 Vascular impedance in the main pulmonary artery of 13 anesthetised open-chest dogs. Calculated resistance 14.2×10^3 dyne sec cm^{-5} kg. (From Bergel and Milnor 1965) with permission American Heart Association Inc.

apparent in the fluctuations in impedance modulus, which show a minimal value at around 3 Hz and a subsequent maximum at around 6 Hz in medium sized dogs. From these figures, and Attinger's (1963) estimation of pulse wave velocity at 200 cm sec^{-1}, Bergel and Milnor (1965) calculated the functional reflecting site to be some 17 cms from the main pulmonary artery, and to represent the resultant of all arterial terminations in the lungs.

Bergel and Milnor (1965) also determined pulmonary vascular impedance during infusion of serotonin, a potent pulmonary vasoconstrictor. Infusion of this drug led to doubling of pulmonary arterial mean pressure as well as vasoconstriction and resulted in a shift in the minimum of impedance modulus and phase crossover from approximately 3 to nearly 6 Hz. There was no apparent change in characteristic impedance. Bergel and Milnor attributed this change in pulmonary vascular impedance to arterial constriction so that reflection sites had moved closer to the heart. This explanation seems unlikely. Subsequently, Bargainer (1967) in Milnor's laboratory showed that serotonin infusion leads to marked increase in pulmonary artery pulse wave velocity, largely (or perhaps completely) as a result of its gross distension at high mean pressure. The effects of serotonin on pulmonary arterial impedance thus appear to be almost identical to the effects of noradrenaline on ascending aortic impedance (p. 107) and to be explicable on the basis of unchanged site of wave reflection, but more rapid travel of the pressure wave. Even the apparent failure of characteristic impedance to change with serotonin infusion is explicable on the basis of the pulmonary artery being constrained by a cuff type probe so that a real increase in characteristic impedance (expressed as dyne sec cm^{-3}) was hidden (p. 108). In humans with pulmonary vascular hypertension, characteristic impedance (determined with a catheter flow technique) is increased to the same degree as pulse wave velocity (Milnor et al 1969).

Technical considerations in determination of vascular impedance

Terminal impedance

The concept of input impedance assumes that pulsatile blood flow enters a vascular bed, and from this bed blood flows in a steady stream at negligible hydrostatic pressure back to the heart. In such a system both resistance and impedance can be calculated by relating arterial pressure to arterial flow, while neglecting venous pressure and venous flow. This is a reasonable presumption for the systemic circulation under normal circumstances, since right atrial pressure is normally close to zero, and venous pressure and flow waves are transmitted back from the heart (Gabe et al 1959) and not through the arterioles. In the pulmonary system, the position is less simple. Left atrial pressure is considerably higher than right atrial pressure and certainly not negligible in relation to mean pulmonary artery pressure (normally being some 25–35 percent of this). It is not reasonable to neglect this in calculation of pulmonary vascular resistance which is determined as (mean pulmonary artery minus mean left atrial pressure) ÷ cardiac output. Because of pulmonary arteriolar vasodilation, pulmonary capillary flow is pulsatile (Karatazas et al 1970, Reuben et al 1971) and some of this pulsation

is transmitted through to the veins. Since this is only some five percent of pulmonary arterial pulsation (Morris 1965, Bergel and Milnor 1965) it is considered reasonable for it to be neglected in calculation of impedance. Thus in determining vascular impedance, pulsatile arterial pressure and flow are related directly, and venous pulsations are ignored; in calculating the resistive component of impedance it is not reasonable to neglect mean left atrial pressure, even under normal circumstances, nor mean right atrial pressure if this is elevated under abnormal circumstances.

The theory of vascular impedance has been studied in depth by Taylor (1957a, b, 1959, 1964, 1965, 1966a, b). He has shown that terminal impedance at zero frequency is indeed the peripheral resistance, and demonstrated this experimentally by showing that the frequency–dependent components of impedance increase gradually and progressively towards the peripheral resistance at frequencies as low as 0.01 Hz. He calculated reflection coefficient using resistance as terminal impedance and emphasised that this is higher than had been calculated previously by McDonald (1960) and by Bergel and Milnor (1965). McDonald conceded this point in the second (1974) edition of his monograph. Taylor further showed that the impedance curves obtained experimentally were readily explained from modelling studies only when very high reflection coefficients were assumed, as determined by considering peripheral resistance to be the terminal impedance.

Characteristic impedance

Characteristic impedance is input impedance in the absence of wave reflection. Since some degree of wave reflection is present under normal circumstances, this can only be estimated, and not measured directly. When using frequency spectrum analysis and with the heart beating irregularly, (Taylor 1966a) it is possible to obtain impedance values up to 25 Hz, at which frequency fluctuations due to reflection have been completely attenuated. In our studies with this technique (O'Rourke 1965, Taylor 1966a, O'Rourke and Taylor 1967) the average value of modulus between 15–25 Hz was taken to represent characteristic impedance. In other studies, where impedance has been determined only up to 12 Hz, characteristic impedance has been gauged as the average value of modulus between 2–12 Hz (Bergel and Milnor 1965, Milnor et al 1969), above 2 Hz (Nichols et al 1977, Murgo et al 1980), or above the frequency of the first minimum (McDonald 1974). It is important to appreciate that these techniques of assessment are arbitrary and provide estimates only. In averaging impedance modulus over a band of frequencies, one hopes to include as much fluctuation above the true characteristic impedance value as there is below. Obviously, how successful this is will depend on the band of frequencies selected, and the position of impedance maxima and minima. In Figure 8.11, (dog 34) characteristic impedance was 340 dyne sec cm^{-5} by the first method and 250 dyne sec cm^{-5} by the second. In Figure 8.15 at mean pressure 150 mm Hg, the difference was even greater–300 dyne sec cm^{-5} by the first method and 170 dyne sec cm^{-5} by the second. It should be apparent that characteristic impedance cannot be measured precisely, and that current methods of estimation, particularly those that average impedance modulus over a band where it may still be fluctuating greatly, are at best just approximations.

Expression of impedance modulus

Impedance modulus is pressure ÷ flow. Flow can be expressed in terms of volume flow (ml sec^{-1}) or in terms of linear flow velocity (cm sec^{-1}), so that impedance modulus takes the units of dyne sec cm^{-5} (volume flow) or dyne sec cm^{-3} (linear flow velocity). In the literature, and indeed in this book, some results are expressed in the one unit, and some in the other. Still others have been expressed in terms of volume flow divided by weight (Bergel and Milnor 1965, Milnor et al 1966) while others have been normalised in relation to peripheral resistance (Patel et al 1963, Murgo et al 1980) or in relation to characteristic impedance (Murgo et al 1980). Clearly, some standardisation is desirable.

Volume flow (ml sec^{-1}) has the benefit of familiarity and appears to make more sense in calculating peripheral resistance than flow velocity (cm sec^{-1}). However, volume flow varies by several orders of magnitude in different arteries of the same animal, and in the same artery of different animals, while linear flow velocity, like pressure, is similar in different arteries and in different species. Impedance modulus expressed as dyne sec cm^{-3} (i.e. from flow velocity) can be compared on the same graph for different arteries of the same animal (Fig. 8.9), and for the same artery of different animals (Fig. 8.17). This is not possible when modulus is expressed in terms of volume flow unless a logarithmic scale is employed (Cox and Pace 1965). Thus, comparisons between different arteries and between different animals can best be made when impedance is expressed in terms of linear flow velocity. The same argument applies when comparisons are made in the same artery under different circumstances. Reference has been made (p. 108) to the finding that characteristic impedance, expressed in terms of volume flow, did not increase as expected under experimental circumstances when mean arterial pressure was elevated by noradrenaline or serotonin wheras pulse wave velocity increased markedly. Use of volume flow under these circumstances fails to take account of the change in arterial calibre which accompanies a change in mean pressure. When characteristic impedance is expressed in terms of velocity flow in the unconstrained artery, characteristic impedance increases to the same degree as pulse wave velocity (Merillon et al 1980, Murgo et al 1980).

This subject is discussed also by McDonald (1974) who pointed out that the correct expression of acoustic and hydraulic impedance in physics is as dyne sec cm^{-3} (linear flow velocity) and advised that vascular impedance be expressed in the same way. The relationship between characteristic impedance and pulse wave velocity has been discussed by Bargainer (1967) and by Taylor (1965). The 'waterhammer formula'

$$p = \rho.c.v \qquad (\text{p. 40})$$

which relates pressure fluctuation to flow fluctuation in the absence of wave reflection refers to linear flow velocity, not volume flow. This can be arranged as

$$\frac{p}{v} = \rho.c$$

The first term p/v is characteristic impedance in dyne sec cm^{-3}; ρ is density of blood and c is wave velocity. Thus characteristic impedance (in dyne sec cm^{-3}) varies directly with pulse wave velocity and so is a measure of arterial distensibility. Since density of blood is approximately 1.05 gram cm^{-3}, these values are numerically very close. At a pulse wave velocity of 400 cm/sec in the ascending aorta, one would expect characteristic impedance to be 420 dyne sec cm^{-3}.

Normalisation of impedance modulus (in terms of volume flow) to body weight, surface area, peripheral resistance, or characteristic impedance represents an attempt to allow for diffferences in body size. In expressing impedance modulus in terms of linear velocity, one is accomplishing the same thing, by normalising volume flow to arterial cross sectional area. In so doing, one has a term in the same units as used in the physical sciences, which is directly and numerically comparable to pulse wave velocity, and which is an index of arterial distensibility. This:—impedance modulus as dyne sec cm^{-3} – appears preferable to all other units.

Measurement of pressure – end on or side on to the direction of flow

The theory that was developed by Womersley, McDonald and Taylor to describe pressure-flow relationships as vascular impedance (Ch. 4) ap-

plies only to arteries in which peak flow velocity is low and so kinetic energy insignificant, so that lateral pressure is a measure of the total energy of blood in the vessel. When venous pressure is negligible and flow velocity is low, the lateral pressure is equivalent to the energy per ml expanded in driving blood through the peripheral vascular bed. In the ascending aorta and pulmonary artery however, peak flow velocity during ventricular systole is so high that kinetic energy represents a significant fraction (some 10–15 percent – O'Rourke 1967, Milnor et al 1966) of the total pulsatile energy under basal circumstances, and substantially more when flow velocity is increased (Elkins and Milnor 1968, Hopkins et al 1979). As a result, lateral pressure is not a complete measure of the total energy lost in the vessels downstream. The question thus arises as to how one should determine impedance in these large vessels – as the relationship between lateral pressure and flow (and so ignore kinetic energy) or as the relationship between total energy (expressed as pressure) and flow.

This subject is discussed by Burton (1965) in relation to calculation of peripheral resistance. He argues for use of total energy expressed as pressure, and not lateral pressure alone. The subject is also discussed in detail by O'Rourke (1968, 1981, 1981) where the argument is advanced that impedance should be determined from pressure measured end-on to the direction of flow so that this

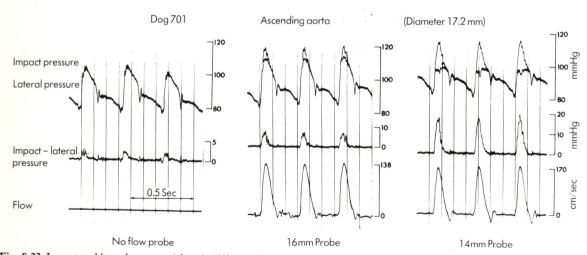

Fig. 8.22 Impact and lateral pressure (above), difference between impact and lateral pressure (centre) and linear flow velocity (below) in the ascending aorta of a dog under three different conditions. (From O'Rourke, 1968)

includes the kinetic energy imparted to blood at high flow velocity. Such has been the routine practice of Taylor and myself since 1964 (O'Rourke and Taylor 1966, 1967).

The difference between impact★ and lateral pressure in an artery is totally dependent on the square of linear flow velocity, and can be calculated from the Bernouilli formula (Ch. 4). Flow velocity depends on both volume flow and on the extent of arterial narrowing by a cuff-type flow transducer. The greatest differences between impact and lateral pressure are likely to arise when volume flow is high (as in an unanesthetised animal when exercising or in the presence of arteriovenous shunt) and when an artery is narrowed by a flow transducer. Figure 8.22 shows the difference between impact and lateral pressure waves measured downstream from a cuff-type flow transducer when the artery was slightly (7 percent) and moderately (19 percent) narrowed. Presence of the flow transducer caused no perceptible change in the contour of flow and impact pressure waves, but considerable alteration in the contour and amplitude of the lateral pressure wave. Figure 8.23 shows impedance modulus and phase determined from the same flow waves, and simultaneously-recorded impact and lateral pressure waves. Impedance modulus determined from lateral pressure was lower than that determined from impact pressure while phase was more negative.

The difference between impedance modulus measured from impact and from lateral pressure depends on the magnitude of linear flow velocity. When this exceeded 90 cm sec^{-1} peak in the pulmonary artery or 120 cm sec^{-1} peak in the ascending aorta, impedance modulus determined from lateral pressure was often well below half of that determined from impact pressure (O'Rourke 1968).

This subject warrants more attention than it has in the past received, since the results obtained at high flow velocities are dependent on the technique of pressure (and flow) measurement. Few studies of vascular impedance discuss the technique of pressure measurement in interpretation of results obtained. In a recent report Hopkins et al (1979) showed marked reduction in modulus of pulmonary vascular impedance in the presence of arteriovenous shunt, and attributed this to increase in arterial distensibility. Since pressure was measured side-on to the direction of flow in an artery with very high flow velocity, the observations could have been due to underestimation of energy in the pulmonary artery through use of lateral rather than impact pressure (O'Rourke 1980).

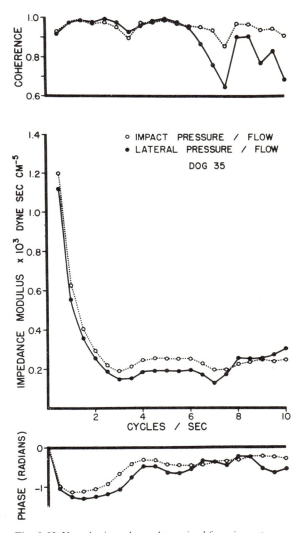

Fig. 8.23 Vascular impedance determined from impact pressure (open circles, dotted line) and from lateral pressure (closed circles, solid line) in the ascending aorta of a dog. (From O'Rourke, 1968)

★ Pressure measured end-on to the direction of flow

As with the method for calculating characteristic impedance, and with the units used for expression of impedance modulus, standardisation in the technique for pressure measurement in determining impedance is most desirable. From theoretic and practical considerations, I remain convinced that this pressure should represent the total energy of blood in an artery – the pressure that would be measured in all directions if blood had no kinetic energy – and so this should be measured in a vessel with flat velocity profile, end-on to the direction of flow.

VASCULAR IMPEDANCE IN MAN

There is less detailed information available on vascular impedance in man than in experimental animals. This is not surprising since data must be obtained during invasive procedures – with flow measured by a cuff type flow transducer from an exposed artery at surgery or through a catheter during a diagnostic procedure. In either case records must be taken promptly so that the research procedure does not delay or prejudice patient care. At surgery there is often insufficient time for the cuff type transducer to become properly seated, so that signal/noise ratio is usually greater than in the experimental laboratory; additionally, with the interface of a sterile field, the presence of others who are uninterested in a research procedure, and in an atmosphere of haste, some compromise often has to be made by the researcher in other respects such as the frequency response of the manometric system. With the electromagnetic flow catheter (currently the best catheter technique for measuring flow) noise is considerably greater than with the larger cuff-type transducer at the same site, partly because of the weaker magnetic field that can be generated by the small coils and partly as a result of catheter movement.

These technical considerations explain some of the variability in results obtained from humans. Another source of variation is the presence of vascular disease. All humans from whom measurements of pressure and flow have been taken were at the time undergoing a diagnostic or therapeutic procedure for a real or suspected medical problem. Those in whom no specific disease is demon-strated are often regarded as 'normal', but one cannot really be certain of this since diagnostic procedures such as cardiac catheterisation and coronary arteriography do not exclude the presence of atheroma or arterial degeneration in other parts of the arterial tree. In contrast to experimental animals, most humans have from early adult life some degree of arterial degeneration, and this progresses as age advances, even in the absence of symptoms (Stehbens 1979). Such asymptomatic progression of arterial degeneration is manifest as increase in pulse wave velocity (Bramwell and Hill 1922, Schimmler 1965), alteration in pressure pulse contour (Freis et al 1966) and change in pulse wave transmission characteristics (O'Rourke et al 1968) with advancing years (See Ch. 12).

These matters must be taken into consideration when interpreting human data. As will be explained, many of the differences in impedance patterns and wave contour between 'normal' man and experimental animals can be explained on the basis of unsuspected arterial degeneration.

Femoral vascular impedance in 'normal' man

This has been determined by Patel et al (1964, 1965) in patients undergoing open heart surgery, by Farrar et al (1977) in patients undergoing operative procedures on the thigh, and (in the iliac artery) by Mills et al (1970) with an electromagnetic flow/pressure catheter during diagnostic cardiac catheterisation. Results are similar to but less regular than, those noted in experimental animals (Fig. 8.24). As expected, the minimum of impedance modulus and phase crossover occur at a lower frequency than in dogs, doubtless because the human leg is longer so that the femoral or iliac artery is at a greater distance from arterial terminations downstream. Patel et al (1964, 1965) studied the effects of an intra-arterial infusion of norepinephrine and of reactive hyperemia on femoral vascular impedance. As with dogs, (p. 101), no change in frequency-dependent components of impedance was noted with the vasopressor, but with reactive hyperemia, there was a fall in terminal impedance and a reduction in impedance phase, as had been noted in dogs. (Scatter was such in experimental results as

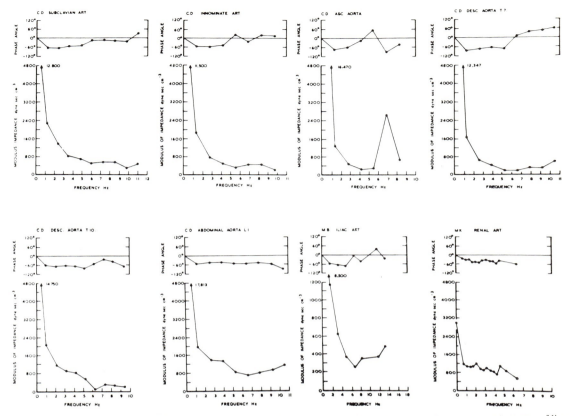

Fig. 8.24 Vascular impedance in different arteries of conscious human subjects. Impedance modulus expressed in terms of linear flow velocity (From Mills et al, 1970)

displayed by Patel et al that no definite effects on modulus could be determined). Similar results for reactive hyperemia as seen in the dog were obtained by Farrar et al (1977).

Vascular impedance in different systemic arteries of 'normal' man

Mills et al (1970) in a classic study, used their newly-developed electromagnetic velocity/pressure catheter to measure flow and pressure wave forms in different arteries, and from these, calculated vascular impedance. Impedance plots, and data from which they were obtained are shown in Figures 8.24 and 8.25. The impedance patterns are similar to those in dogs and other experimental animals (Figs. 8.9, 8.17). As in these animals impedance modulus in man fell from an initially high value at zero frequency to a minimal value, then increased again; phase was initially negative, then

crossed zero (usually) at about the frequency of this minimum of modulus. The minimal value of modulus and phase cross-over occurred at a lower frequency in the ascending aorta than in other arteries. The frequency of the minimal value increased as expected in more peripheral arteries, occurring at around 10 Hz in the subclavian artery at the axillary level, and was still not reached at 8.5 Hz in the renal artery. As for experimental animals, these patterns can be explained on the basis of wave travel and reflection in the systemic circulation.

Two points of difference should be noted at this stage when comparing data from humans with those from experimental animals. Firstly (Fig. 8.25), the pressure wave in proximal arteries is different. Murgo and colleagues (Murgo et al 1980 ab, Westerhof et al 1979) have drawn particular attention to this. In humans there is often no diastolic pressure wave; instead there is a late

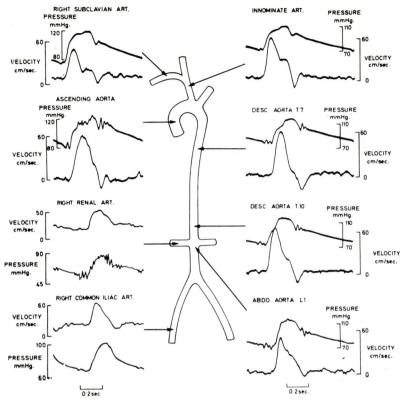

Fig. 8.25 Pressure and flow waves recorded from various arteries of conscious human subjects, pressure with a hydraulic catheter system and flow with a catheter mounted electromagnetic flowmeter (From Mills et al, 1970)

systolic 'hump' on the aortic pressure wave. This can be explained on the basis of early return of wave reflection from upper and lower body sites; it is not seen in children and probably is a manifestation of arterial degeneration acting through increase in pulse wave velocity (O'Rourke et al 1968). The second point probably has the same explanation – that minima of impedance modulus occur at higher frequencies than would be expected from the dimensions of the human body. In Figure 8.24, the minimum of impedance modulus and associated phase cross-over in the ascending and upper descending thoracic aorta occur between 4–7 Hz, considerably higher than the corresponding frequency in dogs and sheep (Figures 8.11, 8.12, 8.17), even though bodily dimensions in these animals are considerably shorter. The implications of these matters are profound and will be discussed in detail later: – that 'normal' man is quite different to experimental animals; that the difference is of considerable im-

portance with respect to arterial efficiency and cardiac function, and that the difference is attributable completely to unsuspected and asymptomatic arterial degeneration.

Ascending aortic impedance in 'normal' man

Ascending aortic impedance has been determined by Gabe et al (1964) using a differential pressure technique for measuring flow, by Patel et al (1964, 1965) and by O'Rourke and Avolio (1980) using a cuff type electromagnetic transducer for flow measurement at cardiac surgery, and most recently and most successfully by Murgo and colleagues in San Antonio (Murgo et al 1977, 1978, 1980ab, Westerhof et al 1979), by Nichols and colleagues in Gainesville (Nichols et al 1977, Pepine at al 1978, 1979), and by others including Merillon et al (1980) in Paris, and Yaginuma et al (1979) in Japan, all using the multi-sensor pressure/electromagnetic flow catheters developed by Murgo and

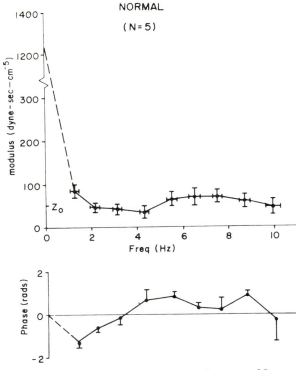

Millar (Murgo and Millar 1972, Murgo 1975). Earlier detailed work with the original electro-magnetic catheter constructed in London (Mills and Shillingford 1969) has been referred to on the previous page. Impedance has been studied in patients with heart failure, hypertension, coronary artery disease, and during vasodilator therapy. These studies will be referred to in subsequent chapters; only those in apparently 'normal' subjects will be referred to here.

Figure 8.26 shows representative results of ascending aortic impedance in apparently normal subjects, as determined by Nichols et al (1977). In this there is a minimal value of modulus at around 4 Hz, corresponding to a cross-over of phase, and a maximal value at around 8 Hz with a second phase cross-over at a slightly higher frequency. Results similar to these have been reported by others including Mills et al (1970), Murgo et al (1980), and from my own department (O'Rourke and Avolio 1980). These findings are different from those reported in dogs, and have been interpreted (Mills et al 1970, Murgo et al 1980, Westerhof et al 1979) to indicate the presence of only one functionally discrete reflecting site in the systemic arterial tree. Murgo and colleagues however

Fig. 8.26 Vascular impedance in the ascending aorta of five apparently normal human adult subjects (From Nichols et al 1977) with permission American Heart Association Inc.

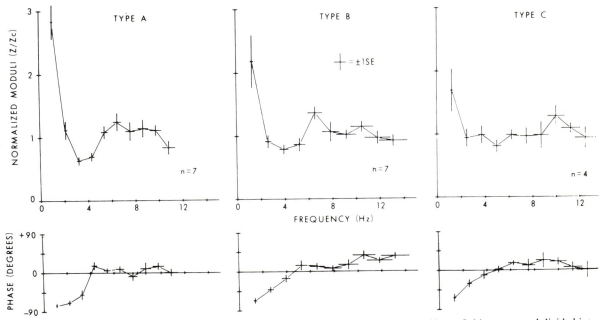

Fig. 8.27 Vascular impedance in the ascending aorta of 18 apparently normal human adult subjects. Subjects were subdivided into three different groups according to the contour of the ascending aortic pressure wave. (From Murgo et al, 1980) with permission American Heart Association Inc.

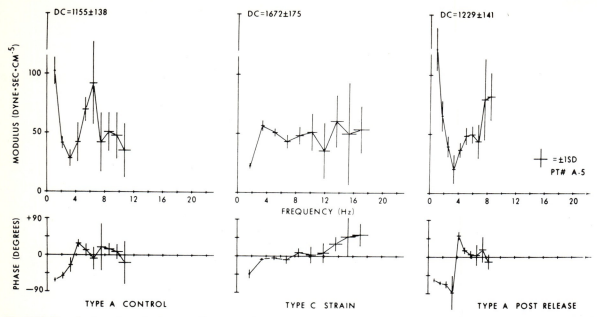

Fig. 8.28 Vascular impedance in the ascending aorta of 8 human subjects before, during, and after a Valsalva manouver. Impedance modulus normalised in relation to calculated characteristic impedance. From Murgo et al (1981) with permission American Heart Association Inc.

in their detailed and careful studies have pointed out that quite different patterns of impedance are seen in different subjects, and that the type of impedance pattern can be predicted from the contour of the aortic pressure wave (Fig. 8.27). When the aortic pressure wave shows a late systolic peak, as in Figure 8.25, the impedance pattern shows fluctuations in modulus and phase which suggest the presence of a single functionally-discrete reflecting site; when the aortic pressure wave resembles that seen in dogs, with an early peak in systole, and with a secondary fluctuation following or superimposed on the incisura, the ascending aortic impedance shows far less fluctuation with frequency, and resembles that seen in dogs (Figs. 8.11, 8.12). Murgo (1978, 1981) has extended these studies to investigate the effects of the Valsalva manouver on pressure wave contour and ascending aortic impedance. In the interests of preserving continuity, I will describe the effects of the Valsalva manouver on the arterial pulse in the next chapter, where a full explanation for phenomena observed by Murgo and others will be offered. With respect to aortic impedance however, Murgo et al found that during Valsalva strain, the fluctua-

tions of modulus which had been prominent under control conditions all but disappeared, leaving impedance modulus virtually flat over a broad band of frequencies; these patterns reverted back to normal immediately the manouver was terminated (Fig. 8.28). Thus the impedance pattern changed from that seen in most 'normal' human subjects, through that seen in dogs, and back to that seen originally in man. Murgo initially (1978) explained this on the basis of decreased arterial reflection during the Valsalva manouver. A better, and more plausible explanation (which in a sense means the same thing) is that there is more interaction and cancellation of reflected waves from different sites during the Valsalva manouver.

On the basis of data published by Murgo and others, and having obtained similar results ourselves, we were anxious to find an explanation which would reconcile all results, including the observed pressure and flow waveforms in man in different arteries under different conditions, with the general principles and concepts that had been developed for experimental animals. The mathematical model of the arterial system was developed by Avolio (1976, 1980) for this purpose. As pre-

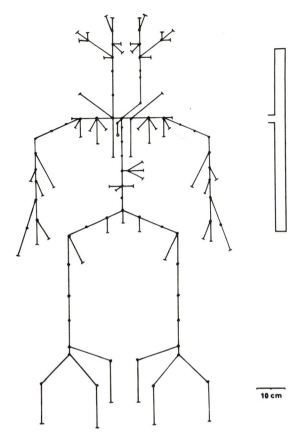

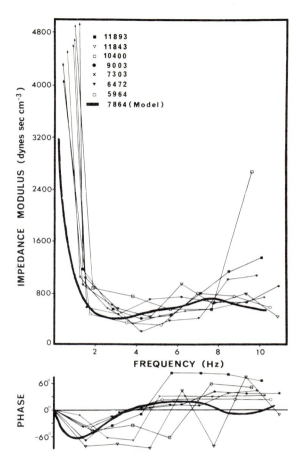

Fig. 8.29 Avolio's multi-branched model of the systemic arterial system in man (left), and its equivalent asymmetric T tube model, both drawn to scale. The open circle in the branched model and the open base of the T in the simple model represent the aortic valve. From O'Rourke and Avolio (1980) with permission American Heart Association Inc.

Fig. 8.30 Ascending aortic impedance in 7 human subjects and in the multi-branched model. Values of peripheral resistance are given at upper left (From O'Rourke and Avolio, 1980) with permission American Heart Association Inc.

viously explained (p. 112), this model provides a general algorithm of the systemic arterial tree; when measured dimensions of arterial segments and branches are used, together with experimentally-determined values of arterial distensibility, and of blood viscosity and density, the impedance in different arteries of different animals can be calculated; these are in excellent agreement with experimentally determined values in sheep, rabbits, and guinea pigs (Fig. 8.20). This same model was used to calculate ascending aortic impedance in humans, using arterial dimensions and branching patterns taken from an anatomical atlas, and from published work of Noordergraaf et al (1963) and Westerhof et al (1969) together with realistic values of arterial distensibil-

ity, blood viscosity and density, and of peripheral reflection coefficient. The multi-branched model as used for simulation of the human arterial tree is shown in Figure 8.29. Figure 8.30 shows results obtained, and compares impedance in the model with that determined from pressure and flow waves recorded at surgery from the ascending aorta in seven human subjects. There is good agreement between human and modelling results. Avolio was able further to show that by delaying return of wave reflection from the lower part of the body – either by increasing segment length or by increasing distensibility of lower body arteries so that wave velocity in these was decreased – impedance fluctuations could be reduced, while by speeding up wave reflection from the lower body, the fluctuations could be increased. By calculating impedance at the origin of the descending aorta and brachiocephalic artery of the model, Avolio determined the distance to functional reflecting site in the upper part of the body as 25.7 cm, and to that in the lower body as 39. 8 cm. These figures compare with values of 29 cm determined by Mills et al (1970) for the brachiocephalic bed, and 44 cms determined by both Mills et al and by Murgo et al (1980 a) for the lower body bed (as seen from the ascending aorta). These dimensions suggested that the arterial system in man can be represented by an asymmetric T tube just as in experimental animals (Fig. 8.29). The essential difference between humans and dogs (against which most comparisons of ascending aortic impedance have been made) is that the lower body reflecting site is only about 1.5 times (instead of twice) as far distant as the upper, so that there is less interaction and less cancellation of reflected waves from the upper and lower parts of the body.

One can easily explain on the basis of this model, impedance patterns in man under normal circumstances, the difference in impedence patterns between man, dogs and other experimental animals and also the changes in impedance patterns which accompany the Valsalva manouver. The flattening of impedance modulus during strain is attributable to decrease in transmural pressure across the thoracic and abdominal aorta so that wave velocity in these vessels is decreased, and the lower body reflecting site behaves as though it were further away in relation to the upper body site, so that cancellation of wave reflection is more complete (O'Rourke and Avolio 1980).

Ascending aortic impedance during exercise in 'normal' man

Murgo and colleagues (1980 b) have recently reported studies of ascending aortic impedance in man during supine exercise (Fig. 8.31). With exercise, cardiac output rose from 6.8 to 12.8 litre min^{-1}, mean pressure rose from 96 to 111 mm Hg, and peripheral resistance fell from 1142 to 712 dyne sec cm^{-5}. With exercise, characteristic impedance expressed as dyne sec cm^{-5} (i.e.

in terms of volume flow) did not change, but when expressed in terms of linear velocity (as dyne sec cm^{-3}), increased to the same degree as pulse wave velocity (i.e. by 20–25 percent). The fluctuations in modulus and phase of impedance were preserved, but the frequencies of impedance minima shifted to the degree that would have been expected from the concomitant increase in pulse wave velocity.

These changes with exercise are readily explained on the basis of vasodilation in the legs and increase in mean arterial pressure. One might have expected an apparent decrease in reflection coefficient to accompany the peripheral vasodilation. There was no evidence of this in the aortic impedance plots. However if vasodilation were confined to a relatively small vascular bed (that of the quadriceps muscles) the presence of high arteriolar tone elsewhere may have prevented this from becoming apparent. In other studies of the effects of peripheral vasodilation (p. 97), tone was reduced in most or all arterioles of the vascular bed through infusion of a vasodilator drug or through induction of reactive hyperemia. With generalised vasodilation, reflection coefficient is clearly reduced and fluctuations of modulus and phase of impedance are decreased. The situation with exercise seems to resemble that in arteriovenous shunt (Mang and O'Rourke 1976, Mang et al 1980) when the resistive component of impedance is decreased, but the frequency-dependent components are unchanged.

Characteristic impedance in the ascending aorta of man

There is considerable interest in characteristic impedance in the ascending aorta as an index of aortic distensibility, and an important factor in determining cardiac load. There is however considerable variation in reported values, both within the one study and between different reports. Comparisons are not easy because of the different units in which impedance has been expressed. In Table 8.1, published values have been compared in the same units (dyne sec cm^{-3}) by using measured aortic radius or if this was not stated, assuming radius to be 1.3 cm (the average of values reported

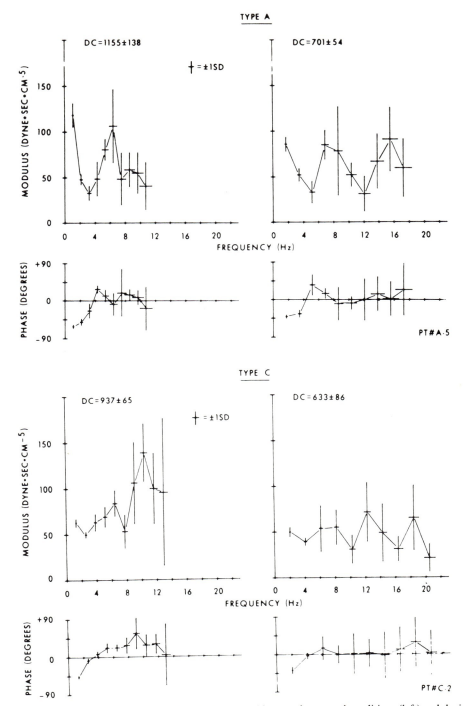

Fig. 8.31 Vascular impedance in the ascending aorta of 13 human subjects under control conditions (left) and during mild supine leg exercise (right). As for Fig. 8.27, modulus is normalised in relation to calculated characteristic impedance and subjects were sub-divided into two groups according to the contour of the ascending aortic pressure wave under control conditions (From Murgo et al, 1980b) with permission American Heart Association Inc.

Table 8.1

Author	Calculation	Characteristic Impedance Value	Subjects
Patel et al (1965)	—	700*cm H_2O(cm³/sec) *700* dyne sec cm⁻³*	Various (n = 3)
Gabe et al (1964)	—	100* dyne sec cm⁻⁵ *531* dyne sec cm⁻³*	Various (n = 3)
Mills et al (1970)	—	*700* dyne sec cm⁻³*	Various (n = 5)
Nichols et al (1977)	$\bar{Z}o$ (2 – 12 Hz)	53 ± 4 dyne sec cm⁻⁵ *(426 dyne sec cm⁻³)*	'Normal' (n = 5)
		95 ± 12 dyne sec cm⁻⁵ *575 dyne sec cm⁻³*	C.A.D. (n = 7)
		202 ± 32 dyne sec cm⁻⁵ *1244 dyne sec cm⁻³*	C.A.D. & hypertension (n = 4)
Pepine et al (1978)	$\bar{Z}o$ (2 – 12 Hz)	89 ± 8 dyne sec cm⁻³ *530 dyne sec cm⁻³*	'Normal' (n = 10)
		131 ± 9 dyne sec cm⁻⁵ *875 dyne sec cm⁻³*	Cardiac failure (n = 10)
Murgo et al (1980)	$\bar{Z}o > 2Hz$	47 ± 4 dyne sec cm⁻⁵ *212 dyne sec cm⁻³*	'Normal' (n = 18)
O'Rourke/Avolio (1980)	—	*500* dyne sec cm⁻³*	Various (n = 7)
Merillon et al (1980)	$\bar{Z}o > 2Hz$	82 ± 30 dyne sec cm⁻⁵ *435 dyne sec cm⁻³*	'Normal' (n = 9)
		147 ± 61 dyne sec cm⁻⁵ *780 dyne sec cm⁻³*	Hypertension (n = 7)

* Approximate; C.A.D. – Coronary artery Disease; SD – Standard deviation

by Murgo (1980) and Nichols (1977). It is of course possible that some of the reported values such as those found in patients with cardiac failure, hypertension, and coronary artery disease are affected by arterial degeneration and so are above the 'normal' range. However there seems to be a disparity between some of the lower values published by Nichols et al (1977) and Murgo et al (1980a) in relation to the value of pulse wave velocity in the ascending aorta. Murgo and colleagues determined ascending aortic pulse wave velocity as 6.68 ± 0.32 metre sec⁻¹ in the ascending aorta of 'normal' subjects. Their value of characteristic impedance was 47 ± 4 dyne sec cm⁻⁵ or 212 dyne sec cm⁻³ when this was expressed in terms of linear flow, using the measured value of aortic radius. From the 'waterhammer' formula (p. 117) one would calculate characteristic impedance as 668 × 1.05 or 701 dyne sec cm⁻³. The reason for the large discrepancy between observed (212) and predicted (701) values for characteristic impedance is unclear.

Characteristic impedance appears to be an unreliable guide to aortic distensibility. Its determination requires measurement of the aortic flow wave which always has a lower signal/noise ratio than the aortic pressure wave, especially when this can be measured with a miniature catheter-mounted transducer. Additionally, characteristic impedance cannot be measured directly, but is estimated by averaging impedance modulus over an arbitrary band of frequencies (p. 116). Further, in inferring arterial distensibility (p. 29), one must express impedance in terms of velocity flow – which varies with diameter along the ascending aorta as it tapers down from the sinuses of Valsalva.

Pulse wave velocity is a well established index of arterial distensibility. It can be easily and accurately measured with the modern multisensor catheters, and is not influenced by variation in aortic diameter. It is probably preferable to characteristic impedance as an index of aortic distensibility.

Impedance in the main pulmonary artery of 'normal' human subjects

Input impedance in the main pulmonary artery of man (Fig. 8.32) has been determined by Mills et al (1970) using an electromagnetic velocity cathe-

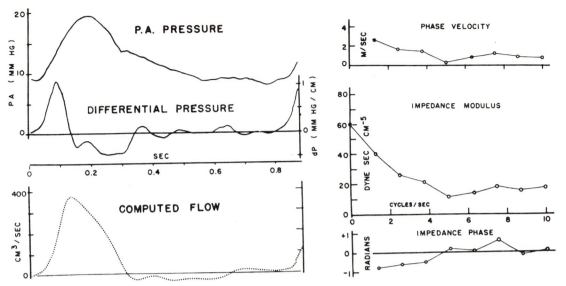

Fig. 8.32 *Right:* Apparent phase velocity (top) and impedance modulus (centre) and phase (below) in the main pulmonary artery of a human subject.
Left: Pulmonary artery pressure, differential pressure and computed flow in this subject. (From Milnor et al, 1969) with permission American Heart Association Inc.

ter to measure flow, and by Milnor et al (1969) using the differential pressure technique for flow measurement. Results obtained are similar to those in dogs, with a relatively low value of terminal and characteristic impedance, a less steep fall of modulus than in the ascending aorta, a minimal value of modulus and phase cross-over at 3–5 Hz and a maximal value of modulus at twice this frequency, and with impedance phase showing less fluctuation than in the ascending aorta. Results are explicable, as in dogs, on the basis of low pulmonary arteriolar tone, high pulmonary arterial distensibility, a low reflection coefficient in the pulmonary vascular bed, and an apparently single functional reflection site in the lungs. Milnor and colleagues (1969) determined pulmonary vascular impedance in pulmonary hypertension. The results are explicable on the basis of increased pulmonary vascular resistance and decreased pul-

monary distensibility. These will be discussed in Chapter 14.

Input impedance from non-invasively recorded pulses

Good quality sphygmograms and Doppler ultrasonic flow pulses have been obtained transcutaneously by Pasch et al (1977) in Erlangen, and from these, impedance spectra have been determined. The patterns of impedance modulus and phase are similar to those obtained from pressure and flow pulses recorded directly from the artery, but of course since indirectly-determined pressure and flow pulses cannot be calibrated, modulus must be expressed in arbitrary units. Further improvements in methodology for indirect recording of pressure and flow pulses will doubtless see this important work extended.

REFERENCES

Abel FL 1971 Fourier analysis of left ventricular performance. Circulation Research 28: 119–135
Anliker M, Histand MB, Ogden E 1968 Dispersion and attenuation of small artificial pressure waves in the canine aorta. Circulation Research 23: 539–551
Attinger EO 1963 Pressure transmission in pulmonary arteries related to frequency and geometry. Circulation Research 12: 623–641
Attinger EO, Sugawara H, Navarro A, Riccetto A, Martin R 1966 Pressure/flow relations in dog arteries. Circulation Research 19: 230–246
Avolio AP 1976 Hemodynamic studies and modelling of the

mammalian arterial system. Ph D Thesis University of New South Wales Sydney

Avolio AP 1980 Multi-branched model of the human arterial system. Medical and Biological Engineering and Computing 18: 709–718

Avolio AP, O'Rourke MF, Mang K, Bason PT, Gow BS 1976 A comparative study of pulsatile arterial hemodynamics in rabbits and guinea pigs. American Journal of Physiology 230: 868–875

Avolio AP, O'Rourke MF, Webster M 1980 Pulsatile hemodynamics in the arterial system of the snake. Proceedings 28th International Congress and Physiological Sciences Budapest p. 306

Bagshaw RJ 1976 Assessment of cerebrovascular hydraulic input impedance. IEEE Transactions in Biomedical Engineering BME 23: 412–417

Bargainer JD 1967 Pulse wave velocity in the main pulmonary artery of the dog. Circulation Research 20: 630–637

Bergel DH, McDonald DA, Taylor MG 1958 A method for measuring arterial impedance using a differential manometer. Journal of Physiology (London) 141: p 17–18

Bergel DH, Milnor WR 1965 Pulmonary vascular impedance in the dog. Circulation Research 16: 401–415

Bramwell JC, Hill AV 1922 Velocity of transmission of the pulse wave and elasticity of arteries. Lancet 1: 891–892

Burton A 1965 Physiology and biophysics of the circulation. Year Book Medical Publishers Chicago p 102–105

Caro CG, McDonald DA 1961 The relation of pulsatile pressure and flow in the pulmonary vascular bed. Journal of Physiology 157: 426–453

Caro CG, Pedley TJ, Schroter RC, Seed WA 1978 The mechanics of the circulation. Oxford University Press New York

Cox RH 1974 Determinants of systemic hydraulic power in unanesthetised dogs. American Journal of Physiology 226: 579–587

Cox RH, Pace JB 1975 Pressure-flow relations in the vessels of the canine aortic arch. American Journal of Physiology 228: 1–10

Dujardin JP, Stone DN, Paul LT, Peiper HP 1980 Effect of acute volume loading on aortic smooth muscle activity in intact dogs. American Journal of Physiology 238: H379–H383

Dujardin JP, Stone DN, Paul LT, Pieper HP 1980 Response of systemic arterial input impedance to volume expansion and hemorrhage. American Journal of Physiology 238: H902–H908

Elkins RC, Milnor WR 1971 Pulmonary vascular response to exercise in the dog. Circulation Research 29: 591–599

Elkins RC, Peyton MD, Greenfield LJ 1974 Pulmonary vascular impedance in chronic pulmonary hypertension. Surgery 76: 57–64

Elzinga G, Westerhof N 1973 Pressure and flow generated by the left ventricle against different impedances. Circulation Research 32: 178–186

Farrar DJ, Malindzak GS, Johnson G Jr 1977 Large vessel impedance in peripheral atherosclerosis. Circulation 56 (Supplement 11): 171–178

Fries ED, Heath WC, Luchsinger PC, Snell RE 1966 Changes in the carotid pulse which occur with age and in hypertension. American Heart Journal 71: 757–765

Gabe IT, Gault JH, Ross J Jr., Mason DT, Mills CJ, Shillingford JP, Braunwald E 1969 Measurements of instantaneous blood flow velocity and pressure in conscious man with a catheter tip velocity probe. Circulation 40: 603–614

Gabe IT, Karnell J, Porje IG, Rudewald B 1964 The measurement of input impedance and apparent phase velocity in the human aorta. Acta Physiologica Scandinavica 61: 73–84

Gessner U 1972 Vascular input impedance. In: Bergel DH (ed) Cardiovascular fluid dynamics Academic Press London 315–349

Giolma J, Murgo J, Altobelli S 1977 Aortic input impedance in man during rest and exercise. Circulation 55 (Supplement 111) 111–234

Gow BS 1980 Circulatory correlates; impedance, resistance and capacity. In: D. Bohr and D. Somlyo (eds) 'Handbook of Physiology' Section 2 The Cardiovascular System; Vol 2 Vascular Smooth Muscle. The American Physiological Society, Maryland, 1980 p. 353–408.

Greenfield JC, Cox RL, Hernandez RR, Thomas C, Schoonmaker FW 1967 Pressure-flow studies in man during the Valsalva manouver with observations on the mechanical properties of the ascending aorta. Circulation 35: 653–661

Greenfield JC Jr., Gribbs DM 1963 Relation between pressure and diameter in main pulmonary artery of man. Journal of Applied Physiology 18: 557–559

Hamilton WF 1944 The patterns of the arterial pressure pulse. American Journal of Physiology 141: 235–241

Hernandez RR, Greenfield JC, McCall BW 1964 Pressure-flow studies in hypertrophic subaortic stenosis. Journal of Clinical Investigation 43: 401–407

Hopkins RA, Hammon JW, Hale PA, Smith PK, Anderson RW 1979 Pulmonary vascular impedance analysis of adaption to chronically elevated blood flow in the awake dog. Circulation Research 45: 267–274

Karatzas NB, Noble MIM, Saunders KB, McIlroy MB 1970 Transmission of the blood flow pulse through the pulmonary arterial tree of the dog. Circulation Research 27: 1–9

Kenner T 1972 Flow and pressure in the arteries. In: Fung YC, Peronne N, Anliker M(eds) Biomechanics: its foundations and objectives Prentice Hill New Jersey p. 381–434

Kenner T 1978 Models of the arterial system. In: Bauer RD, Busse R(eds) The arterial system, Springer Berlin 80–88

Kouchoukos NT, Sheppard IC, McDonald DA 1970 Estimation of stroke volume in the dog by a pulse contour method. Circulation Research 26: 611–623

Lambert R, Tessier G 1927 Theorie de la similitude biologique. Annals de Physiologie 3: 212–246

Little RC 1977 Physiology of the heart and circulation. Year Book Medical Publishers Chicago

Mang K, O'Rourke MF 1976 Input impedance of the systemic circulation in the presence of arteriovenous shunt. Proceedings of the Australian Physiologial Society 7: 44

Mang K, O'Rourke MF, Avolio AP 1980 Input impedance of the systemic circulation in the presence of arteriovenous shunt. Proceedings of the 28th International Congress of Physiological Sciences Budapest p. 563

McDonald DA 1960 Blood flow in arteries. 1st Edition Arnold London

McDonald DA 1974 Blood flow in arteries. 2nd Edition Arnold London

McDonald DA, Taylor MG 1956 An investigation of the arterial system using a hydraulic oscillator. Journal of Physiology (London) 133: 74–75

McDonald DA, Taylor MG 1959 The hydrodynamics of the

arterial circulation. Progress in Biophysics and Biophysical Chemistry 9: 107–173

Merillon JP, Motte G, Aumont MC, Masquet C, Lecarpentier Y, Gourgon R 1979 Post-Extrasystolic left ventricular peak pressure with and without left ventricular failure. Cardiovascular Research 13: 338–344

Merillon JP, Motte G, Fruchaud J, Masquet C, Gourgon R 1978 Evaluation of the elasticity and characteristic impedance of the ascending aorta in man. Cardiovascular Research 12: 401–406

Merillon JP, Fontenier G, Chastre J, Lerallut JF, Jaffrin MY, Gourgon R 1980 Etude du spectre d'impédance chez l'homme normal et hypertendu. Effets de l'accroissement de fréquence cardiaque et des drogues vasomotrices. Archives des Maladies de Coeur 73: 83–90

Mills CJ, Gabe IT, Gault JH, Mason DT, Ross J Jr, Braunwald E, Shillingford JP 1970 Pressure/flow relationships and vascular impedance in man. Cardiovascular Research 4: 405–417

Mills CJ, Shillingford JP 1967 A catheter tip electromagnetic velocity probe and its evaluation. Cardiovascular Research 1: 263–273

Milnor WR 1975 Arterial impedance as ventricular afterload. Circulation Research 36: 565–570

Milnor WR 1974 The circulation. In: Mountcastle VB (ed) Medical Physiology Mosby St. Louis p. 839–1026

Milnor WR 1979a Aortic wavelength as a determinant of the relation between heart rate and body size in mammals. American Journal of Physiology 237: R3–R6

Milnor WR 1979b Influence of arterial impedance on ventricular function. In Bauer RD, Busse R (eds) The arterial system Springer Berlin p. 227–235

Milnor WR, Bergel DH, Bargainer JD 1966 Hydraulic power associated with pulmonary blood flow and its relation to heart rate. Circulation Research 19: 467–480

Milnor WR, Conti CR, Lewis KB, O'Rourke MF 1969 Pulmonary arterial pulse wave velocity and impedance in man. Circulation Research 25: 637–649

Morris MJ 1965 Pressure and flow in the pulmonary vasculature of the dog. Thesis for BSc Med University of Sydney Sydney

Morris MJ, O'Rourke MF 1965 Steady and pulsatile work of the left and right ventricles. Proceedings of the Australian Physiological Society p. 35

Murgo JP 1975 Multisensor cardiac catheterisation. New methods to study cardiovascular dynamics in man Proceedings 28th ACEMB New Orleans p. 503

Murgo JP, Millar H 1972 A new cardiac catheter for high fidelity differential pressure recordings. 25th ACEMB Bal Harbour Florida p. 303

Murgo JP, Westerhof N, Giolma JP, Altobelli SA 1980a Aortic input impedance in normal man; relationship to pressure waveshapes. Circulation 62: 105–116

Murgo JP, Westerhof N, Giolma JP, Altobelli SA 1980b Effects of exercise on aortic input impedance and pressure waveforms in normal man. Circulation Research 48: 334–343

Murgo JP, Westerhof N, Giolma JP, Altobelli SA 1981 Manipulation of ascending aortic pressure and flow wave reflections with the Valsalva manouver; relationship to input impedance. Circulation 63: 122–132

Nichols WW, Conti CR, Walker WW, Milnor WR 1977 Input impedance of the systemic circulation in man. Circulation Research 40: 451–458

Noble MIM 1979 Left ventricular load, arterial impedance and their relationship. Cardiovascular Research 13: 183–198

Noble MIM, Gabe I, Trenchard D, and Guz A 1967 Blood pressure and flow in the ascending aorta of conscious dogs. Cardiovascular Research 1: 9–20

Noordergraaf A, Verdouw PD, Boom HB 1963 Analog computer in a circulation model. Progress in Cardiovascular Diseases 5: 419–439

O'Rourke MF 1965 Pressure and flow in arteries. M.D. Thesis University of Sydney Sydney

O'Rourke MF 1967a Pressure and flow waves in systemic arteries and the anatomical design of the arterial system. Journal of Applied Physiology 23: 139–149

O'Rourke MF 1967b Steady and pulsatile energy losses in the systemic circulation under normal conditions and in simulated arterial disease. Cardiovascular Research 1: 313–326

O'Rourke MF 1968 Impact pressure, lateral pressure and impedance in the proximal aorta and pulmonary artery. Journal of Applied Physiology 25: 533–541

O'Rourke MF 1969 Effects of major artery occlusion on pressure wave transmission along the human aorta. Proceedings of the Australian Physiological and Pharmacological Society p. 24

O'Rourke MF 1970 Arterial hemodynamics in hypertension. Circulation Research 26 Supplement 11: 123–133

O'Rourke MF 1971 The arterial pulse in health and disease. American Heart Journal 82: 687–802

O'Rourke MF 1976 Pulsatile arterial hemodynamics in hypertension. Australian and New Zealand Journal of Medicine 6 Supplement 2: 40–48

O'Rourke MF 1980 Comments on pulmonary vascular impedance analysis of adaptation to chronically elevated blood flow in the awake dog. Circulation Research 46: 731, 1980

O'Rourke MF 1981a Vascular impedance: A call for standardisation. in Kenner T, Hinghoffer-Szalkay. Berlin Plenum (in press)

O'Rourke MF 1981b Vascular impedance in studies of cardiac and arterial function. Physiological Reviews (in press)

O'Rourke MF, Avolio AP 1980 Pulsatile flow and pressure in human systemic arteries; studies in man and in a multi-branched model of the human systemic arterial tree. Circulation Research 46: 363–372

O'Rourke MF, Blazek JV, Morreels CL, Krovetz LJ 1968 Pressure wave transmission along the human aorta; changes with age and in arterial degenerative disease. Circulation Research 23: 567–579

O'Rourke MF, Cartmill TB 1971 Influence of aortic coarctation on pulsatile hemodynamics in the proximal aorta. Circulation 44: 281–292

O'Rourke MF, Milnor WR 1971 Relation between differential pressure and flow in the pulmonary artery of the dog. Cardiovascular Research 5: 558–565

O'Rourke MF Taylor MG 1966 Vascular impedance of the femoral bed. Circulation Research 18: 126–139

O'Rourke MF, Taylor MG 1967 Input impedance of the systemic circulation. Circulation Research 20: 365–380

Pasch Th, Bauer RD, Busse R 1976 Determination of arterial input impedance spectra from non-invasively recorded pulses. Basic Research in Cardiology 71: 229–242

Patel DJ, DeFreitas FM, Mallos AJ 1962 Mechanical function of the main pulmonary artery. Journal of Applied Physiology 17: 205–208

Patel DJ, DeFreitas FM, Fry DL 1963 Hydraulic input impedance to aorta and pulmonary artery in dogs. Journal of Applied Physiology 18: 134–140

Patel DJ, Austen WG, Greenfield JC, Tindall GT 1964 Impedance of certain large blood vessels in man. Annals of the New York Academy of Sciences 115: 1129–1139

Patel DJ, Greenfield JC, Austen WG, Morrow AG, Fry DL 1965 Pressure-flow relationships in the ascending aorta and femoral artery of man. Journal of Applied Physiology 20: 459–463

Pepine CJ, Nichols WW, Conti CR 1978 Aortic input impedance in heart failure. Circulation 58: 460–465

Pepine CJ, Nichols WW, Curry RC Jr, Conti CR 1979 Aortic input impedance during nitroprusside infusion; a reconsideration of afterload reduction and beneficial action. Journal of Clinical Investigation 64: 643–654

Porjé IG 1965 Hemodynamics of the ascending aorta. In: Attinger EO (ed) Pulsatile blood flow McGraw Hill New York p. 237–245

Randall JE, Stacy RW 1956 Mechanical impedance of the dog's hind leg to pulsatile blood flow. American Journal of Physiology 187: 94–98

Randall JE 1958 Statistical properties of pulsatile pressure and flow in the femoral artery of the dog. Circulation Research 6: 689–698

Remington JW 1963 The physiology of the aorta and major arteries. Handbook of Physiology American Physiological Society Washington D.C. Volume 2, Circulation 2: 799–838

Remington JW, Hamilton WF 1947 Evaluation of the work of the heart. American Journal of Physiology 150: 292–298

Reuben SR, Swadling JP, Gersh J, Lee G de J 1971 Impedance and transmission properties of the pulmonary arterial system. Cardiovascular Research 5: 1–9

Reuben SR, Swadling JP, Lee G de J 1970 Velocity profiles in the main pulmonary artery of dogs and man, measured with a thin-film resistance anemometer. Circulation Research 27: 995–1001

Schimmler, W 1965 Untersuchungen zum elastizitaetsproblem der aorta (Statistische Korrelation der Pulswellengeschwindigkeit zu Alter, Geschlecht und Blutdruck). Archiv KreislForsch 47: 189–233

Sipkema P, Westerhof N, Randall OS 1980 The arterial system characterised in the time domain. Cardiovascular Research 4: 270–290

Stehbens WE 1979 Hemodynamics of the blood vessel wall. Thomas Springfield

Taylor MG 1957b An approach to an analysis of the arterial pulse wave 1. Oscillations in an attenuating line. Physics in Medicine and Biology 1: 258–269

Taylor MG 1957a An approach to an analysis of the arterial pulse wave 2. Fluid oscillations in an elastic pipe. Physics in Medicine and Biology 1: 321–329

Taylor MG 1959 An experimental determination of the propogation of fluid oscillations in a tube with a visco elastic wall; together with an analysis of the characteristics required in an electrical analogue. Physics in Medicine and Biology 4: 63–82

Taylor MG 1964 Wave travel in arteries and the design of the cardiovascular system. In: Attinger EO (ed) Pulsatile Blood Flow McGraw New York p. 343–372

Taylor MG 1965 Wave travel in a non-uniform transmission line, in relation to pulses in arteries. Physics in Medicine and Biology 10: 539–550

Taylor MG 1966a Use of random excitation and spectral analysis in the study of frequency – dependent parameters of the cardiovascular system. Circulation Research 18: 585–595

Taylor MG 1966b The input impedance of an assembly or randomly branching elastic tubes. Biophysical Journal 6: 29–51

Taylor MG 1966c An introduction to some recent developments in arterial hemodynamics. Australasian Annals of Medicine 15: 71–86

Taylor MG 1969a The optimum elastic properties of arteries. In: Wolstenholme GEW, Knight J (eds) Ciba Foundation Symposium on Circulatory and Respiratory Mass Transport Churchill London p. 136–147

Taylor MG 1969b Arterial impedance and distensibility. In: Fishman AP, Hecht HH (eds) The pulmonary circulation and interstitial space, The University of Chicago Chicago p. 341–354

Thompson D'A 1917 On growth and form. Abridged edition edited by Bonner JT 1961 Cambridge University Press

Urshel CW, Covell JW, Sonnenblick EH, Ross J Jr, Braunwald E 1968 Myocardial mechanics in aortic and mitral valvular regurgitation; the concept of instantaneous impedance as a determinant of the performance of the intact heart. Journal of Clinical Investigation 47: 867–883

Walker WE 1975 The influence of changes of aortic input impedance on the dynamics of left ventricular performance. Ph D Thesis Johns Hopkins University Baltimore

Westerhof N, Bosman F, deVries CJ, Noordergraaf A. 1969 Analog studies of the human systemic arterial tree. Journal of Biomechanics 2: 121–143

Westerhof N, Elzinga G, Van Den Bos GC 1973 Influence of central and peripheral changes on the hydraulic input impedance of the systemic arterial tree. Medical and Biological Engineering 11: 710–723

Westerhof N, Sipkema P, Elzinga G, Murgo JP, Giolma JP 1979 Arterial impedance. In: Hwang HC, Gross DR, Patel DJ (eds) Quantitative cardiovascular studies University Park Baltimore Ch 3 p. 111–150

Wetterer E 1954 Flow and pressure in the arterial system, their hemodynamic relationship and the principles of the measurement. Minnesota Medicine 37: 77–86

Wetterer E, Kenner T 1968 Grundlagen der dynamik des arterienpulses. Springer Verlag, Berlin

Yaginuma T, Hosoda S, Tsuchiya M, Miyatak. Analysis of left ventricular performance in relation to the aortic impedance in man. Abstracts: Seventh Asian-Pacific Congress of Cardiology, Bangkok p. 71

9

Contour of the arterial pulse and its interpretation

Having considered the physical properties of blood and arteries, wave transmission and reflection, frequency components of the pulse, – and pressure/flow relationships expressed as vascular impedance, it is now appropriate to describe and explain the contour of pressure and flow pulses in different systemic arteries. Since the pattern of ventricular ejection is remarkably similar in different mammals (Fig. 9.1) and under different conditions, it is in terms of vascular, not cardiac properties, that such an explanation must be offered. Features of pressure and flow waves in systemic arteries have been pointed out already, and are shown in Figures 2.1, 2.5, 7.12 and 8.25. Changes in pressure and flow waves between the

heart and lower body arteries are summarised in Figure 9.2, and are seen to be a progressive rise in amplitude of the pressure wave, and a progressive fall in amplitude of flow, together with appearance of prominent diastolic fluctuations in each. It will be useful to describe pressure and flow waves separately, taking the archetypal patterns to be those recorded in dogs, discussing later the differences in patterns of other mammals and of normal man. A simple all-embracing explanation can be offered which appears to account for patterns of pressure and flow waves in terms of interpretations that have already been made from consideration of vascular impedance.

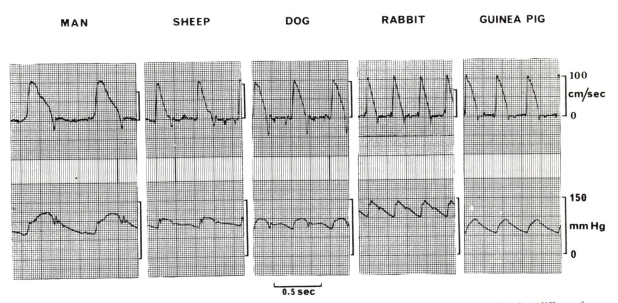

Fig. 9.1 Flow (above) and pressure (below) waves in the ascending aorta of five different mammals. Flow calibration (different for each animal) is 100 cm sec^{-1} in each case. Pressure calibration (0–150 mmHg) and time scale are the same for each animal

PRESSURE WAVES

In the ascending aorta (Figs. 9.1, 9.2) the systolic part of the pressure wave is broadened, and the peak value of pressure is reached after the peak of flow. The incisura indents the pressure wave and marks the end of ventricular systole. In diastole, a secondary pressure wave is seen, superimposed on a general decline in pressure before the next heart beat. Contour of the pressure wave is unchanged in the proximal descending aorta and in the proximal brachiocephalic and left subclavian arteries, but in more distal arteries successive changes are seen. As the pressure pulse is transmitted down the aorta (Fig. 9.2, 9.3) amplitude of the diastolic wave first decreases, so that in the mid descending thoracic aorta, pressure appears to fall exponentially during diastole. (This region was described by Hamilton and Dow (1939) as the 'node' of the aortic 'standing wave'). Below the mid-thoracic aorta, the diastolic wave reappears, and usually becomes very prominent, particularly in the most peripheral arteries. In these vessels, reappearance and increased prominence of the diastolic wave is accompanied by amplification of the systolic peak. In the femoral artery, pulse pressure may be 50

percent or more than in the ascending aorta. These changes in the systolic and diastolic parts of the wave are accompanied by progressive delay of the foot of the wave (a manifestation of finite wave velocity – p. 41) and disappearance of the incisura in more peripheral arteries. It is important to note that the incisura is represented by a short sharp inflection, which is best seen in the proximal aorta. This usually occurs close to the foot of the diastolic wave, but does not bear a constant relationship to it in different arteries (Fig. 9.3) or under different conditions, since the incisura is caused by cardiac relaxation and the diastolic wave by vascular wave reflection. Another point should be noted in illustrations of pressure wave reflection such as Figure 9.3 – that whereas the foot of the pressure wave is progressively delayed in more peripheral arteries, the peaks of both systolic and diastolic waves are not delayed to nearly the same extent, and may indeed as in Figure 9.3 appear to occur simultaneously. Such an appearance in dogs prompted Hamilton and Dow in 1939 to invoke the concept of aortic 'standing waves'.

As the aortic pressure wave is transmitted to arteries in the upper part of the body, similar changes are seen to those already noted in the lower part of the body (Meisner and Remington 1962, Remington and Wood 1956, O'Rourke 1970), with progressive delay in the foot of the wave, disappearance of the incisura, amplification of the systolic peak, and exaggeration of the diastolic wave. When pressure waves in the upper part of the body are compared to those in the lower part of the body (Figs. 9.3, 9.4), one notes that the diastolic fluctuations are reciprocally related – i.e. that the diastolic peak in upper body arteries corresponds with a dip in lower body arteries, and that the subsequent dip in upper bodly arteries corresponds to the peak of the diastolic wave in the lower part of the body. This point too was highlighted by Hamilton and Dow in their description of the aortic 'standing wave'.

These features of the arterial pressure wave have been known since accurate pressure waves were first recorded by Otto Frank in the nineteenth century. Frank (1899) referred to the 'Grundform' or basic shape of the arterial pressure wave, and the 'Grundschwingung' or reflected wave which was superimposed on this and which was responsible

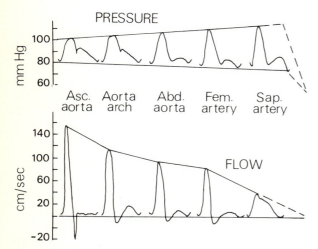

Fig. 9.2 Diagrammatic representation of change in pressure (above) and flow (below) patterns between the ascending aorta and peripheral arteries. The most distal pressure and flow patterns illustrated are those in the saphenous artery. Beyond this site, dotted lines indicate the steep fall in systolic pressure, diastolic pressure and pulse pressure, and further attenuation of pulsatile flow within the arterioles downstream. From McDonald (1960)

for amplification of the pressure wave and for the prominent diastolic wave in arteries at the extremities of the body (Frank 1905, 1930). In his monograph, Wiggers (1928) explained changes in pressure wave shape during transmission as resulting from:–

1. Damping or attenuation of the wave in travel,
2. Dispersion of the wave due to different frequency components travelling at different velocities,
3. Reduction or amplification of components of the pulse wave by reflected waves,
4. The occurrence of natural vibrations or resonance in various parts of the arterial tree, to which McDonald (1960) added
5. The progressive increase in stiffness of peripheral arteries.

The principal changes in contour of pressure waves between the heart and periphery are attributable to factors 3, 4, and 5, all of which are part

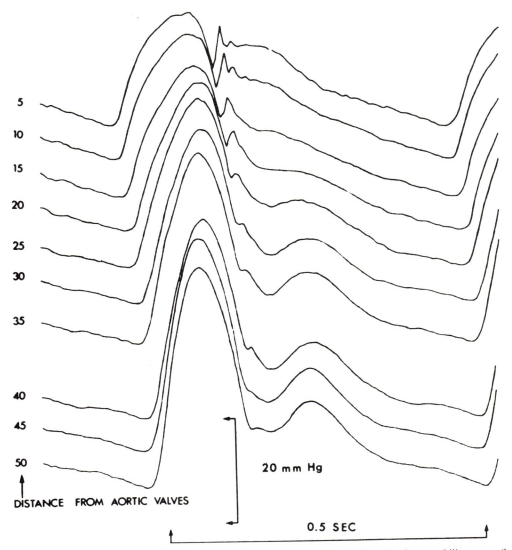

Fig. 9.3 Pressure waves recorded successively at 5 cm intervals between the aortic arch (above) and external iliac artery (below) in a 16.5 kg wombat, through a catheter inserted in the femoral artery. The wombat (*Wombatus hirsuitis*) is a native Australian marsupial, similar in size to a dog, but having a thick head, and short, stubby limbs. From O'Rourke (1967) (Fig. 6.7 compares harmonic components of these waves.

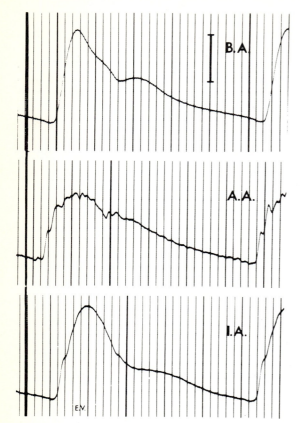

Fig. 9.4 Pressure waves recorded at short time intervals apart, and displayed as though recorded simultaneously, from the brachial artery (B.A, above), ascending aorta (A.A. centre) and iliac artery (I.A., below) of a normotensive human subject without evidence of arterial disease. Pressure calibration; 25 mmHg, Time lines 0.04 sec. From O'Rourke (1970) with permission American Heart Association Inc.

and parcel of wave reflection (Ch. 7). Damping of the pressure wave is relatively low, amounting in a vessel such as the carotid artery for a decrease in amplitude of the major components of the pressure wave (up to 8 Hz) of only about five percent over a 10 cm interval (Busse et al 1979) – and in the aorta to considerably less than this. The high frequency components of the pulse i.e. those above 25 Hz which make up the incisura are damped more heavily – by about 25 percent over a 10 cm length of the carotid artery. This damping is responsible for disappearance of the incisura along the length of the aorta, and for ultimate disappearance of diastolic fluctuations over a longer distance – sometimes the distance represented by

two or more round trips of the arterial tree (Fig. 7.13). Dispersion of the pressure wave accounts for a single discrete pulse becoming broadened as it travels – as does that in an elastic tube (Fig. 7.5). In the arterial tree such dispersion is very small indeed, and is a minor factor in modification of the arterial pulse (Anliker et al 1968, McDonald 1960, 1974).

It is generally agreed that wave reflection is the major factor responsible for change in shape of the pulse in systemic arteries. There is still some dispute as to where most reflection arises, and still no agreement as to how much reflection of the pulse occurs after its initial reflection (Ch. 7). The account given here is my own, but I am persuaded that it is correct because it adds to and fills in the gaps of classical theories, while providing explanations not only for arterial pressure wave transmission, but also for flow wave contour and for pressure/flow relationships expressed as vascular impedance in different arteries and under different conditions. There is no other single explanation that can account for all observed phenomena.

Frank (1905, 1930) believed that the arterial pulse was reflected between sites in the periphery of the body and the closed aortic valve. Hamilton (1944) stressed that peripheral reflecting sites represent the systemic arterioles whose effects summate to present a single functionally discrete reflecting site in the systemic circulation, so that the arterial pressure pulse bounces back and forth between this site and the closed aortic valves. Having recorded pressure pulses similar to those in Figure 9.3, he described his concept of aortic 'standing waves'. Literally speaking, this concept is erroneous as McDonald (1960) stressed, since for 'standing waves' to be generated – as they are in an organ pipe and in a violin string, there must be complete reflection and no attenuation of the wave in travel. This subject is discussed in Chapter 7. In any case other investigators have not been able to reproduce the precise findings of Hamilton and Dow (1939) in dogs or in other species (except the Australian wombat – Fig. 9.3) unless major peripheral arteries are occluded, and so peripheral reflection is exaggerated. It now appears that the dog preparation used by Hamilton and Dow had three major arteries – carotid, subclavian and femoral – occluded when pressure records were

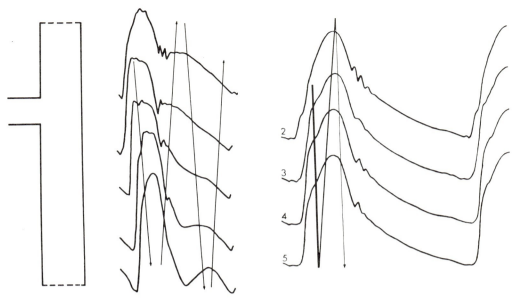

Fig. 9.5 The asymmetric T model of the systemic arterial system with pressure waves in a dog (left) and in a patient with arterial degeneration (right) recorded in the aortic arch (top) iliac artery (below), and intermediate points. A line is drawn parallel to the foot of the wave indicating reflection at arterial terminations in the lower and upper parts of the body. Wave contour in all arteries in both cases can be explained on the basis of reflection and re-reflection of the initial impulse generated by ventricular ejection. Differences between dog (left) and elderly human (right) are readily explained on the basis of more rapid wave velocity in the human's stiffened arteries. From O'Rourke (1971) The arterial pulse in health and disease American Heart Journal 82: 687–702

taken. Nonetheless I believe that McDonald's criticism was too strong – that Hamilton and Dow did not wish their concept to be taken literally and that the concept of 'standing waves' is as defensible as other terms – anemia, anoxia, agranulocytosis etc. which have common use in physiology and medicine, and which do not imply total lack of red cells, oxygen or white cells. It is true that pressure wave peaks do not occur simultaneously below the mid-thoracic aorta in most animals, and that the diastolic pressure fluctuations are not precisely 180° out of phase in upper and lower body arteries, but they are close enough to these figures for the concept of Hamilton and Dow to be regarded as useful in stressing reflection and re-reflection of the pulse as the mechanism for pressure wave peaking and diastolic pressure fluctuations in peripheral arteries. As discussed in Chapter 7, McDonald up to the time of his death would not concede that rereflection of the pulse was a practical physical possibility; he offered no other explanation for the diastolic wave in the time domain. I subscribe to the view of Hamilton and Dow that reflection and rereflection of the arterial

pulse is the major factor determining pulse wave contour.

Frank (1905, 1930), Hamilton and Dow (1939), Wetterer (1954), Wetterer et al (1977), Busse et al (1975) and others have considered that pressure waves are reflected between the multiple reflecting sites in the peripheral circulation and the closed aortic valve, with the resultant of peripheral reflecting sites behaving as though located in the pelvic area. There are two aspects of this explanation which do not fit comfortably. Firstly, Hamilton and Dow found the 'node' of the aortic 'standing wave' – taken to be the region where diastolic pressure fluctuations were minimal – was in the mid-descending thoracic aorta, much closer to the aortic valve than the apparent distal site in the pelvis. Secondly, Kapal et al (1951) and others (see Busse et al 1975) found that the period between the peaks of systolic and diastolic waves in peripheral arteries was greater than twice the transit time between the ascending aorta and pelvic vessels, suggesting that the effective resonating system was between the aortic valve and arterioles in the distal part of the leg.

An explanation for these findings has already been proposed (p. 90, Fig. 7.13) and is illustrated in Figure 9.5 that pressure waves are reflected back and forth, not between all peripheral reflecting sites and the closed aortic valve, but between the resultant of all reflecting sites in the lower part of the body and all reflecting sites in the upper part of the body (only one of which is the closed aortic valve). Such an explanation accounts for the relatively proximal position of the aortic node, and the relatively long resonating system as suggested by Kapal et al (1951) and Busse et al (1975), though this is taken to represent a distance from pelvic region in the lower body to the mid upper arm, rather than from distal leg to aortic valve. Such an explanation, while compatible with older theories, earlier findings of pressure wave transmission, and our observations on pressure wave contour in different arteries under different conditions, appears to provide the only possible explanation for the contour of arterial flow waves in vessels supplying the upper and lower parts of the body, as described below.

FLOW WAVES

Instruments for recording details of pulsatile flow were not available when Frank, Wiggers and Hamilton undertook their pioneering work, and introduced the concepts of arterial reflection and resonance. Such instruments were introduced in the late 1930s (electromagnetic flowmeter), 1940s (thermostromuhr) and 1950s (ultrasonic devices) – see Chapter 2. At the time (1960) that McDonald published the first edition of his monograph, there was still contention as to the pattern of flow waves in different arteries. Only more recently (Spencer and Denison 1963, O'Rourke 1967, Mills et al 1970, Wetterer et al 1977, O'Rourke and Avolio 1980, Murgo et al 1980) have attempts been made to reconcile patterns of flow waves with concepts of pressure wave reflection.

The main features of flow waves between the ascending aorta and lower body vessels are shown in Figure 9.2, and comprise a decrease in peak velocity, appearance of diastolic flow fluctuation (which is greatest in the mid descending thoracic aorta, and decreases thereafter in more peripheral

arteries (O'Rourke 1967)), and absence of backflow in the smallest distal arteries. The progressive decrease in amplitude of flow waves is readily explained on the basis of two factors – increased cross sectional area of the vascular bed (Schleier 1918, McDonald 1974, Ch. 1) – which causes decrease in velocity without altering wave contour –, and closer proximity to peripheral reflection sites – which decreases fluctuation around the value of mean flow. Peripheral reflecting sites act simultaneously as an antinode for pressure and as a node for flow (Ch. 7); thus peripheral wave reflection accounts for both the *increase* in pressure fluctuation around the mean value in peripheral arteries, and the *decrease* in flow fluctuation around its mean value in the same vessels. Diastolic fluctuations of flow, while least in the smallest peripheral arteries, are usually very prominent in the mid-descending aorta, as would be expected from the concept of aortic 'standing waves', since the 'node' of the 'standing' pressure wave should correspond with an antinode (point of maximal oscillation) of flow (Ch. 7). Thus, flow patterns in vessels to the lower part of the body are just what one would expect on the basis of Hamilton and Dow's theory, though, as with pressure, there are two hitches:– the antinode of flow is closer to the presumed upper reflecting site (closed aortic valve) than to the lower (region of the pelvis), and the period between systolic and diastolic peaks is greater than would be expected on the basis of wave travel to and fro between these sites.

The comprehensive explanation for these patterns of both pressure and flow appears to be given by consideration of flow wave contour in arteries supplying the upper part of the body (brachiocephalic and left subclavian vessels). In these, the flow pattern is quite different to that in the descending aorta which supplies the lower part of the body. In these arteries systolic forward flow is markedly abbreviated (Figs. 9.6–9.8), and indeed there is often backflow down into the descending aorta while the left ventricle is still contracting. When brachiocephalic backflow is pronounced (as in Fig. 9.6), there is often a second 'hump' which widens the peak of the descending thoracic flow peak. This is a most curious phenomenon. It means that during systole, blood flow down the descending thoracic aorta may be

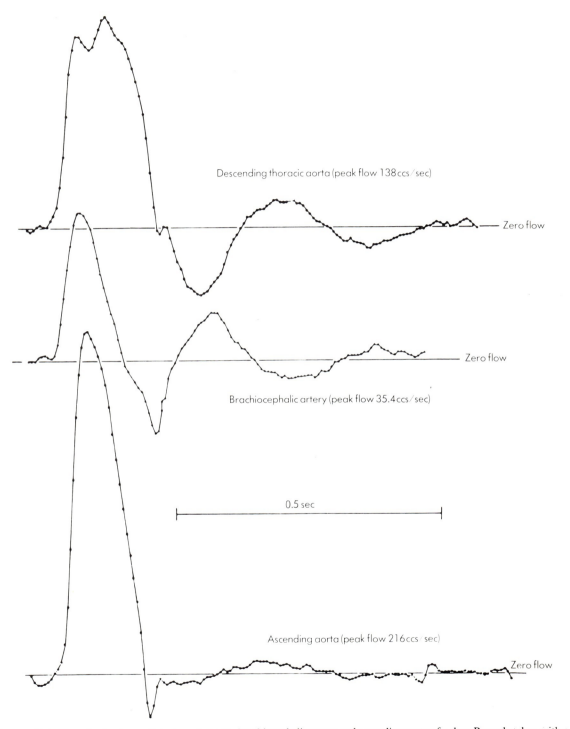

Descending thoracic aorta (peak flow 138 ccs/sec)

Zero flow

Zero flow

Brachiocephalic artery (peak flow 35.4 ccs/sec)

0.5 sec

Ascending aorta (peak flow 216 ccs/sec)

Zero flow

Fig. 9.6 Flow waves in the descending thoracic aorta, brachiocephalic artery and ascending aorta of a dog. Records taken with a single channel flowmeter at intervals of approximately 15 seconds. Waves drawn from the digital voltmeter output and displayed as though recorded simultaneously. From O'Rourke (1967)

coming not only from the heart, but also from backflow down the brachiocephalic and left subclavian arteries. The abbreviated systolic flow wave in upper body branches of the aortic arch is usually followed by a secondary systolic or very early diastolic wave which occurs simultaneously with backflow in the descending thoracic aorta. Thus, there appears to be a sloshing of blood to and fro between the upper and lower parts of the body, through the branches of the aortic arch, and commencing in the mid-late part of systole, and continuing through diastole. While such a finding may initially come as a surprise, on full consideration it just has to be so. If there is considerable backflow in the descending thoracic aorta close to the heart during diastole, this has to go somewhere. If the aortic valve is shut, and there is no flow in the ascending aorta during diastole, then there is only one place for this blood to go – up into the brachiocephalic and subclavian arteries; the diastolic flow waves in these will be greater than in the descending aorta, since the same volume of blood is channeled into vessels of smaller calibre.

It would be tempting to challenge or even discount upper body flow waves such as those displayed in Figures 9.6–9.8. Yet these constitute the normal flow patterns in the brachiocephalic and subclavian arteries, and have been recorded by ourselves in a variety of animals including dogs, sheep, wombats, kangaros, and rabbits (O'Rourke 1965, Avolio 1976, O'Rourke 1967), and by others in dogs (Cox and Pace 1975), and in humans (Kalmanson et al 1968, Gault et al 1966, Mills et al 1970, Wetterer et al 1977, O'Rourke and Avolio 1980).

These flow patterns can readily be explained on the basis of early return of wave reflection from the upper part of the body. Such a retrograde pressure wave would decelerate flow during systole. The late positive systolic or early diastolic flow wave is explained on the basis of later wave reflection from the lower part of the body. This type of flow wave pattern is precisely what one would predict in the simple asymmetric T model previously proposed to represent the systemic arterial tree. Its presence in different animals and in man lends further credence to the model.

This explanation for flow wave contour (O'Rourke and Avolio 1980) appears perfectly logical but it has not gained general acceptance. Kalmanson et al (1968) and Gault et al (1966) offered no explanation. Mills et al (1970) suggested that in some but not all humans, the secondary flow wave in the brachiocephalic artery is due to wave reflection returning from the lower body. They were unwilling to take this explanation further in giving an account of the systolic part of the wave, even though their impedance data gave clear evidence of a reflecting site in the upper body much closer than the reflecting site in the lower part of the body. Figure 9.8 shows flow

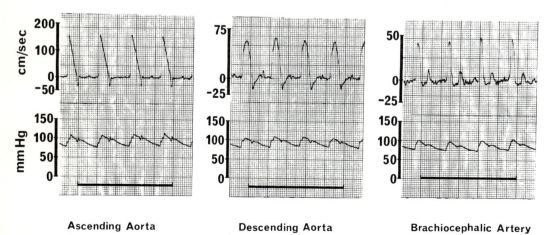

Ascending Aorta   **Descending Aorta**   **Brachiocephalic Artery**

Fig. 9.7 Flow (above) and pressure (below) in the ascending aorta, upper descending thoracic aorta and proximal brachiocephalic artery of a rabbit. Pressure waves are similar at all locations, but flow waves are quite dissimilar, indicating reciprocal flow fluctuations during late systole and early diastole in the latter two vessels. From Avolio et al (1976)

waves recorded by Mills et al (1970), together with (below) the suggested mechanism. Mills et al noted three different patterns of brachiocephalic flow which they designated type I, II and type III. (These different patterns of brachiocephalic flow correspond to three different patterns of ascending aortic pressure which Murgo et al (1980) independently designated as type A, B, and C; their mechanism is identical (p. 145, Fig. 9.9)). Mills et al found type I patterns most commonly in older patients, and type III most commonly in the younger. They found that type I and type II patterns changed into type III patterns during the Valsalva manouver when duration of systole was shortened and pulse wave velocity in the lower body decreased. The suggested explanation for these wave patterns (Fig. 9.8) is that they all result from early wave reflection from the upper part of the body (which decelerates flow) and later reflection from the lower body which accelerates flow, and that the difference in wave contour depends on the timing of these backward and forward waves in relation to aortic valve closure. In all, the backward wave returns during systole, though progressively later from type I to type III, while in types I and II, the

forward reflected wave returns from the lower body before or as the aortic valve is shutting whereas the type III pattern results from this wave returning after the aortic valve has shut. More common observation of type III patterns in younger subjects is attributable to lower wave velocity in the aorta, and so later return of lower body reflection. Change from type I or II to type III patterns during the Valsalva manouver is readily explained on the basis of the lower body reflected wave returning after the incisura because of shortening of systole, and decreased wave velocity in the lower part of the body resulting from low transmural aortic pressure. (O'Rourke and Avolio 1980). Change in shape of pressure waves during the Valsalva manouver (Kroeker and Wood 1967, Salans et al 1951, Greenfield et al 1967, Murgo et al 1981) is completely consistent with this explanation.

Avolio's (1976) model of the systemic arterial tree gives further support to this explanation (O'Rourke and Avolio 1980). The model was activated with a realistic ascending aortic flow wave, and flow patterns were determined at the origins of the brachiocephalic artery and descending thoracic aorta. The flow patterns (Fig. 9.10) were very

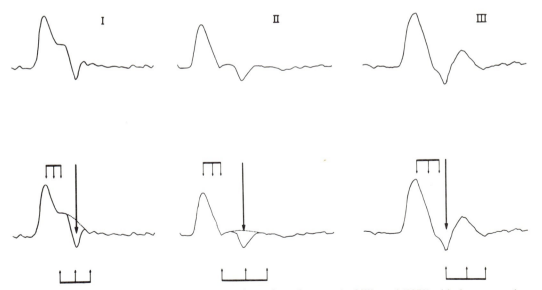

Fig. 9.8 Types I, II and III brachiocephalic flow waves redrawn from the paper by Mills et al (1970) with the suggested mechanism outlined below. The single arrow represents aortic valve closure and the triple arrow represents the timing of early wave reflection from the upper part of the body and later wave reflection from the lower part of the body. The dotted line indicates the expected wave pattern in the absence of an incisura caused by backflow through the aortic value. From O'Rourke and Avolio (1980) by permission American Heart Association Inc.

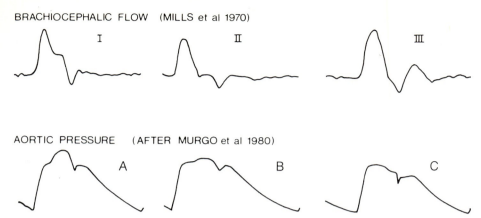

Fig. 9.9 Comparison of types I, II and III brachiocephalic flow waves as recorded by Mills et al (1970) with corresponding ascending aortic pressure waves recorded by Murgo et al (1980). Explanations are identical. The different flow and pressure patterns are attributable to differences in timing of wave reflection from the lower part of the body, with the reflected wave returning before aortic valve closure in type I, during valve closure in type II, and after valve closure in type III

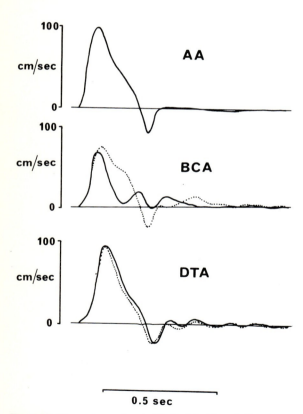

Fig. 9.10 Flow waves generated in the brachiocephalic artery (BCA) and descending thoracic aorta (DTA) of Avolio's model of the human systemic arterial tree, using the ascending aortic flow wave as input. Dotted lines indicate altered flow patterns when lengths of all arterial segments in the upper part of the body were doubled. (From O'Rourke and Avolio 1980) with permission American Heart Association Inc.

similar to those observed in patients, with, in the brachiocephalic artery, an abbreviated systolic wave and a second positive wave superimposed on the incisura. In this model (p. 125), the average distance to reflection sites in the upper body was 26.7 cm, and to reflecting sites in the lower body, 39.8 cm. When the upper body arteries were doubled in length (a manouver that could never be accomplished in life!) so that the average distance to upper body reflecting sites was 53.4 cms (Fig. 9.10) the brachiocephalic flow wave came to resemble that previously seen in the descending thoracic aorta, while the systolic flow pulse in this vessel was abbreviated. This can only be interpreted as indicating that the abbreviated systolic wave normally seen in the brachiocephalic artery results from close proximity to upper body reflecting sites. The effects of decreasing ejection period (Fig. 9.11) and of decreasing wave velocity (Fig. 9.12) were also simulated in the model. Both caused the original 'type II' brachiocephalic flow pulse in this vessel to change to 'type III', as predicted. These modelling studies are supported by those of Busse et al (1977) which showed that the typical human brachiocephalic and subclavian wave contour is dependent on the presence of a shorter sidebranch from the single tubular model of the arterial system.

These explanations of pulse wave contour are further supported by recent studies of Sipkema et al (1980) who have succeeded in characterising the

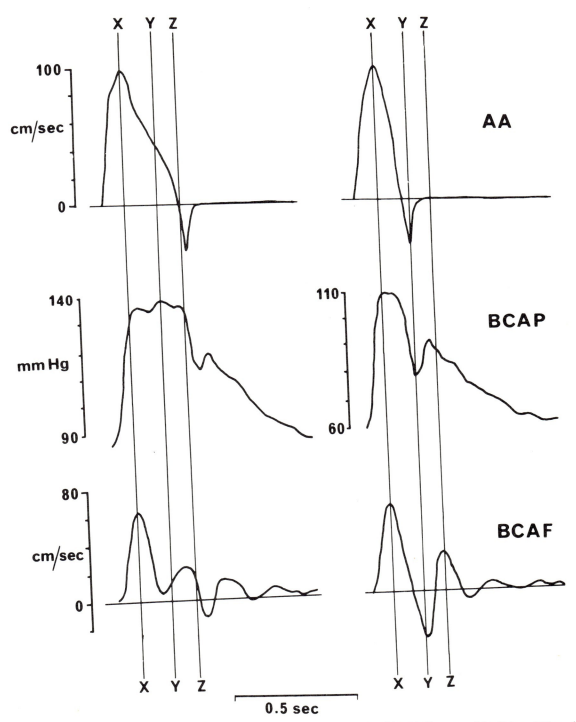

Fig. 9.11 Effects of change in ejection period on pressure and flow waves in the brachiocephalic artery of Avolio's multi-branched model of the human systemic arterial tree. Ascending aortic flow (A.A.) (top) was input and brachiocephalic pressure (BCAP) (Centre) and flow (BCAF) (bottom) were generated in the model. The line XX corresponds to the peak of ventricular ejection, the line YY corresponds to the calculated time for peak reflection from the upper part of the body, and the line ZZ to the calculated time for peak reflection from the lower part of the body. From O'Rourke and Avolio (1980) with permission American Heart Association Inc.

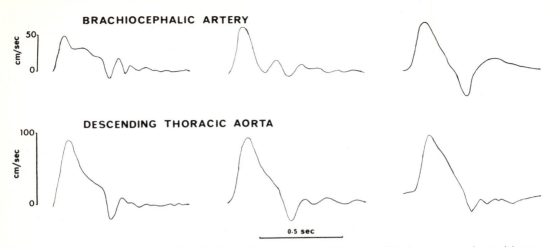

Fig. 9.12 Effects of alteration in arterial distensibility on flow waves in Avolio's model of the human systemic arterial tree. Brachiocephalic artery (above) and descending thoracic aortic (below) flow waves are shown under control conditions (centre), and with increase in pulse wave velocity by $\sqrt{2}$ (left) and decrease in wave velocity by $\sqrt{2}$ (right). From O'Rourke and Avolio (1980) with permission American Heart Association Inc.

arterial system in the time domain. After exciting the arterial system with a short, sharp impulse, there was clear evidence of early discrete reflection from the upper part of the body followed by later discrete reflection from the lower part.

PARTICULAR FEATURES OF PRESSURE AND FLOW CONTOUR IN HUMAN SYSTEMIC ARTERIES

The archetypal patterns of pressure and flow waves as described here have been taken from the dog, in which most experimental data have been obtained. It is clear however that pressure and flow waves in human arteries are often different to those recorded in dogs. Nonetheless these differences appear to have a simple explanation. Pressure (and probably flow) patterns in children and in many young adults are similar to those seen in dogs. In all adult humans, (Salans et al 1951, Greenfield et al 1967, Kroeker and Wood 1967, Mills et al 1970, Murgo et al 1981) pressure and flow patterns taken during the Valsalva manouver (in which aortic pulse wave velocity falls) are similar to those seen in dogs. With advancing years there is a gradual increase in pulse wave velocity, especially in the lower aorta and vessels to the lower limbs (O'Rourke et al 1968); wave velocity in upper limb vessels does not appear to alter to the

same degree (O'Rourke 1971). This increase in pulse wave velocity appears to be due to unsuspected and asymptomatic arterial degeneration (O'Rourke et al 1968). It is associated with alteration in pulse wave contour to that which has come to be regarded as the 'normal' pattern in adult man (Remington and Wood 1967, Freis et al 1966, Puls et al 1967, Luchsinger et al 1964, Murgo et al 1980), with pressure in the ascending aorta rising to a late systolic peak, then falling smoothly during diastole with little or no diastolic fluctuation, and with little amplification of the pressure wave between the proximal aorta and peripheral arteries, and little diastolic pressure (or flow – Mills et al 1970) fluctuation in these. In elderly humans, and in those with severe hypertension and/or arteriosclerosis the pressure and flow waves show little or no diastolic fluctuation at all (Goodman 1968 – personal communication, Farrar et al 1977) and little or no amplification of pressure between the proximal aorta and iliac artery (Fig. 9.5, O'Rourke et al 1968). This will be discussed again under aging and arterial degeneration in man (Ch. 12). Suffice is to say that the contour of pressure and flow waves in 'normal' humans, and derived impedance patterns differ from those seen in experimental animals in a way that can best be explained on the basis of increasing wave velocity as caused by progressive arterial stiffening with advancing years. Thus the type III brachiocephalic artery flow pattern is similar to that normally seen in dogs, sheep and rabbits, and the types I and II are similar to those seen in these animals when arterial pressure (and so, wave velocity) are abnormally elevated. The type I and II patterns as normally seen in man are attributable to earlier return of wave reflection from upper and lower (but particularly lower) body. Murgo et al (1980) have recently drawn attention to inflections and secondary systolic fluctuations in pressure waves recorded in the ascending aorta of 'normal' humans, and have (like Mills et al) but quite independently designated these as type A, type B and type C patterns (Fig. 9.9). These appear to correspond exactly to the brachiocephalic flow patterns described by Mills et al, and to have the same explanation. The type C aortic pressure pattern is similar to that normally seen in dogs, sheep, and rabbits under basal conditions while the type A and type B patterns are similar to those seen in these animals when arterial pressure and wave velocity are abnormally elevated. The type A and B aortic pressure patterns as described by Murgo et al are, like the corresponding flow patterns described by Mills et al, attributable to earlier return of wave reflection from lower body sites, consequent on increased pulse wave velocity caused by arterial degeneration.

With this one proviso – that pressure and flow wave patterns in 'normal' human adults appear to show evidence of arterial degeneration – human findings are explicable on the same basis as previously proposed for experimental animals.

PRESSURE WAVE TRANSMISSION TO FEMORAL AND TO BRACHIAL AND RADIAL ARTERIES IN MAN

Femoral artery

As mentioned on page 144, pressure wave transmission to the lower limb arteries in children is similar to that seen in dogs and other experimental animals, with some 50 percent or more amplification of pulse pressure between the ascending aorta and femoral artery. This is associated with appearance and exaggeration of diastolic waves in peripheral arteries; both phenomena are attributable to wave reflection. As in experimental animals,

both amplification of pulse pressure and amplitude of diastolic waves are markedly reduced when vasodilation is induced in the lower limbs (Hamilton 1944, Kroeker and Wood 1955, Busse et al 1977). Amplification of the femoral pulse falls progressively with advancing years (Fig. 9.13) as does amplitude of the diastolic wave; as discussed, this is associated with increased pulse wave velocity in the lower body arteries and is attributable to arterial degeneration. This will be discussed further in Ch. 12. Peak femoral artery pressure is sometimes related to left ventricular systolic pressure in assessment of pressure gradient across the aortic valve. It is clear that this must be done with caution because of the variable increase in systolic pressure between the ascending aorta and femoral artery in different patients, and at different ages.

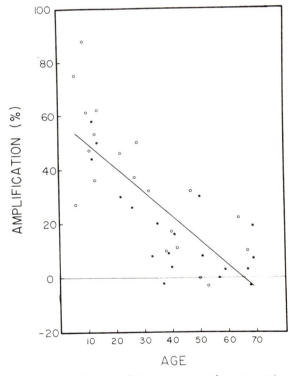

Fig. 9.13 Amplification of the pressure wave between aortic arch and iliac artery ((iliac artery pulse pressure – aortic arch pulse pressure) ÷ aortic arch pulse pressure) in human subjects, plotted against age. Open circles indicate patients without clinical evidence of any vascular lesion, and closed circles indicate patients with known vascular lesions (from O'Rourke et al 1968) with permission American Heart Association Inc.

Brachial and radial arteries

This subject is of major clinical importance since arterial pressure is conventionally recorded from the brachial artery; values of systolic and diastolic pressure obtained are usually taken to represent those to be found in the proximal aorta, and indeed throughout the arterial system. Differences in amplification of the pulse to the brachial artery under different conditions must be considered in interpretation of brachial artery blood pressure recordings.

Studies of pressure wave transmission to the brachial artery have been reported by Salans et al (1951), Remington and Wood (1956), Kroeker and Wood (1955, 1956), Rowell et al (1968) and O'Rourke (1970). Kroeker and Wood studied wave transmission in 'normal' man – the authors themselves and their colleagues – and found that amplification of the pressure pulse between the aortic arch and brachial artery under basal conditions averaged 31 percent (while amplification to the radial artery averaged 46 percent, and to the femoral artery averaged 39 percent). In a similar study, but on patients undergoing cardiac catheterisation, O'Rourke (1970) found average amplification of 18 percent to the brachial artery (while amplification to the iliac artery averaged 24 percent). O'Rourke found no consistent relationship between age and brachial amplification in contrast to the definite relationship previously shown (Fig. 9.13) between age and femoral amplification. Both Kroeker and Wood (1955, 1956) and O'Rourke (1970) found that brachial amplification was markedly dependent on the duration of ventricular systole, being decreased when systole was lengthened (as in aortic valve disease), and increased when systole was shortened (as by head-up tilt, prolonged expiration, and during the Valsalva manouver (Fig. 9.14). These changes were often quite marked, with amplification of pulse pressure to the radial artery increasing to almost 200 percent during the Valsalva manouver. During leg exercise, amplification of the brachial artery pulse is often increased (Rowell et al 1968) as systole shortens. This is attributable to change in ejection pattern and not to alteration in properties of arteries in the upper limb (O'Rourke 1970). As with amplification to the femoral artery, brachial amplification is dependent on wave reflection in the peripheral vascular bed and virtually disappears when vasodilation is induced in the upper limb (Rowell et al 1968).

Kroeker and Wood (1955, 1956) explained in-

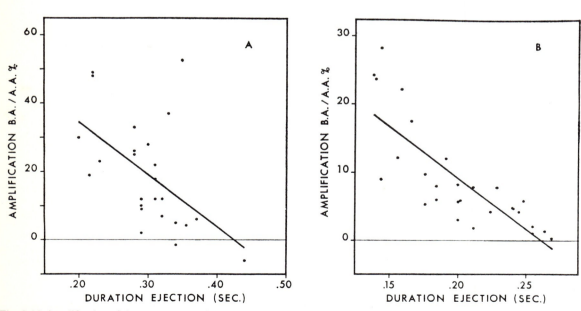

Fig. 9.14 Amplification of the pressure wave between aortic arch and brachial artery, plotted against ejection period, (A) in 25 patients studied at diagnostic cardiac catheterisation, and (B) for individual beats in a patient with atrial fibrillation (From O'Rourke, 1970)

creased amplification with decreased ejection period on the basis of resonance:– apparent exaggeration of wave reflection when the frequency of the driving function (ventricular ejection) corresponded to the resonant frequency of the arterial system in the upper limb (Ch. 7). Kroeker and Wood found maximal amplification of the pulse to the radial artery when duration of ejection was around 200 m sec. O'Rourke (1970) obtained similar results. He expressed amplification in terms of frequency by relating corresponding frequency components of simultaneously-recorded brachial and central aortic pressure pulses, and showed that peak amplification occurred at 4– 5 Hz, whereas peak amplification to the iliac artery, determined in similar fashion, occurred at a lower frequency – around 2–3.5 Hz. Differences in the frequency of peak amplification between the proximal aorta and brachial artery on the one hand, and between central aorta and iliac artery on the other are due to the different lengths of vascular segments, and explain the different degrees of amplification under different circumstances. This is discussed more fully in O'Rourke (1970).

Pressure pulse transmission to the brachial artery must be considered in interpreting directly recorded brachial artery pressure waves. It is clear that brachial artery tracings may give a falsely high measure of systolic pressure and falsely low measure of diastolic pressure in the ascending aorta and the rest of the arterial tree under conditions when duration of systole is shortened or resonant frequency of the whole arterial system or of specific vascular segments is decreased (as when blood pressure, and so, wave velocity, are decreased). When shortened systole and hypotension are combined, as in clinical shock (Fig. 9.15) these differences may be markedly altered. Strangely, such differences in arterial pressure are usually overlooked in descriptions of arterial pressure in clinical conditions, including shock, where criteria for different interventions are usually given on the basis of *the* systolic and *the* diastolic pressure as though these were the same in all arteries. When, under clinical conditions these differences may be large or crucial to management, pressure should be monitored in the proximal aorta.

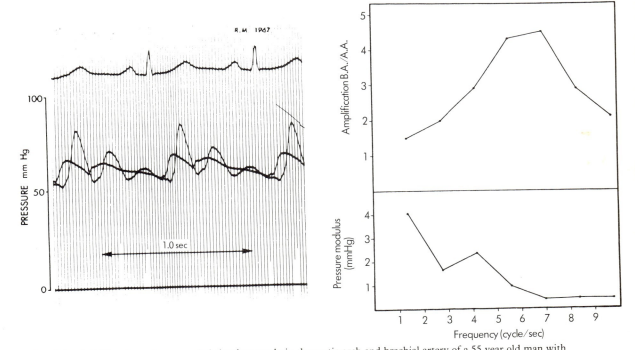

Fig. 9.15 *Left* Pressure waves recorded simultaneously in the aortic arch and brachial artery of a 55 year old man with hypotension and clinical features of peripheral vasoconstriction.
Right Ratio of corresponding harmonics of these brachial and aortic pressure waves (above), and modulus of the harmonics of the aortic pressure waves (below). From O'Rourke (1970)

No mention has been made of the relationship between direct and indirectly recorded brachial artery pressure. There is far more variation in this relationship under basal conditions (and more so under abnormal conditions) than most are aware of (Floras et al 1981). The Korotkov sounds do not accurately identify systolic and diastolic pressure – especially diastolic pressure. Variations are such that there is no internationally accepted standard for determining diastolic pressure, with some taking this to be cuff pressure at muffling of sound (phase 4) and some at disappearance of sound (phase 5). Our own results (Breit and O'Rourke 1974) support the latter. I would regard this uncomfortable but important topic as outside the scope of this book. The variable relationship between indirectly and directly recorded brachial artery pressure, and between directly recorded brachial artery pressure and aortic pressure underlines the importance of direct central aortic pressure monitoring under such conditions as cardiogenic shock, where cardiac function must be assessed accurately, and intra-aortic balloon pumping timed correctly.

RELATIONSHIP BETWEEN THE ARTERIAL PULSE AND BODY SIZE AND SHAPE

A detailed discussion of comparative physiology will be given in Chapter 11. It is relevant however to mention briefly at this stage the relationship between pulse contour and body size and shape. The explanation given for pressure and flow wave contour in dogs appears to be applicable throughout the animal kingdom. Since mean arterial pressure and pulse wave velocity are similar in different animals (not only mammals but in others including reptiles as well), and since wave reflection from peripheral arterioles is the major factor determining wave contour, one would expect that the length and shape of different animals would also be a major factor in determination of wave contour, with length determining 'natural frequency' and shape determining the degree of dispersion of reflecting sites and so the intensity of wave reflection. This appears to be the case. The

resonant frequency (measured from the period between peaks of systolic and diastolic waves in peripheral arteries) is higher in smaller than in larger animals. Additionally, the intensity of reflection appears to depend on body shape. Under basal conditions, phenomena attributable to wave reflection are more marked in the Australian wombat than in any other species studied, and least apparent in snakes (Figs. 6.7, 9.3, 11.1). The wombat is a native marsupial about the size of a dog, but having a relatively long body, thick head, and short, stubby limbs, (Fig. 9.16). In this animal there appears to be less dispersion of peripheral arterioles at both ends of the body than in any other. The exaggerated diastolic pressure and flow waves in this animal are similar to those recorded in dogs when both femoral, subclavian and carotid arteries are occluded. Chance findings of exaggerated reflection phenomena in this animal first suggested to Michael Taylor and myself a relationship

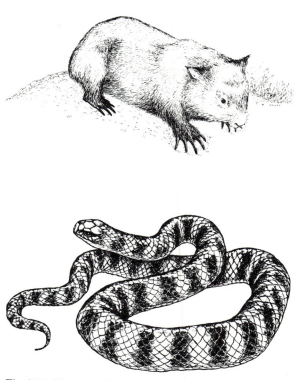

Fig. 9.16 The Australian wombat (Wombatus hirsuitis), a nocturnal burrowing marsupial. See also Fig. 11.4. Body shape of this animal is contrasted with that of a snake (Bottom). Courtesy of Geoffrey Molloy.

between arterial dispersion, body shape, and wave reflection. The snake represents the opposite extreme, with a long thin body and tapering ends, and with multiple arterial terminations widely spread over a great distance. In the snake (Avolio et al 1980), phenomena attributable to discrete wave reflection are completely absent, and arterial pressure waves show an exponential decline without secondary waves after even the shortest perturbation. Man and all other animals studied show pressure and flow patterns intermediate between those of the snake and wombat.

A SIMPLE MODEL OF THE ARTERIAL SYSTEM IN DIFFERENT SPECIES – THE CATHEDRAL

In man and all other animals, the heart is eccentrically placed, closer to arterial terminations in the upper than in the lower parts of the body. A possible benefit of this with respect to cardiac performance is discussed in the next chapter. This

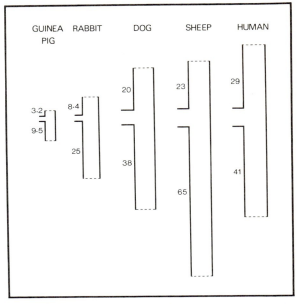

Fig. 9.17 Asymmetric T tube models of the systemic arterial tree in a variety of mammals and calculated from determination of impedance in the ascending aorta, brachiocephalic artery and descending thoracic aorta

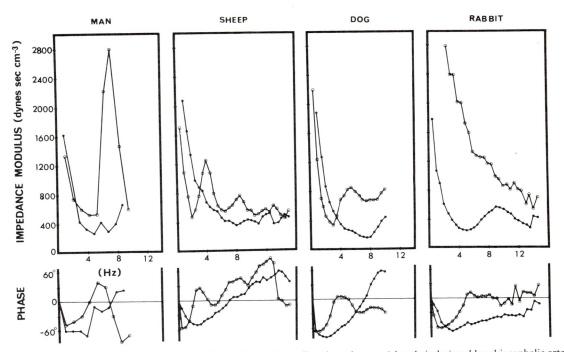

Fig. 9.18 Typical results for impedance determination in the descending thoracic aorta (closed circles) and brachiocephalic artery (open circles) of a man, sheep, dog, and rabbit. After Avolio (1976), with human values from Mills et al (1970)

arrangement results in the arterial system acting like an asymmetric T, with the short limb representing the average distance to reflecting sites in the upper part of the body, and the long limb, the average distance to reflecting sites in the lower part of the body. Figure 9.17 shows the asymmetric T models suggested for different mammals from values of impedance determined in the brachiocephalic artery, and ascending and descending aorta (Fig. 9.18). These models are similar, but with overall length being related to body size, and the relative lengths of the limbs of the T to the relative length of the trunk and lower limbs to the length of neck, head, and arms. (The inappropriately short length of the long limb in man is explicable on the basis of unsuspected arterial degeneration and wave velocity higher than presumed in the lower part of the body). These models explain not only impedance patterns (from which they were calculated), but also the main features of pressure and flow wave contour in different major systemic arteries. This model appears to have general application throughout the mammalian and perhaps the whole animal kingdom.

The term asymmetric T model was coined by McDonald in 1966 (see McDonald 1968). Possibly a more appropriate, and certainly more elegant model is a cathedral (Fig. 9.19) whose apse (behind the altar) represents the short limb of the T and whose nave (in front) represents the long limb of the T. Different cathedrals have different lengths (corresponding to different body lengths) and different relative lengths of apse to nave (corresponding to different relative lengths of upper to lower parts of the body). Ely cathedral (with apse almost as long as nave) provides a good representation of the human body, while Strasburg (with a very short apse) probably provides a good representation of the kangaroo (Fig. 9.19). Salisbury cathedral is a good general model for the dog, and Westminster Abbey for rabbit or sheep.

While the design of different cathedrals can be taken to represent relative differences in mammalian shape, the whole subject of pressure wave reflection in mammals is similar to that of sound reflection in cathedrals. Cathedrals have many nooks, crannies and pillars which partially disperse reflected sound waves, as do the many distributed reflecting sites in mammals, but most

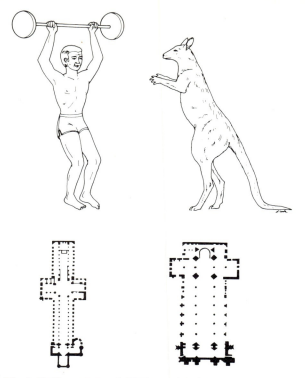

Fig. 9.19 The asymmetric T tube model of the systemic arterial system can be likened to a cathedral. That for man can be likened to Ely Cathedral whose floor plan is shown below, while Strasburg Cathedral (with relatively short apse, and whose floor plan is shown below) appears an appropriate representation for the kangaroo

sound reflection occurs between the front and rear wall at the end of apse and nave respectively. Even the timing and periodicity of resonance in cathedrals is similar to that in mammals. With apparent length of human or sheep arterial resonating system of – say 75 cms, and wave velocity of – say 7 metre sec^{-1}, the resonant frequency will be 700 ÷ 150 or 4.6 sec^{-1}. In a cathedral of length 300 feet, and with velocity of sound in air 1100 feet sec^{-1}, resonant frequency will be 1100 ÷ 600 or 1.9 sec^{-1}.

Other similes with the cathedral appear appropriate as well, such as how discrete or diffuse echos appear to be under different circumstances. The long organ chord in the cathedral with intermingled reflections and slow gradual decay represents the arterial pulse in the adult human, where ventricular ejection is so long in relation to wavelength that reflections are fused with the original wave and with each other so that none are separately identifiable (Fig. 9.5). The short, sharp shock of a bible dropped, with its successive echos represents the initial and subsequent discrete fluctuations in the pulse as observed when duration of ventricular ejection is short in relation to wavelength – as during the Valsalva manouver, prolonged expiration, or shock (Fig. 9.15). Even the position of the pulpit, from which the bishop speaks, at the junction of apse and nave corresponds to the site of activation – the heart – in the mammalian body.

In earlier days of learning, when theology was part of contemporary science, other comparisons between the animal body and God's temple might have been inferred. Lack of competence in the first discipline, infrequent visitation, and the added complexities of modern ecclesiastical loudspeaker systems prevent me at present from seeing (or hearing) any further.

REFERENCES

Avolio AP 1976 Hemodynamic studies and modelling of the mammalian arterial system. Ph D Thesis University of New South Wales, Sydney

Avolio AP, O'Rourke MF Mang K, Bason PT, Gow BS 1976 A comparative study of pulsatile arterial hemodynamics in rabbits and guinea pigs. American Journal of Physiology 230: 868–875

Avolio AP, O'Rourke MF, Webster M 1980 Pulsatile hemodynamics in the arterial system of the snake. Proceedings, 28th International Congress of Physiological Sciences Budapest p. 306

Bramwell JC, Hill AV 1922 Velocity of transmission of the pulse wave and elasticity of arteries. Lancet 1: 891–892

Breit SN, O'Rourke MF 1974 Comparison of direct and indirect arterial pressure measurements in hospitalised patients. Australian and New Zealand Journal of Medicine 4: 485–491

Busse R, Bauer RD, Schabert A, Summa Y, Wetterer E 1979 An improved method for the determination of the pulse transmission characteristics of arteries in vivo. Circulation Research 44: 630–636

Busse R, Bauer RD, Schabert A, Summa Y, Zinecker U, Wetterer E 1977 Principles of the genesis of pressure and flow pulse contours of the human carotid artery. Basic Research in Cardiology 72: 611–618

Busse R, Wetterer E, Bauer RD, Pasch Th, Summa Y 1975 The genesis of pulse contours of the distal leg arteries in man. Pflugers Archives 360: 63–79

Cox RH, Pace JB 1975 Pressure – flow relations in the vessels of the canine aortic arch. American Journal of Physiology 228: 1–10

Floras JS, Jones JV, Hassan MO, Osikowska B, Sever PS, Sleight P 1981 Cuff and ambulatory blood pressure in subjects with essential hypertension. Lancet 2: 107–109

Farrar DJ, Malindzak GS, Johnson G Jr. 1977 Large vessel impedance in peripheral atherosclerosis. Circulation 56 (Supplement 11): 171–178

Frank O 1899 Die Grundform des arteriellen Pulses. Erste Abhandlung. Mathematishe Analyse. Zeitschrift für Biologie 37: 483–526

Frank O 1905 Der Puls in den Arterien. Zeitschrift für Biologie 46: 441–553

Frank O 1930 Schätzung des Schlagvolumens des menschlichen Herzens auf Grund der Wellenund Windkesseltheorie. Zeitschrift für Biologie 90: 405–409

Freis ED, Heath WC, Luchsinger PC, Snell RE 1966 Changes in the carotid pulse which occur with age and hypertension. American Heart Journal 71: 757–765

Gault JH, Ross J Jr, Mason DT 1966 Patterns of brachial arterial flow in conscious human subjects with and without cardiac dysfunction. Circulation 34: 833–848

Greenfield JC, Cox RL, Hernandez RR, Thomas C, Schoonmaker FW 1967 Pressure-flow studies in man during the Valsalva manouver with observations on the mechanical properties of the ascending aorta. Circulation 35: 653–661

Hamilton WF 1944 The patterns of the arterial pressure pulse. American Journal of Physiology 141: 235–241

Hamilton WF and Dow P 1939 An experimental study of the standing waves in the pulse propogated through aorta. American Journal of Physiology 125: 48–59

Kalmanson D, Veyrat C, Chiche P 1968 Aspects morphologiques de l' onde de flux artérial enrigestrée par voie transcutanée chez le subject normal. Bulletins et Memoires de la Society Medicale des Hopitaux de Paris 119: 743–752

Kapal E, Martini F, Wetterer E 1951 Untersuchung über die Länge der stehenden Welle im arteriellen Systems des Menschen. Zeitschrift fur Biologie 104: 256–284

Kroeker EJ, Wood EH 1955 Comparison of simultaneously recorded central and peripheral arterial pressure pulses during rest, exercise and tilted position in man Circulation Research 3: 623–632

Kroeker EJ, Wood EH 1956 Beat-to-beat alterations in the relationship of simultaneously recorded central and peripheral arterial pressure pulses during Valsalva manouver and prolonged expiration in man Journal of Applied Physiology 8: 483–494

Luchsinger PC, Snell RE, Patel DJ, Fry DL 1964 Instantaneous pressure distribution along the human aorta. Circulation Research 15: 503–510

McDonald DA 1968 Hemodynamics. Annual Review of Physiology 30: 525–556

McDonald DA 1974 Blood flow in arteries. 2nd edition Arnold London

Meisner JE, Remington JW 1962 Pulse contour changes in carotid and foreleg arterial systems. American Journal of Physiology 202: 527–535

Mills CJ, Gabe IT 1972 Pulsatile blood velocity and pressure and the computer analysis of cardiovascular data. In: Snellen HA, Hemker HC, Hugenholtz PG, Van Bemmel JH (eds) Quantitation in Cardiology Leiden University Leiden

Mills CJ, Gabe IT, Gault JH, Mason DT, Ross J Jr,

Braunwald E, Shillingford JP 1970 Pressure-flow relationship and vascular impedance in man. Cardiovascular Research 4: 405–417

Murgo JP, Westerhof N, Giolma JP, Altobelli SA 1980 Aortic input impedance in normal man: relationship to pressure waveshapes. Circulation 62: 105–116

Murgo JP, Westerhof N, Giolma JP, Altobelli SA 1981 Manipulation of ascending aortic pressure and flow wave reflections with the Valsalva manouver: relationship to input impedance. Circulation 63: 122–132

O'Rourke MF 1967 Pressure and flow waves in systemic arteries and the anatomical design of the arterial system. Journal of Applied Physiology 23: 139–149

O'Rourke MF 1969 Effects of major artery occlusion on pressure wave transmission along the human aorta. Proceedings of the Australian Physiological and Pharmacological Society p. 24

O'Rourke MF 1970 Influence of ventricular ejection on the relationship between central aortic and brachial pressure pulse in man. Cardiovascular Research 4: 291–300

O'Rourke MF, Avolio AP 1980 Pulsatile flow and pressure in human systemic arteries; studies in man and in a multi-branched model of the systemic arterial tree. Circulation Research 44: 363–372

O'Rourke MF, Blazek JV, Morreels CL, Krovetz LJ 1968 Pressure wave transmission along the human aorta; changes with age and in arterial degenerative disease. Circulation Research 23: 567–579

Puls RJ, Heizer KW 1967 Pulse wave changes with aging. Journal of the American Geriatrics Society 15: 153–165

Remington JW 1963 The physiology of the aorta and major arteries. Handbook of Physiology, American Physiological Society Washington D.C. Volume 2 Circulation 2 p. 799–838

Remington JW, Wood EH 1956 Formation of peripheral pulse contour in man. Journal of Applied Physiology 9: 433–442

Rowell LB, Brengelmann GL, Blackmon JR, Bruce RA, Murray JA 1968 Disparities between aortic and peripheral pulse pressures induced by upright exercise and vasomotor changes in man. Circulation 37: 954–964

Salans AH, Katz LN, Graham GR, Gordon A, Elisberg EI, Gerber A 1951 A study of the central and peripheral arterial pressure pulse in man. Correlation with simultaneously recorded electrokymograms. Circulation 4: 510–521

Schleier J 1918 Der energieverbrauch in der Blutbahn Pflugers Archives Gesamte physiologie 173: 172–223

Sipkema P, Westerhof N, Randall OS 1980 The Arterial system characterised in the time domain. Cardiovascular Research 14: 270–279

Spencer MP, Denison AB 1963 Pulsatile blood flow in the vascular system. Handbook of Physiology American Physiological Society Washington D.C. Volume 2 Circulation 2 : 839–864

Taylor MG 1966 The input impedance of an assembly of randomly-branching elastic tubes. Biophysical Journal 6: 29–51

Watt TB, Burrus CS 1976 Arterial pressure contour analysis for estimating human vascular properties. Journal of Applied Physiology 40: 171–176

Wetterer E 1954 Flow and pressure in the arterial system, their hemodynamic relationship and the principles of their measurement. Minnesota Medicine 37: 77–86

Wetterer E, Bauer RD, Busse R 1977 Arterial dynamics. INSERM Euromech 92 Cardiovascular and Pulmonary Dynamics 71: 17–42

Wetterer E, Kenner TH 1968 Grundlagen der Dynamik des Arterienpulses. Springer Berlin

Wiggers CJ 1928 The pressure pulses in the cardiovascular system. Longmans London p. 65–90

10

Vascular impedance and cardiac function

In the ascending aorta, the left ventricular ejection (flow) wave is determined by the pattern of ventricular ejection, while the resulting pressure wave is determined both by this and by the properties of the vascular system, principally distensibility of the aorta, the tone of arterioles and the timing of reflections from different parts of the arterial tree, as described previously (Chs. 7, 8, 9). The relationship between pressure and flow in the ascending aorta is characterised by ascending aortic impedance; while vascular properties remain constant, this remains constant, so that there is a unique relationship between pressure and flow, and for any flow ejection pattern, the contour of the resulting pressure wave can be determined precisely. For this reason, ascending aortic impedance is quite properly regarded as an expression of left ventricular hydraulic load; for the same reason, impedance in the main pulmonary artery is a proper expression of right ventricular hydraulic load (Patel et al 1963, O'Rourke and Taylor 1967, Milnor 1975, 1979).

While ascending aortic and pulmonary artery impedance can be taken to characterise the hydraulic load presented to the respective ventricle, there are problems in applying these terms in studies of cardiac function, as well explained by Noble (1979). These problems include: 1. the fact that impedance is a complex quantity, having both modulus and phase, both of which vary with frequency, so that there is no possibility of expressing this as a single number, and so saying that this or that intervention increases or decreases impedance to ventricular ejection by this or that degree; 2. the fact that there is an inverse relationship between ventricular ejection (flow) and generated pressure so that the relationship between the two is determined by cardiac as well as vascular properties (Wilcken et al 1963, Weber et al 1974, Elzinga and Westerhof 1979); and 3. the fact that indices of cardiac function and efficiency – output, generated pressure, oxygen consumption etc can only be expressed in terms of time and not of frequency. The subject of hydraulic load in relation to cardiac performance – the interface between heart and vascular system – is a difficult conceptual and analytical matter. It is however extremely important, being fundamental to such problems as development of hypertrophy in hypertension, the mechanisms responsible for myocardial ischemia and cardiac failure, and modern therapies for these.

This subject is best addressed by considering arterial and vascular function – first ascending aortic and pulmonary artery impedance and the factors which determine these, then the relationship between impedance and the frequency components of the ventricular ejection wave, then the steady and pulsatile components of external heart work i.e. the energy generated by the heart which is lost in the circulation (p. 46). These subjects give insight into design and efficiency of arteries as these relate to cardiac performance. The main role of vascular impedance is to give information on vascular and particularly arterial function, and so, the contribution of these vascular and arterial properties to the amplitude and contour of pressure waves in the ascending aorta and main pulmonary artery. When it comes to specific consideration of ventricular afterload, ventricular output, performance and perfusion, this, — the generated pressure wave i.e. the time course of pressure in the aorta, pulmonary artery and respective ventricle — is the decisive factor.

ARTERIAL AND VASCULAR FUNCTION

Vascular impedance as hydraulic load

Vascular impedance in the ascending aorta describes the relationship between the steady and pulsatile components of the left ventricular ejection (flow) and resulting pressure wave, with the opposition to steady flow being represented by impedance at zero frequency and to pulsatile flow by the frequency-dependent terms. It is clear (Fig. 10.1) that the opposition to pulsatile flow is far less than the opposition to steady flow:– impedance modulus falls steeply from its value at zero frequency to a minimal value which is lower than, and occurs at a lower frequency than that in any other artery. This is most desirable – the opposition to the pulsatile components of flow from the heart (which are a consequence of a limitation in organic pump design i.e. that it must pump intermittently) is very small in relation to opposition to the steady component (which is necessary for body perfusion).

The magnitude of benefit, and underlying mechanisms, can be determined from the impedance curves. In dogs (O'Rourke and Taylor 1967, Noble et al 1967), man (Mills et al 1970, Nichols et al 1977, O'Rourke and Avolio 1980, Murgo et al 1980) and in a variety of experimental animals (Avolio et al 1976, Avolio 1976), impedance modulus above heart rate frequency averages some 5 percent of the peripheral resistance. This level – the characteristic impedance (p. 116) is determined by the distensibility of the aorta and proximal arteries. Thus, high distensibility of these vessels is an important factor in reducing characteristic impedance, and so the amplitude of pulsatile pressure that results from intermittent ventricular ejection. But there is another factor – wave reflection – that causes impedance modulus to fall even further, below characteristic impedance, over a band of frequencies which is determined by wave velocity and the distance to peripheral reflecting sites (p. 112). Over this frequency band in dogs, man, and various experimental animals, modulus may be only one half of the characteristic impedance, and so in the region of 2.5 percent of peripheral resistance. In addition, arterial distensibility and wave reflection have a further effect on impedance:– by causing a

phase delay between pressure and flow (the impedance phase angle), these factors reduce the component of pulsatile pressure that is in phase with pulsatile flow. This in-phase impedance or Z cosine φ (impedance modulus at a given frequency multiplied by cosine of impedance phase at the same frequency) is usually less than two percent of peripheral resistance over that frequency band (see below) which normally contains most of the energy of the left ventricular ejection wave (O'Rourke 1967, McDonald 1974, Fig. 10.1)

In using vascular impedance in ascending aorta or main pulmonary artery to describe ventricular load, we are apt to assume that ejection patterns are similar under different conditions and that

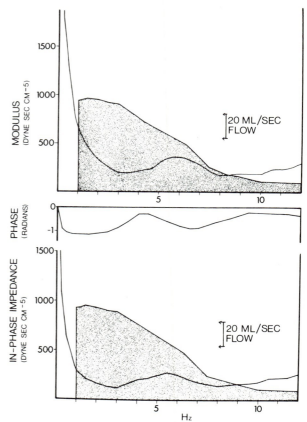

Fig. 10.1 *Top*: Relationship between impedance modulus in the ascending aorta of a dog and amplitude of harmonics of ventricular ejection (flow) waves (stippled area, as determined in an animal of similar size – see Fig. 10.3). Contrast with Fig. 13.11 *Bottom*: Relationship between in-phase impedance (Z cosine φ) in the ascending aorta of the same dog and amplitude of harmonics of ventricular ejection (flow) waves (stippled area) (From O'Rourke, 1981)

pressure varies only as does impedance under different conditions. This is not strictly true. In making this assumption we assume that the ventricle is a flow source and ejects the same volume of blood in the same way irrespective of the pressure generated. There is however no truly independent variable. Pressure and flow are dependent on each other according to the strength of ventricular contraction (Reichel and Baumann 1978, Elzinga and Westerhof 1979, Noble 1979); but they are also related to each according to vascular properties expressed as impedance. Ventricular factors in ventricular load are discussed on page 164.

Input impedance and ventricular ejection

The relationship between ascending aortic impedance and ventricular ejection (flow) wave is illustrated in Figures 10.1–10.3. Figure 10.2 shows an ascending aortic flow wave from a dog at heart

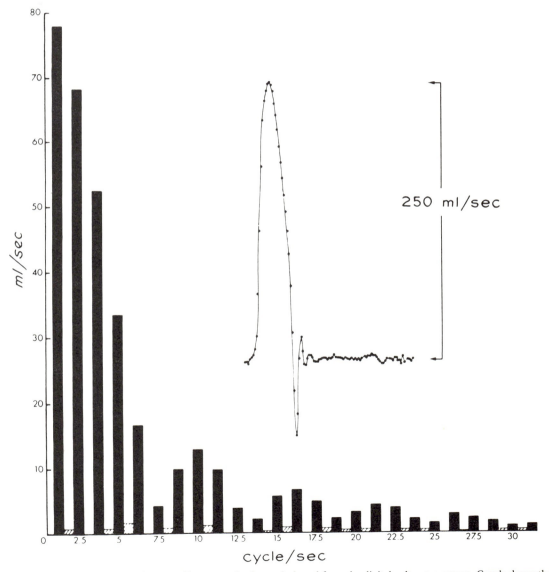

Fig. 10.2 A flow wave recorded in the ascending aorta of a dog and plotted from the digital voltmeter output. Graph shows the first 25 harmonics of this wave after correcting each for instrumental errors. Approximate noise level indicated by the diagonally striped bars. (From O'Rourke and Taylor, 1967) with permission American Heart Association Inc.

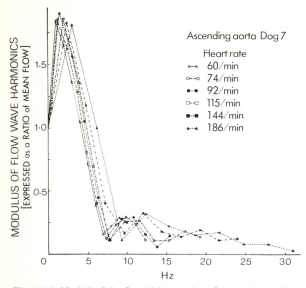

Fig. 10.3 Moduli of the first 10 harmonics of ascending aortic flow waves at heart rates between 60 and 186 minute⁻¹. Data obtained from a dog with surgically-induced heart block, and an electrically paced heart. Despite changes in heart rate, the highest harmonic flow content was contained in the frequency band 1–7 Hz. (From O'Rourke and Taylor, 1967) with permission American Heart Association Inc.

rate 1.25/sec, together with the moduli of its first 25 harmonic components. The amplitude of the first five harmonics (up to 7 hz) is far greater than the amplitude of the sixth and higher harmonics. Even with changes in heart rate (Fig. 10.3), moduli of flow harmonics remains concentrated in this frequency band. This is due to diastolic period becoming shorter in relation to systolic period as heart rate increases (Morris 1965, O'Rourke and Taylor 1967), so that energy of the flow wave shifts into the lower harmonics. Figure 10.1 relates energy of the flow wave within this frequency band to ascending aortic impedance and its in-phase component (Z cosine φ), determined in a dog of similar size. It is apparent that there is favourable matching between energy of the flow wave and ascending aortic impedance. Energy of the ventricular ejection (flow) wave is greatest over the frequency band at which impedance modulus is least. This shows how input impedance characteristics of the systemic circulation – determined by arterial distensibility, wave velocity and wave reflection in the vascular system-are favourably adapted to the pattern of left ventricular ejection. Relationship between aortic impedance and ven-

tricular ejection pattern is an expression of the interface between heart and vascular system, and illustrates arterial structure well adapted to its function of receiving blood in spurts from the heart.

The relationship between harmonic components of the left ventricular ejection wave and favourable aortic input impedance characteristics appears to be a general phenomenom in nature, with a few exceptions (Taylor 1967c, O'Rourke 1965, O'Rourke and Taylor 1967, Avolio et al 1976, Milnor 1979) and to explain the inverse relationship between heart rate and body length within the mammalian kingdom. This is discussed further in Chapter 11. As discussed later in this chapter, and in Chapters 12 and 13, apparent divergence of man from this favourable relationship is explicable on the basis of asymptomatic arterial degeneration.

The same considerations of pulsatile flow into the systemic circulation apply also to the pulmonary circulation. However since pulmonary vascular resistance is only about one sixth of systemic resistance, and pulmonary artery characteristic impedance, one half of ascending aortic impedance, the difference between resistive and frequency-dependent modulus terms is only about one third of that in the ascending aorta (Patel et al 1963, Bergel and Milnor 1965). Since lower wave velocity compensates for shorter length to arterial terminations, minima of impedance modulus in the main pulmonary artery occur at much the same frequency as in the ascending aorta, and the same relationship is seen between impedance modulus and frequency components of the right ventricular ejection (flow) wave (Morris 1965, Patel et al 1963, Bergel and Milnor 1965).

Figure 10.4 summarises the effects of various vascular abnormalities, and of peripheral vasodilation on ascending aortic impedance, and shows how all disturb the normally favourable relationship between input impedance characteristics and frequency components of the left ventricular ejection wave. These will be discussed again in Chapters 12 and 13. It will be seen that ill effects of hypertension (which shifts impedance curves to the right) coarctation of the aorta (which causes loss of the first impedance minimum) and arteriosclerosis (which increases characteristic impe-

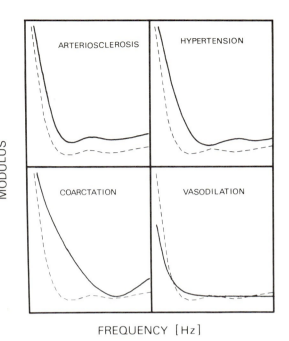

Fig. 10.4 Schematic diagram representing the effects of simulated disease and of vasodilation on impedance modulus in the ascending aorta. Dashed line indicates impedance modulus under control conditions. See text.

dance) can be explained on the basis of increased impedance modulus at low frequencies where moduli of the ventricular ejection wave are greatest. As a result of increase in impedance modulus, pressure pulsation generated by flow pulsation is greater, and for the same ventricular ejection wave, amplitude of the aortic pressure wave is increased. The effects of peripheral vasodilation are less apparent and more subtle. By decreasing peripheral reflection coefficient, this causes a lesser fall in modulus below characteristic impedance than under control conditions, together with reduction in impedance phase, so that the inphase component of impedance (Z cosine ϕ) is increased. A favourable effect of nitroprusside on ascending aortic impedance in man has been described (Pepine et al 1979), but this appears to be due to the fall in resistance and so, in mean pressure, with corresponding decrease in characteristic impedance. A reduction of characteristic impedance independent of pressure alteration would be desirable in vasodilator therapy; this however has not been convincingly demonstrated. This subject is discussed in Chapter 16.

Steady and pulsatile components of external heart work (see also p. 46)

Favourable characteristics of the arterial system in accepting pulsatile flow from the heart can be quantified in terms of steady and pulsatile components of external heart work. This is a useful concept with respect to arterial function because it separates energy losses in the vascular system into those associated with steady flow through the small resistance vessels, and those associated with pulsatile flow and lost mainly in the large arteries. The first component may be viewed as that which is physiologically useful because it is lost as blood is driven forward (*i.e.* is related to conduit function of the whole circulation), while the second simply represents energy wasted in vascular pulsations (*i.e.* is related to cushioning function of the arteries).

Total External Work = Steady External Work + Pulsatile External Work

External heart work was first calculated by Evans and Matsuoka (1915). Steady and pulsatile components of external heart work were first referred to by Bramwell and Hill (1922) and later by Remington and Hamilton (1947); both identified the pulsatile component to represent energy lost in arterial pulsations, and the steady component to represent energy lost in steady flow through the peripheral resistance. Bramwell and Hill referred to the pulsatile component in terms of the 'amount of unproductive work the heart is called on to perform' in relation to the 'efficiency' of the 'arterial mechanism'. Further studies of pulsatile and steady components of external left ventricular work have been reported by Porje (1967) and O'Rourke (1967), and of right ventricular work by Morris and O'Rourke (1965) and by Milnor et al (1966).

In discussing the components of external heart work, it is desirable to make two points, the first in relation to ventricular function, and the second to kinetic and potential energy as components of ventricular work.

The first point is that external ventricular work is the hydraulic work imparted to blood by the heart, and which is lost as blood flows through the systemic (for left ventricular work) and pulmonary (for right ventricular work) circulations. This work bears no constant relationship to total heart work or to myocardial oxygen needs; these are determined by the pressure the heart needs generate (Sarnoff et al 1958), and so the tension developed and sustained by the ventricular muscle during systole (Braunwald 1968, Weber and Janicki 1977). Since external ventricular work represents energy lost within the vascular system, it is more relevant to the circulation than to the heart. Since the steady component represents useful ventricular work while the pulsatile component is expended without purpose in pulsations, the ratio of pulsatile to total external ventricular work has been taken to represent an index of arterial efficiency in accepting pulsatile flow from the heart – the higher the efficiency, the lower the index, and *vice versa*.

The second specific technical point about external heart work relates to its potential and kinetic components. The magnitude of these depends on the technique of flow measurement (Evans 1918, Katz 1931, Remington and Hamilton 1947). A number of authors (Milnor et al 1966, Elkins et al 1974) have separated both pulsatile and steady components of external heart work into potential and kinetic components. This I believe is confusing, unnecessary and artificial:– confusing because one needs to describe four components of external heart work instead of two, unnecessary because the kinetic is included with the potential component if pressure is measured end-on to the direction of flow (see p. 46), and artificial because values obtained depend on the degree of arterial constriction. The latter point was discussed at length by Remington and Hamilton (1947) in relation to the work of Evans (1918) and Katz (1931). Taking the data of Milnor et al (1966), with the degree of constriction by the flow transducer (as stated) to be between 10 and 20 percent of lumen diameter (Bergel and Milnor 1965), the values of kinetic energy obtained would have been excessive by at least 50 percent, and at most 143 percent. It is I believe completely satisfactory to express ventricular work in terms only of steady and pulsatile components, including kinetic energy in determinations by measuring pressure end–on to the direction of flow.

Under basal conditions, the ratio of pulsatile to total external left ventricular work is around 10 percent (O'Rourke 1967), and of pulsatile to total external right ventricular work, around 25 percent (Milnor et al 1966). This ratio depends on heart rate, cardiac output and peripheral resistance. The ratio increases as heart rate decreases (Fig. 10.5) and tends to settle at a low constant value at very fast heart rates. This has been taken to indicate that the arterial system becomes very inefficient as heart rate slows, and that the optimal range of heart rates is set at its lower limit by arterial design. This is precisely what one would conclude from consideration of impedance curves. For other reasons (Taylor 1964), it is concluded that the upper limit of optimal heart rates is set by the heart itself.

With changes in mean pressure, the value of *pulsatile* external left ventricular work usually remains relatively constant, while, with cardiac output constant, *steady* external work increases or decreases in proportion to the change in mean pressure; thus the ratio of pulsatile to total work tends to fall with increasing pressure, and to rise when pressure decreases. With a fall in peripheral resistance, there is normally an increase in pulsatile external left ventricular work, and in the ratio of pulsatile to total external work; again this is as predicted from consideration of impedance curves and harmonic components of the left ventricular ejection wave.

The relatively high value of pulsatile to total right ventricular work is predictable from pulmonary artery impedance curves; the actual magnitude of pulsatile right ventricular work is less than that of pulsatile left ventricular work.

The ratio of pulsatile to total external left ventricular work appears to be higher in man than in experimental animals (O'Rourke 1967, Porjé 1967, Nichols et al 1977); as with impedance curves (p. 122) and pressure wave contour (p. 144) this is attributable to unsuspected arterial degeneration. As discussed in Chapters 12 and 13, the ratio of pulsatile to total external ventricular work is markedly increased in simulated arterial disease in experimental animals (O'Rourke 1967, O'Rourke and Cartmill 1971) and in patients with arterial disease (Porje 1967, Milnor et al 1969, Nichols et al 1977) indicating reduced arterial efficiency in accepting pulsatile flow from the heart. These ill effects of arterial disease are worsened, as predicted from consideration of impedance curves,

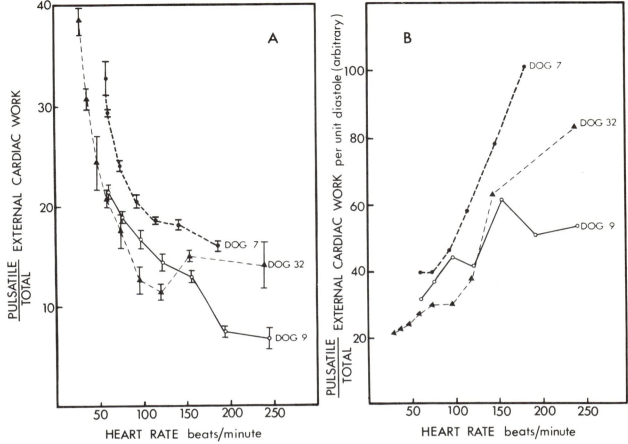

Fig. 10.5 The effects of heart rate on the ratio of pulsatile to total left ventricular work in three dogs with chronic surgically-induced heart block and whose hearts were paced electrically.
A. The ratio of pulsatile to total external left ventricular work plotted against heart rate.
B. The ratio of pulsatile to total external left ventricular work expressed as a function of diastolic time and plotted against heart rate (from O'Rourke, 1967)

during vasodilation or in extreme bradycardia. These matters are pursued and extended in chapters 12, 13 and 16.

Input impedance, arterial design, and arterial models

That the arterial system is well designed is obvious from the relationship of ascending aortic impedance curves to harmonic components of the left ventricular ejection wave (Figs. 10.1, 10.3). This is an expression of a favourable 'match' between the heart and vascular system, and it results under normal circumstances in the ventricle having to generate only 10 percent extra external work than

if its output were continuous. But what is adapted to what – arterial system to heart or heart to arterial system? There is no simple answer to this; each appears to be is adapted to the other. In chapter 11 the relationship between heart rate and body size, is discussed; data and arguments are presented which suggest that body length is an evolutionary determinant of optimal heart rate. The impedance curves illustrate quite clearly that the arterial system is well adapted to the demands of the heart.

Factors determining optimal arterial design and function have been discussed in detail by Taylor (1964, 1966ab, 1967, 1969ab). His ideas are summarised with the models shown in Figure

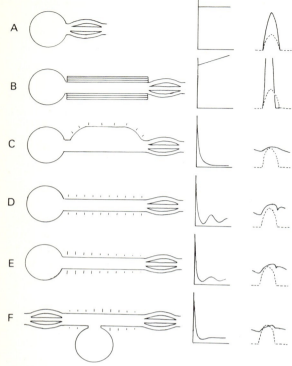

Fig. 10.6 Ascending aortic impedance presented by and pressure waves generated in the ascending aorta of different models of the systemic arterial tree, for the same ventricular ejection wave. At left, the model; in centre, modulus of ascending aortic impedance, at right the ventricular ejection (flow) wave (broken line) and resulting pressure wave (solid line)

A: The arterial system does not exist and the ventricle pumps directly into the peripheral resistance

B: The arterial system is represented by a rigid tube

C: The arterial system contains a large distensible reservoir

D: The arterial system is represented by a single distensible tube with homogenous elastic properties

E: The arterial system is a single tube whose proximal segment is very distensible but which becomes progressively stiffer towards the periphery

F: The arterial system is a tube as in case E but is connected to the heart approximately one third of the way along its length

10.6. In the first model (A) there is no arterial system and the heart is connected directly to the peripheral resistance. If this occurred (and of course it could never be), frequency-dependent components of impedance would be the same as peripheral resistance, and impedance phase would remain near zero at all frequencies. The magnitude of pressure generated by pulsatile flow would be more than twenty times that seen in life. The heart would be faced by an extremely high press-

ure against which to pump during systole, and the arteries would have to bear enormous stresses. In addition, pressure would fall to zero during diastole, and coronary perfusion could not occur. Clearly, for both anatomical and physiological reasons, this situation is impossible, but it is helpful to consider it if only to show how important the arterial system is in 'decoupling' the heart from the peripheral resistance.

The second model (B) is worse. Here, the heart is connected to the peripheral resistance by a rigid tube. With each stroke, the heart would have not only to pump blood through the resistive vessels, but also overcome the momentum of blood contained in the rigid tube. From its value at zero frequency impedance modulus would increase rather than decrease with frequency; phase would be positive because of inertial effects of blood in the tube. At the beginning of ventricular ejection, both aortic and ventricular pressure would be higher than the previous case.

The third model (C) is the *Windkessel*, which can very effectively decouple the heart from the peripheral resistance through damping of flow pulsations in the large elastic chamber. This is the simplest conceptual model to explain cushioning function of the arterial system. In the Windkessel model, impedance modulus falls steeply with frequency to a steady low value, and phase is near 90° at high frequencies. The practical problem with such a system is its anatomical size, and its adaptability under different physiological conditions. To be effective in damping pressure fluctuations, the *Windkessel* has to be large, and to have a very distensible wall. The changes in mean pressure which accompany bodily activity such as exercise would be associated with large shifts of blood into the *Windkessel*, and so away from the capillaries and veins, with the attending danger of less nutrient flow, and a fall in venous pressure and venous return to the heart.

The fourth model is an elastic tube which terminates at the peripheral resistance. This has many of the desirable features of the *Windkessel*, but the presence of a single peripheral reflecting site causes instability, with impedance modulus rising and falling to successive maxima and minima at frequencies determined by the wave velocity and length of the tube. This could be desirable if all energy of the ventricular ejection wave occurred at or near the frequency of the first minimum. However with a compound wave containing many harmonics, this cannot occur, and in any case changes in heart rate would alter the relationship between energy of the ventricular ejection wave and the impedance minimum. Perhaps one would think it desirable to have a very distensible elastic tube with wave velocity so low that the heart could only operate about the first impedance minimum. This however would have the same disadvantage as the Windkessel, and another to boot:– if ventricular flow velocity were to exceed pulse wave velocity, high pressure shock waves would be developed, as when an aeroplane crosses the 'sound barrier', and the system could behave paradoxically like the second model (p. 42).

The fifth model resembles the fourth, but with the elastic tube becoming progressively stiffer towards the periphery. This has several major advantages over the simple elastic tube. The low impedance modulus is preserved, since this is determined by the first part of the tube, but successive maxima of modulus are markedly reduced (Taylor 1964). In addition, since total compliance of the system is low, large shifts of blood are avoided from veins to arteries with changes in mean pressure. This model combines some of the advantages of the Windkessel (model C) with the only benefit of the rigid tube (model B).

The sixth model (F) is like the fifth, but the tube has more than one end joining to the peripheral resistance. In this model, the first impedance minimum (caused by the furthest reflecting site) is preserved but the later maximum and subsequent fluctuations of modulus are markedly attenuated. This model combines all the advantages of the other tubular models, with none of the disadvantages.

The systemic circulation behaves like the sixth model (F). Favourable impedance characteristics are maintained at rest and with different levels of activity. The heart reaps the benefit of low arterial distensibility, with few of the disadvantages, and the benefit of wave reflection without the problems. Favourable impedance characteristics result from graded distensibility of the aorta and arteries and from the site and dispersion of arterial terminations.

The sixth model (F) is not as good a representation of the pulmonary as of the systemic arterial tree. Peripheral reflecting sites here are dispersed in two discrete networks, but not with the same different spatial relationships as in the systemic circulation. Further, the pulmonary arterial tree does not show the elastic non uniformity which is evident in the systemic circulation. These points help explain why the pulmonary arterial tree does not display as favourable impedance characteristics to pulsatile flow as does the systemic. With regard to evolutionary pressures and survival advantage, this is probably not as important as in the systemic circulation, where a more complex system must be perfused at much higher pressure, and where there seems to be more opportunity for small aberations to impair cardiac performance and so slow down an animal when chasing prey or escaping from predators.

Ventricular afterload and input impedance

Ventricular afterload is a term used to describe the external factors which oppose ventricular ejection. There is dispute as to how this can be best characterised. Milnor (1975, 1979) has suggested that input impedance to the respective circulation is an appropriate term for ventricular afterload. There is a good argument to be made for this; input impedance is completely independent of cardiac properties, and it does determine what pressure is generated by any given ventricular ejection. But there are difficulties (Noble 1979, Pouleur et al 1979 Piene and Sund 1979, Ischide et al 1980) and the concept has not gained popula appeal. Impedance is a complex quantity comprising modulus and phase, both of which vary with frequency so that one cannot say that with different interventions, impedance has increased or decreased without qualifying the answer by specifying at what frequency and with what phase. Additionally, impedance has the units of pressure ÷ flow, while the term afterload, as applied to isolated papillary muscle preparations has the units of force or pressure.

The concept of impedance as ventricular afterload might be more useful if it were possible to describe cardiac function in frequency dependent terms. This has been attempted (Abel 1971,

Elzinga and Westerhof 1973, 1974, Westerhof and Elzinga 1978, Reichel and Baumann 1978) with the heart considered as a flow or pressure generator in series with its own source impedance. This concept has not proved useful, and there has been debate conceptually as to whether the heart is a flow or pressure source (the normal heart at physiological pressures appears to behave as a flow source while the failing heart behaves like a pressure source – Reichel and Baumann 1978), and to what degree the generator and source impedance are altered by changes in myocardial contractility.

Ventricular afterload is usually taken to be a function of pressure generated by the ventricle, and against which it must eject. Obviously, ventricular pressure acts in a complicated way (as determined by myocardial elasticity, dimensions, and ejection pattern) to determine the stress applied to individual myocardial fibres (Noble 1979). There is considerable controversy as to how afterload can be best expressed, and many ostensibly established concepts of afterload are presently under challenge (Abbott and Gordon 1975, Paulus et al 1976, 1979, Brutsaert and Paulus 1977, Elzinga and Westerhof 1979, Noble 1979). Suffice is to say here that arterial and vascular properties (through input impedance characteristics) are one important factor in determining the magnitude and time course of ventricular pressure, the other factor being ventricular ejection itself. Afterload reduction as a therapeutic manouver is always induced by alteration of impedance; one could of course reduce afterload by decreasing stroke volume, but to no useful purpose. Even though impedance may not be a useful expression of ventricular afterload, it is one important determinant of afterload, and the only determinant whose manipulation is therapeutically useful. This is discussed further in Chapter 16.

Input impedance as a determinant of aortic and left ventricular pressure

Input impedance of the systemic circulation determines the contour of the pressure wave generated in the ascending aorta throughout the cardiac cycle, and the pressure generated in the left ventricle as well, when the aortic valve is open. During ventricular ejection, ventricular and aortic pressures

are virtually identical (Fig. 10.7), the slight difference in early systole being attributable to the pressure gradient required to move blood into the aorta (p. 14), and the Venturi effect at peak aortic flow (p. 45).

The influence of ascending aortic impedance on ascending aortic pulse contour has been discussed (Ch. 9), but since this subject is so important in relation to ventricular performance, some additional points are warranted, especially in relation to the timing of wave reflection from peripheral sites. One beneficial effect of wave reflection has already been described – a lowering of impedance modulus below characteristic impedance at those frequencies which normally contain most of the energy of the ventricular ejection wave. This results in a decreased fluctuation of pulsatile aortic pressure, and so that aortic and ventricular pressure are less during systole than in the absence of reflection. Another favourable effect is apparent on inspection of aortic pulse contour – the major reflected wave from the lower part of the body returns after the aortic valve has shut, and so augments pressure during the early part of diastole. So close is the correspondence between foot of the diastolic wave (caused by peripheral reflection) and incisura (caused by aortic valve closure) in experimental animals (Figs. 9.2, 9.3), that the two are often regarded as synonomous. This timing of the diastolic wave is highly desirable. By returning after the aortic valve has shut it adds to diastolic pressure and so augments coronary perfusion pressure. But this favourable timing is critically dependent on wave velocity; if this were to increase, the reflected wave from the lower body would return earlier, and have an adverse effect by increasing ventricular systolic pressure, and so increasing ventricular afterload, and possibly causing premature ventricular relaxation (Brutsaert et al 1978, Housmans et al 1980).

In discussing aortic impedance curves it was noted that the apparent match between impedance minima and harmonic components of the ventricular ejection waves is not as favourable in man as in experimental animals – that the impedance minima in man occur at higher frequencies than one would consider desirable. This is associated (Murgo et al 1980) with ascending aortic pulse wave velocity that is higher than in dogs (6.2 compared with 4.0 M sec^{-1} (Nichols and McDonald 1972)) and with ascending aortic pressure wave contour that is different to that seen in experimental animals. These findings suggest the presence of asymptomatic arterial degeneration.

In children, the ascending aortic pressure wave resembles that seen in experimental animals, with a prominent diastolic wave following the incisura, while, with advancing years, (Fig. 9.5), the reflected wave appears to return earlier and to merge with the systolic component, so that amplitude of the systolic part of the wave increases while the diastolic wave is lost (O'Rourke et al 1968). These changes in pressure contour are associated with increased wave velocity in the aorta and have been attributed to arterial degeneration. The careful and elegant studies of Murgo et al (1980) with

catheter flowmeter/manometer systems have taken this subject one step further. Murgo and colleagues have been able to identify the foot of the lower body reflected wave in the ascending aortic pressure traces. In 18 relatively young human adults (mean age 34 years), apparently free from cardiac and arterial disease, this always preceded aortic valve closure, and indeed was sometimes apparent in the early part of systole so that there was substantial augmentation of pressure in the mid-latter part of systole. Clearly this would be undesirable for the heart, since it increases ventricular load while decreasing coronary perfusion pressure. The frequency of this finding, its interpretation, and its significance in relation to ventricular function appear to have been overlooked in the past.

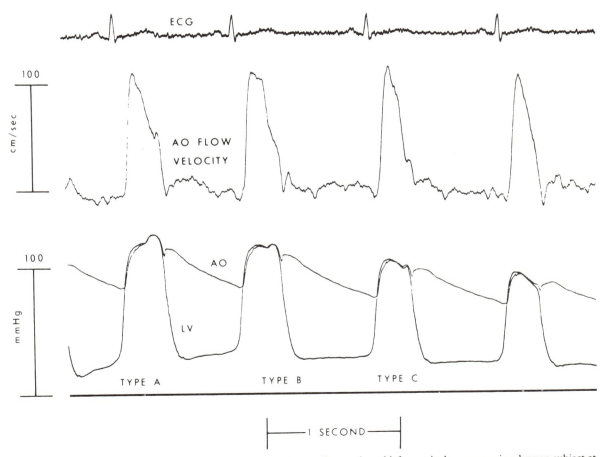

Fig. 10.7 Ascending aortic flow velocity (above) together with ascending aortic and left ventricular pressure in a human subject at the beginning of a Valsalva manouver. Data of Murgo in Westerhof et al (1979)

VENTRICULAR FUNCTION

In a book on arteries it would be inappropriate to delve into the huge and complicated area of myocardial muscle mechanics, especially at the present time when established concepts of cardiac function derived from studies of conventionally-loaded isolated papillary muscle preparations are under fire (Abbott and Gordon 1975, Paulus et al 1977, 1979, Brutsaert and Paulus 1977, Noble 1979). Happily, the most recent concepts of ventricular function (Elzinga and Westerhof 1978, 1979, Noble 1979, Sagawa 1978, Suga et al 1980) relate ventricular pressure directly to ventricular output and oxygen demand, and simplify consideration of interaction between the heart and arterial and vascular system. In using arterial and ventricular pressure in relation to cardiac function, one must consider how this loads myocardial fibres and one must assume that ventricular dimensions and other loading factors remain constant.

Ventricular pressure as a determinant of ventricular output

Studies of isolated papillary muscle (Braunwald 1969) have shown a reciprocal relationship be-

tween shortening and afterload. Likewise, studies of ventricular function have shown a similar relationship between pressure generated and volume of blood ejected. There has been a difference of opinion as to what pressure should most appropriately be related to cardiac output – mean aortic pressure (Elzinga and Westerhof 1973), mean systolic ventricular pressure (Buoncristiani et al 1973), peak ventricular pressure (Weber et al 1974), or mean pressure over the whole cardiac cycle (Elzinga and Westerhof 1978, 1979). Surprisingly, the closest relationship appears to be with mean ventricular pressure over the whole cycle. Using an isolated cat heart preparation, Elzinga and Westerhof (1978) graphed the relationship between mean systolic pressure and ventricular outflow at different values of end-diastolic volume and at different myocardial inotropic states (Fig. 10.8). At any level of end diastolic pressure, and for any inotropic state there was a regular and consistent relationship between mean left ventricular pressure and cardiac output, with output rising as ventricular pressure fell. At different end-diastolic pressures, but with the same inotropic state, the curves were virtually parallel; at the same end diastolic pressure, but with different inotropic states, the curves were regular and reproducible. Simple calibration factors enabled all

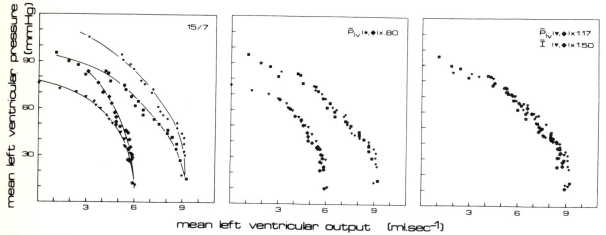

Fig. 10.8 Relationship between mean left ventricular pressure (ordinate), and mean left ventricular output (abscissa) in an isolated heart preparation at two given levels of inotropic state and two levels of left ventricular end-diastolic pressure. Raw data are displayed in left panel. In the centre panel data at the two different inotropic states were superimposable by multiplying values at the enhanced inotropic state by the one factor (0.80). In the right panel, all values in the centre panel were superimposeable by multiplying values at the lower end diastolic pressure by one factor (1.17) for pressure, and another (1.50) for output. From Elzinga and Westerhof (1978) with permission American Heart Association Inc.

curves at different end-diastolic pressures, and different inotropic states to be superimposed. Change in inotropic state could be expressed in terms of a single calibration factor. These graphs (designated pump function graphs) were shown to be similar to those seen in mechanical roller pumps with changes in slope and offset explicable in similar terms.

These concepts are new and challenging, but have yet to be confirmed in intact animals. It is refreshing however to see an apparently simple and comprehensive solution emerge for an old and important problem. With respect to vascular properties, the important point is that through their contribution to aortic impedance, and hence to the aortic pressure wave, arteriolar resistance, arterial distensibility, and the timing of wave reflection are important determinants of ventricular ejection.

The relationship between ventricular pressure and ventricular ejection has been studied in a different but complementary fashion by Suga, Sagawa and colleagues at Johns Hopkins (Sagawa 1978, 1980, Suga et al 1979, 1980). These have shown that the classical Frank-Starling curves can be used not only to describe pressure/volume relationships at end-diastole, but at end-systole as well. At any end-diastole volume, pressure rises as the heart contracts, and would reach the appropriate point on the curve at that volume if ejection were not to occur. However, since the aortic valve does open, blood is ejected and ventricular volume falls; as volume falls, pressure rises at a slower rate, and ejection ceases at a point which represents the pressure that would be generated for an isovolumic ventricular contraction at this volume. In other words, ejection ceases when pressure has risen to reach the Frank-Starling curve (Fig. 10.9). The capacity of Frank-Starling curves to characterise ventricular end-systolic properties and so, ventricular ejection under different conditions is now generally accepted, although there is some argument about what constitutes end-systole and what constitutes end-ejection (Iizuka 1979).

The effect of wave reflection on ventricular ejection can be gauged from the ventricular function curve (Fig. 10.9). With late systolic pressure augmentation, pressure would rise more rapidly and reach the Frank-Starling curve at a higher end-systolic volume. At this point, ejection would

cease and the ventricle would have ejected a lower stroke volume. No specific studies on the adverse effect of wave reflection on ventricular ejection have yet been performed, but there is no reason to believe that these would be different to other in-

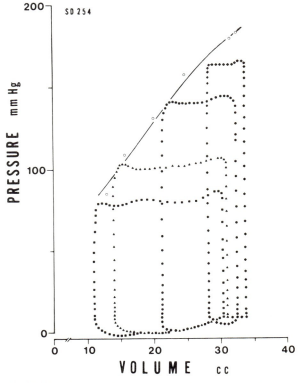

Fig. 10.9 Relationship between ventricular pressure and ventricular volume in an isolated heart preparation. For a given end diastolic volume, volume ejected at different diastolic pressures is determined by the Frank-Starling curve, ejection ceasing when pressure reaches isovolumic pressure normally generated at that given volume (From Weber et al, 1974)

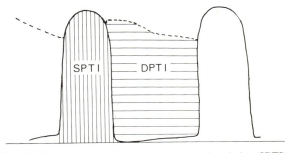

Fig. 10.10 Left ventricular systolic pressure-time index (SPTI) and diastolic pressure-time index (DPTI). 'Endocardial viability ratio' is SPTI ÷ DPTI

terventions, all of which decrease ventricular ejection when late systolic pressure is elevated (Wilcken et al 1964, Reichel and Baumann 1978). Indeed, new concepts of ventricular relaxation suggest an even greater effect of late systolic loading through premature ventricular relaxation (Brutsart et al 1978, Le Carpentier et al 1979, Goethals et al 1980, Housmans et al 1980).

Ventricular pressure as a determinant of ventricular energy utilisation

Sarnoff et al (1958) confirmed that oxygen demands of the heart are determined by the pressure it needs develop, and not at all by the blood it needs eject. This has been repeatedly confirmed (Katz and Feinberg 1958, Katz 1963, Weber and Janicki 1977). Sarnoff and colleagues showed that at the same end-diastolic volume, energy utilisation and oxygen demand were linearly related to the integral of ventricular systolic pressure. They termed this the tension-time index. This corresponds exactly (when diastolic pressure is negligible) to the mean left ventricular pressure used by

Elzinga and Westerhof (1978, 1979) as the determinant of ventricular ejection. Thus the same index is directly related to myocardial oxygen requirement, and inversely to cardiac output. The same vascular factors which are relevant to cardiac output are thus equally relevant to myocardial blood need.

'Subendocardial viability ratio'

Since myocardial blood need is related to pressure maintained during systole, and blood supply to pressure maintained during diastole, Buckberg et al (1972ab) proposed that the ratio of diastolic pressure time index (DPTI) to systolic pressure time index (SPTI) (Fig. 10.10) be used as an expression of myocardial perfusion adequacy. Although Buckberg recognised that this index should express SPTI as pressure under the systolic part of the ventricular pressure curve, and DPTI as the difference between aortic pressure and ventricular pressure when the aortic valve is closed, he showed that little error is introduced by measuring SPTI from aortic pressure (so ignoring

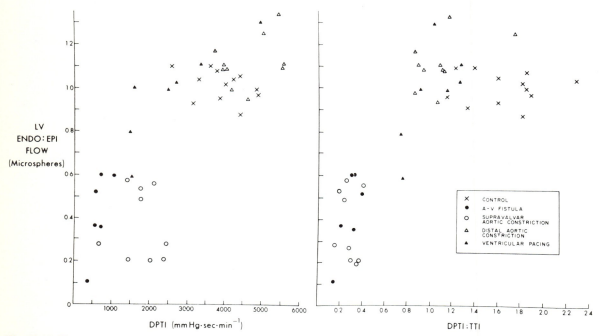

Fig. 10.11 Flow ratio per gram of left ventricular subendocardium to subepicardium, as measured by microspheres, and plotted against DPTI (left) and against the ratio of DPTI to SPTI (From Buckberg et al, 1972) with permission American Heart Association Inc.

isovolumic ventricular pressure rise) and DPTI as aortic diastolic pressure minus left or right atrial pressure, whichever is higher. Using radioactive microspheres, Buckberg et al showed that the ratio of DPTI/SPTI is an important determinant of subendocardial blood flow, this being reduced, often markedly, below blood flow to the outer part of the myocardium when the ratio falls below 0.7 (Fig. 10.11). They showed that this ratio is substantially reduced under different conditions including aortic valve disease, hypotension, tachycardia, and cardiac failure, and that accompanying reduction in blood flow could explain subendocardial ischemia and necrosis under a variety of conditions, even in the absence of coronary artery disease (Buckberg et al 1972 a,b).

Phillips et al (1975) took this concept one step further by developing an analog computer which could calculate the ratio of DPTI/SPTI from arterial and left atrial pressure records by identifying the incisura, integrating pressure during systole and diastole, and subtracting left atrial from diastolic pressure. This analog computer is now commercially available. Phillips et al introduced another assumption by proposing that the ratio of DPTI/SPTI could be measured accurately from pressure recorded in a peripheral artery. Since the ascending aortic pressure wave is amplified, often greatly, in transmission to the brachial artery (especially in the presence of shock (Fig. 9.15)) and since the incisura is lost and substituted by the foot of the diastolic reflected wave in peripheral arteries (p. 135), this presumption is likely to be invalid. In order to determine this index with any accuracy, one must measure pressure close to the aortic valve.

REFERENCES

Abbott BC, Gordon DC 1975 A commentary on muscle mechanics. Circulation Research 36: 1–7

Abel FL 1971 Fourier analysis of left ventricular performance. Circulation Resarch 28: 119–135

Avolio AP 1976 Hemodynamic studies and modelling of the mammalian arterial system. Ph D Thesis University of New South Wales Sydney

Avolio AP, O'Rourke MF, Mang K, Bason PT, Gow BS 1976 A comparative study of pulsatile arterial hemodynamics in rabbits and guinea pigs. American Journal of Physiology 230: 868–875

Bergel DH, Milnor WR 1965 Pulmonary vascular impedance in the dog. Circulation Research 16: 401–415

Bramwell JC, Hill AV 1922 Velocity of transmission of the pulse wave and elasticity of arteries. Lancet 1: 891–892

Braunwald E 1969 The determinants of myocardial oxygen consumption. Physiologist 12: 65–93

Braunwald E, Ross J Jr. 1979 Control of cardiac performance. In: Handbook of Physiology. Section 2 The Cordiovascular System Volume 1 The Heart Berne RM (ed) American Physiologica Society Maryland p. 533–580.

Broemser Ph. 1935 Uber die optimalen Beziehungen zwischen Herztätigkeit und physikalischen Konstanten des Gefä β systems. Zeitschrift für Biologie 96: 1–10

Brutsaert DL, Paulus WJ 1977 Loading and performance of the heart as muscle and pump. Cardiovascular Research 11: 1–16

Brutsaert DL, De Clerk NM, Goethals MA, Housmans PR 1978 Relaxation of ventricular cardiac muscle. Journal of Physiology (London) 283: 469–480

Brutsaert DL, Housmans PR, Goethals MA 1980 Dual control of relaxation. Its role in the ventricular function in the mammalian heart. Circulation Research 47: 637–652

Buckberg GD, Fixler DE, Archie JP, Hoffman JIE 1972a Experimental subendocardial ischemia in dogs with normal coronary arteries. Circulation Research 30: 67–81

Buckberg GD, Towers B, Paglia DE, Mulder DG, Maloney JV 1972b Subendocardial ischemia after cardiopulmonary bypass. Journal of Thoracic and Cardiovascular Surgery 64: 669–685

Buoncristiani JF, Liedtke AJ, Strong RM, Urshel CW 1973 Parameter estimates of a left ventricular model during ejection. IEEE Transactions on Biomedical Electronics 20: 110–114

Elzinga G, Westerhof N 1973 Pressure and flow generated by the left ventricle against different impedances. Circulation Research 32: 178–186

Elzinga G, Westerhof N 1974 End – diastolic volume and source impedance of the heart. In: The Physiological Basis of Starling's Law of the Heart Ciba Foundation Symposium 24 Excerpta Medica Amsterdam p. 242–255

Elzinga G, Westerhof N 1976 The pumping ability of the left heart and the effect of coronary occlusion. Circulation Research 38: 297–302

Elzinga G, Westerhof N 1978 The effect of an increase in inotropic state and end diastolic volume on the pumping ability of the feline left heart. Circulation Research 42: 620–628

Elzinga G, Westerbof N 1980 Pump function of the feline left heart. The value of variables derived from measurements on isolated muscle. Circulation Research 44: 303–308

Elzinga G, Westerhof N 1980 Pump function of the feline lift heart: changes with heart rate and its bearing on the energy balance. Cardiovascular Research 14: 81–92

Elkins RC, Peyton MD, Greenfield LJ 1974 Pulmonary vascular impedance in chronic pulmonary hypertension. Surgery 76: 57–64

Evans CL 1918 The velocity factor in cardiac work. Journal of Physiology (London) 52: 6–14

Farrar DJ, Malindzak GS, Johnson G Jr 1977 Large vessel impedance in peripheral atherosclerosis. Circulation 56 (Supplement 2): 171–178

Ford LE 1980 Effect of afterload reduction in myocardial

energetics. Circulation Research 46: 161–166

Goethals MA, Kersschot IE, Claes VA, Hermans CF, Jageneau AH, Brutsaert DT 1980 Influence of abrupt pressure increments on left ventricular relaxation. American Journal of Cardiology 45: p. 392

Housmans PR, Goethals MA, Brutsaert DT 1980 Double controle de la relaxation du coeur. Archives de Maladies du Coeur 73: 609–616

Huisman RM, Sipkema P, Westerhof N, Elzinga G 1979 Wall stress measurements in non-beating canine hearts; application of a method tested in rubber models. Cardiovascular Research 11: 642–651

Ischide N, Shimizu Y, Maruyama Y, Koiwa Y, Nunokawa T, Isoyama S, Kitaoka S, Tamaki K, Ino-oka E, Takishima T 1980 Effects of change in the aortic input impedance on systolic pressure ejected volume relationship in the isolated supported canine left ventricle. Cardiovascular Research 14: 229–243

Izuka M 1979 Comments on 'The ventricular pressure-volume diagram revisited'. Circulation Research 40: p. 731

Katz LN 1931 Observations on the external work of the isolated turtle heart. American Journal of Physiology 99: 579–597

Katz LN 1963 Recent concepts on the performance of the heart. Circulation 28: 117–135

Katz LN, Feinberg H 1958 The relation of cardiac effort to myocardial oxygen consumption and coronary flow. Circulation Research 6: 656–669

Kenner T, Pfeiffer KP 1980 Studies on the optimal matching between heart and arterial system. In: Baan J, Arntzenius AC, Yellin EL (eds) Cardiac dynamics, Martinus Ni jhoff The Hague p. 261–270

Le Carpentier YC, Chuck LH, Housmans PR, De Clerck NM, Brutsaert DL 1979 Nature of load dependence of relaxation in cardiac muscle. American Journal of Physiology 237: H455–H460

Milnor WR 1975 Arterial impedance as ventricular afterload. Circulation Research 36: 565–570

Milnor WR 1979 Influence of arterial impedance on ventricular function. In: Bauer RD, Busse R (eds) The Arterial System Springer Berlin p. 227–235

Milnor WR, Bergel DH, Bargainer JD 1966 Hydraulic power associated with pulmonary blood flow and its relation to heart rate. Circulation Research 19: 467–480

Mills CJ, Gabe IT, Gault JH, Mason DT, Ross J Jr, Braunwald E, Shillingford JP 1970 Pressure/flow relationships and vascular impedance in man. Cardiovascular Research 4: 405–417

Morris MJ, O'Rourke MF 1965 Steady and pulsatile work of the left and right ventricles. Proceedings, Australian Physiological Society p. 35

Murgo JP, Westerhof N, Giolma JP, Altobelli SA 1980 Aortic input impedance in normal man; relationship to pressure waveforms. Circulation 62: 105–116

Nichols WW, Conti CR, Walker WW, Milnor WR 1977 Input impedance of the systemic circulation in man. Circulation Research 40: 451–458

Noble MIM 1968 The contribution of blood momentum to left ventricular ejection in the dog. Circulation Research 23: 663–670

Noble MIM 1973 Problems in the definition of contractility in terms of myocardial mechanics. European Journal of Cardiology 1: 209–216

Noble MIM 1979a Left ventricular load, arterial impedance and their relationship. Cardiovascular Research 13: 183–198

Noble MIM 1979b The cardiac cycle. Blackwell

O'Rourke MF 1967 Steady and pulsatile energy losses in the systemic circulation under normal conditions and in simulated arterial disease. Cardiovascular Research 1: 313–326

O'Rourke MF, Avolio AP 1980 Pulsatile flow and pressure in human systemic arteries. Studies in man and in a multibranched model of the human systemic arterial tree. Circulation Research 46: 363–372

O'Rourke MF, Blazek JV, Morreels CL, Krovetz LJ 1968 Pressure wave transmission along the human aorta; changes with age and in arterial degenerative disease. Circulation Research 23: 567–579

O'Rourke MF, Taylor MG 1967 Input impedance of the systemic circulation. Circulation Research 20: 365–380

Patel DJ, deFreitas FM, Fry DL 1963 Hydraulic input impedance to aorta and pulmonary artery in dogs. Journal of Applied Physiology 18: 134–140

Patterson SW, Piper W, Starling EH 1914 The regulation of the heart beat. Journal of Physiology (London) 48: 465–513

Patterson SW, Starling EH 1914 On the mechanical factors which determine the output of the ventricles. Journal of Physiology (London) 48: 357–379

Paulus WJ, Claes VA, Brutsaert DL 1979 Physiologic loading of isolated feline cardiac muscle; the interaction between 39: 42–53

Paulus W, Claes VA, Brutsaert DL 1979 Physiologic loading of isolated feline cardiac muscle; the interaction between muscle contraction and vascular impedance in the production of pressure and flow waves. Circulation Research 44: 491–497

Pepine CJ, Nichols WW, Curry RC Jr, Conti CR 1979 Aortic input impedance during nitroprusside infusion; a reconsideration of afterload reduction and beneficial action. Journal of Clinical Investigation 64: 643–654

Pfeiffer KP, Kenner T 1978 Minimisation of the external work of the left ventricle and optimisation of pressure pulses. In: Bauer RD, Busse R The arterial system Springer Berlin p. 216–226

Phillips PA, Marty AT, Miyamoto AM 1975 A clinical method for detecting subendocardial ischemia after cardiopulmonary bypass. Journal of Thoracic and Cardiovascular Surgery 69: 30–39

Piene H, Sund T 1979 Flow and power output of right ventricle facing load with variable input impedance. American Journal of Physiology 237: H125–H130

Porje IG 1967 The energy design of the human circulatory system. Proceedings, 7 th International Conference on Medical and Biological Engineering Stockholm p. 153

Pouleur H, Covell JW, Ross J Jr 1979 Effects of alterations in aortic input impedance on the force-velocity-length relationship in the intact canine heart. Circulation Research 45: 126–135

Reichel H, Baumann K 1979 The effect of systolic rise in arterial pressure on stroke volume and aortic flow. In: Bauer RD, Busse R (eds) The Arterial System Springer Berlin p. 227–235

Remington JW, Hamilton WF 1947 The evaluation of the work of the heart. American Journal of Physiology 150: 292–298

Ross J Jr 1976 Afterload mismatch and preload reserve. Progress in Cardiovascular Diseases 18: 225–264

Sagawa K 1978 The ventricular pressure-volume diagram revisited. Circulation Research 43: 678–687

Sagawa K 1980 Representations of cardiac pump with special

reference to afterload. In: T. Kenner (ed) Cardiovascular System Dynamics; Models and Measurements. (Satellite symposium of the 28th International Congress of Physiological Sciences) Graz. p. 13

Sarnoff SJ, Braunwald E, Welch GH, Case RB, Stainsby WN, Macruz R 1958 Hemodynamic determinants of oxygen consumption of the heart with special reference to the tension-time index. American Journal of Physiology 192: 148–156

Suga H, Kitabatake A, Sagawa K 1979 End-systolic pressure determines stroke volume from fixed end-diastolic volume in the isolated canine left ventricle under a constant contractile state. Circulation Research 44: 238–249

Suga H, Sagawa K, Demer L 1980 Determinants of instantaneous pressure in canine left ventricle; time and volume specifications. Circulation Research 46: 256–263

Taylor MG 1964 Wave travel in arteries and the design of the cardiovascular system. In: Attinger EO (ed) Pulsatile Blood Flow McGraw New York p. 343–372

Taylor MG 1966a The input impedance of an assembly of randomly branching elastic tubes. Biophysical Journal 6: 29–51

Taylor MG 1966b An introduction to some recent developments in arterial hemodynamics. Australasian Annals of Medicine 15: 71–86

Taylor MG 1967 The elastic properties of arteries in relation to the physiological functions of the arterial system. Gastroenterology 52: 358–363

Taylor MG 1969a Arterial impedance and distensibility. In: Fishman AP, Hecht HH (eds) The Pulmonary Circulation and Interstitial Space The University of Chicago Chicago p. 341–354

Taylor MG 1969b The optimum elastic properties of arteries. In: Wolstenholme GEW, Knight J (eds) Ciba Foundation Symposium on Circulatory and respiratory mass transport Churchill London p. 136–147

Urshel CW, Covell JW, Sonneblick EH, Ross J Jr, Braunwald E 1968 Myocardial mechanics in aortic and mitral valvular regurgitation; the concept of instantaneous impedance as a determinant of the performance of the intact heart. Journal of Clinical Investigation 47: 867–883

Vincent WR, Buckberg GD, Hoffman JIE 1974 Left ventricular subendocardial ischemia in severe valvular and supravalvular aortic stenosis; a common mechanism. Circulation 49: 326–333

Walker WE 1975 The influence of changes of aortic input impedance on the dynamics of left ventricular performance. Ph. D Thesis Johns Hopkins University Baltimore

Weber KT, Janicki JS, Reeves RC, Hefner LL, Reeves TJ 1974 Determinants of stroke volume in the isolated canine heart. Journal of Applied Physiology 37: 742–747

Weber KT, Janicki JS 1977 Myocardial oxygen consumption; the role of wall force and shortening. American Journal of Physiology 233 H421–H430

Westerhof N, Elzinga G 1974 The relation between end-diastolic volume and source impedance of the left ventricle. Archives Internationales de Physiologie et Biochemie 82: 326–329

Westerhof N, Elzinga G 1978 The apparent source resistance of heart and muscle. Annals of Biomedical Engineering 6: 16–32

Westerhof N, Sipkema P, Elzinga G, Murgo JP, Giolma JP 1979 Arterial impedance. In: Hwang HC, Gross DR, Patel DJ (eds) Quantitative cardiovascular studies, University Park Baltimore Ch. 3: 111–150

Wilcken DEL, Charlier AA, Hoffman JIE, Guz A 1964 Effects of alterations in aortic impedance on performance of the ventricles. Circulation Research 14: 283–293

11

Comparative physiology of the systemic arterial system

'Two things must be considered in the phenomenon of life: first the fundamental properties of vital units which are general, then arrangements and mechanisms in organisation which give each animal species its peculiar anatomical and physiological form'
Claude Bernard (translation quoted by Gross 1979)

'There are moreover those who cry out that I have striven after the empty glory of vivisections and they disparage and ridicule with childish levity the frogs, snakes, flies and other lower animals that I have brought onto my stage.'
William Harvey 1649 (translated by K.J. Franklin 1957)

GENERAL

Studies of comparative physiology formed some of the vital evidence advanced by Harvey in proposing the circulation of blood. His detractors, such as Jean Riolan – whom he answered forcefully and colorfully – considered these studies irrelevant and unnecessary. There are many today who feel the same way about comparative studies of the vascular system – which may explain the dearth of interest in this subject ·in comparison to the abundant interest in and support for other areas of cardiovascular research. The particular significance of comparative studies of arterial function is the relationship between anatomical and physiological form referred to by Claude Bernard. In contrast to other organ systems, the design of the arterial tree is inextricably linked to body size and shape. Since the geometric pattern of arterial lengths and branchings is a major determinant of vascular impedance, body size and shape are prime determinants of impedance, and so of pressure and flow contour in different arteries and of the hydraulic load presented to the heart. In seeking general principles which can be applied widely and comprehensively in different situations including patients with arterial disease, it seems a logical and useful step to look into nature's own experiments of body design, and to find out how these alter pulsatile pressure and flow phenomena, and car-

diac load. One might hope for insight similar to that already gained for the renal system from studies of the kidneys of primitive fish, and the urine concentrating ability of desert rats.

Various studies of pressure waves, flow waves, and impedance patterns and vascular properties in different species have been reported, as outlined in the bibliography to this chapter, but there have been no large comprehensive detailed investigations of multiple parameters in a wide range of different animals with different size and shape. However, such studies as have already been performed have shown a remarkable degree of uniformity throughout the mammalian (and indeed vertebrate) kingdom. Despite large differences in size and shape, the pattern of ventricular ejection into the aorta of a variety of animals (rats, guinea pigs, rabbits, dogs, sheep, man, and in frogs, turtles, lizards and snakes) is the same (Figs. 9.1, 11.1), and there is no reason to believe that this is different in other species. Systemic arterial pressure varies over a relatively narrow range from a minimal low basal level of 70 mm Hg (mean) in rats and guinea pigs to a maximum of around 200 mm Hg in giraffes and turkeys (Woodbury and Hamilton 1937, Dittmer and Grebe 1959, Warren 1974). Even cold blooded animals such as lizards and snakes at around 25°C. have mean arterial pressure near the lower part of this range (Harrison 1965, Avolio et al 1980). Considerable

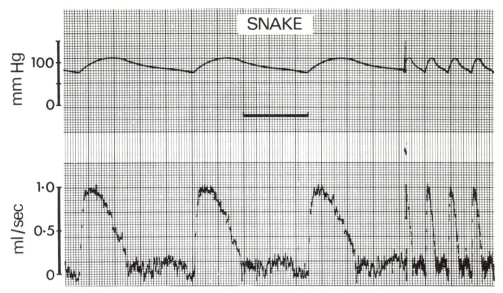

Fig. 11.1 Pressure (above) and flow (below) in the right aortic arch of a snake. Data obtained with M. Webster, A. Avolio, K. Mang and B. Bulliman

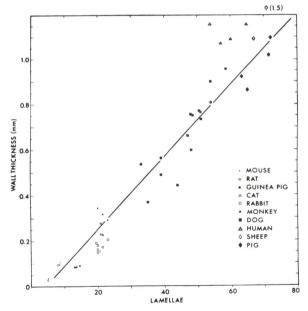

Fig. 11.2 Relationship between thoracic aortic diameter and number of medial lamellar units. The number of units is almost directly proportional to aortic diameter. From Wolinsky and Glagov (1967)

interest has been shown in the arterial pressure of giraffes (Goetz et al 1960, Patterson et al 1965, Van Citters et al 1969, Warren 1974). Although arterial pressure is very high at heart level, it is within the normal range for humans in the upper part of the neck when this is extended. The high arterial pressure in giraffes is considered necessary for cerebral perfusion when the animal is standing erect. Why birds have such high pressures is still not known.

Detailed comparative studies of aortic wall structure have been reported by Wolinsky and Glagov (1967a, 1967b, 1969) who showed that the aortic media of ten different mammals is constructed from individual lamellar units each of which is almost identical in all species, but whose number is related to body size. The number of lamellar units is linearly related to aortic luminal diameter and to wall thickness (Fig. 11.2), ranging from 5 in the thoracic aorta of adult mice to 58 in adult humans and 69 in adult sheep. When tension in the wall was calculated at average mean distending pressure of 100 mm Hg, it was found that despite the wide range of tension in aortas of different size (a consequence of the La Place law), the tension per lamellar unit was relatively constant throughout the whole range, at around 2000 dynes cm^{-1} per lamellar unit (Fig. 11.3). Similar findings obtained for both thoracic and abdominal aorta.

With the similar arterial distending pressures, and similar wall composition and distribution of

Table 11.1 Pulse wave velocities in the thoracic to abdominal aortae of a variety of animals

Animal	Pulse wave velocity m. sec⁻¹	Reference
Guinea Pig	4.1	Avolio et al 1976
Rabbit	4.5	Avolio et al 1976
Dog	5.9	McDonald 1974
Wombat	6.8	O'Rourke 1967
Sheep	6.2	Rollo 1963
Man	5.6	McDonald 1974 (Values for man exclude 'old' subjects)
Goanna	3.2–5.6	Harrison 1965
Snake	4.6	Avolio et al 1980

stress, it is not surprising to find that pulse wave velocity is very similar in different mammals (Table 11.1). No comparable studies of arterial wall structure have been reported for reptiles and birds, but reported wave velocity is similar to that in mammals (Table 11.1).

CONTOUR OF ARTERIAL PRESSURE AND FLOW WAVES

Since the ventricular ejection pattern, wave veloc-

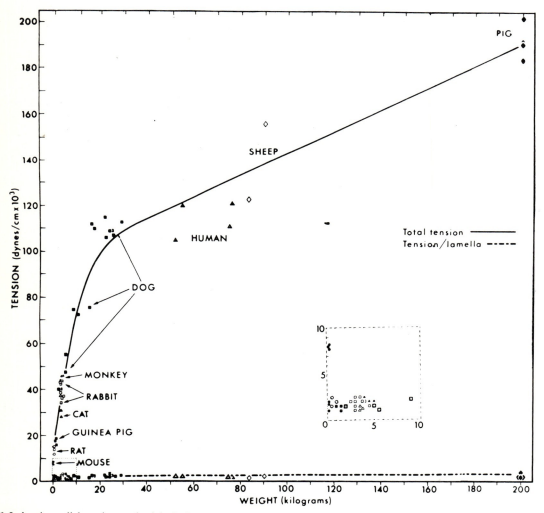

Fig. 11.3 Aortic medial tension at physiological pressure in 10 mammalian species. Total medial tension increases markedly with body weight, (continuous line) but tension per medial lamellar unit is remarkably constant regardless of species (broken line). The insert is an enlargement of the portion of the graph about its origin. From Wolinsky and Glagov (1967) with permission American Heart Association Inc.

ity and arteriolar tone are similar in different animals, one would expect that the geometric pattern of systemic arteries, and so, body size and shape would be the most important factors determining the differences in contour of pressure and flow waves in corresponding arteries of different animals. That body size would determine the timing of wave reflection and so influence wave contour was apparent from the earliest studies of the pulse as recorded with a high-frequency instrument (Frank 1905). That body shape might determine the apparent intensity of wave reflection was suggested by studies of pressure wave transmission in the wombat which were undertaken fortuitously in Taylor's laboratory at the same time that he was conducting theoretic investigations on wave reflection in multi-branched models of the systemic arterial tree (Taylor 1966, O'Rourke 1967, page 100). Taylor's theoretic studies suggested that the intensity of wave reflection as apparent in major arteries would depend on the degree of dispersion of peripheral reflecting sites,

and would be greatest when path lengths to individual sites were nearly equal (i.e. when these were clumped around one region), and least when path lengths to reflecting sites were evenly distributed over a long distance. The wombat has a relatively long body, a thick head, and short, stubby limbs (Fig. 9.16). There is less dispersion of arterial terminations in the upper and lower body than in any other known animal (Fig. 11.4); the prominent diastolic pressure and flow fluctuations in this animal were readily explained on the basis of Taylor's theory. These considerations prompted an investigation of arterial hemodynamics in the snake, which represents the other extreme to the arterial configuration in the wombat:– an animal with a long tapered body and with arterial terminations distributed evenly over a long distance (Fig. 11.4). As expected, (Avolio et al 1980, p. 148), this showed no evidence whatever of discrete wave reflection. All other known animals have body configurations between that of the wombat and snake, and so would be expected to

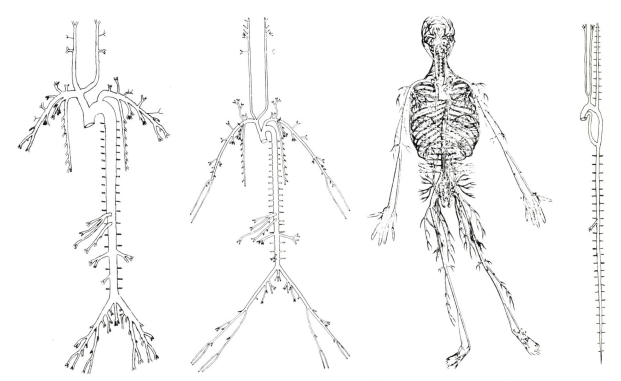

Fig. 11.4 The systemic arterial system of wombat, dog, man and snake. Spatial dispersion of peripheral reflecting sites is extreme in the snake and limited in the wombat, with man and dog occupying intermediate positions

show variable degrees of discrete wave reflection intermediate between that in these two animals.

While body size and shape appear to be the most important variables in determining contour of arterial pressure and flow waves, two other factors must also be considered – the duration of ventricular ejection (i.e. the width of the ventricular ejection wave) and in very small animals, the heavy attenuation of the travelling wave in small blood vessels.

The presence of discrete wave reflection depends on the duration of ventricular ejection in relation to the timing of reflected waves. This was discussed on page 150, where the analogy was made with echoes in a cathedral, these being most obvious when the initial is short and sharp, but merged with the initial impulse when this is prolonged. In humans, and in animals such as sheep, dogs and rabbits, the duration of systole is relatively short in relation to total cycle length whereas in smaller animals such as mice, rats and guinea pigs, duration of ejection is relatively long – 40 percent or more of total cycle length at normal heart rates (Woodbury and Hamilton 1937, Avolio et al 1976).

Attenuation of the pressure wave in travel is critically dependent on arterial calibre (McDonald 1974). McDonald considered this so high, even in the dog or human aorta that he was unwilling to concede that a travelling impulse could be identified as a discrete event after two complete circuits of the aorta. I have challenged this (p. 90), but agree that McDonald's reservations become much more relevant in the narrow aorta and arteries of mice, rats and guinea pigs.

Figure 11.5 shows proximal aortic pressure waves in a variety of mammals, all drawn diagramatically from different published data. The contour of arterial pressure and flow waves in man, sheep, dogs, rabbits and guinea pigs have been explained (Ch. 9) on the basis of wave travel and reflection between functionally discrete reflecting sites in the upper and lower parts of the body. This explanation appears to hold good throughout the mammalian kingdom, though discrete wave reflection, evidenced as obvious diastolic pressure and flow waves, is more apparent in large animals where duration of ejection is relatively short in relation to the whole cardiac cycle than in the small-

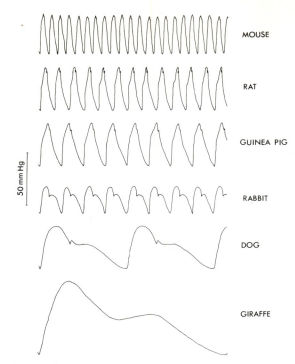

Fig. 11.5 Pressure waves recorded in the carotid artery or proximal aorta of a variety of animals. Redrawn from Avolio et al 1976, Warren 1974, Wiggers 1928, Woodbury and Hamilton 1937

Table 11.2 Approximate 'Resonant Frequency' in a variety of mammals

Mammal	Frequency
Guinea Pig	20 sec^{-1}
Rabbit	7 sec^{-1}
Dog	4 sec^{-1}
Wombat	4 sec^{-1}
Sheep	
Man	3 sec^{-1}
Giraffe	1 sec^{-1}

er animals. Since pulse wave velocity is similar throughout the mammalian kingdom one would expect that the 'resonant frequency', (the reciprocal of the period between the peaks of systolic and diastolic pressure waves in a peripheral artery) would depend on length of the animal. This appears to be the case (Table 11.2), with 'resonant frequency' ranging between approximately 1 sec^{-1} in the giraffe to around 20 sec^{-1} in the guinea pig. Diastolic pressure waves are usually not apparent in guinea pigs but only become evident when duration of ejection is shortened as in an early induced extrasystole.

Woodbury and Hamilton (1937), in studies that have still not been bettered, first noted that small mammals – guinea pigs, rats and mice – have no apparent diastolic wave. Similar findings were noted in birds (McLachlan 1962). Hamilton described the arterial system of these animals as behaving like a capacitative system (a *Windkessel*) without any superadded 'standing' or 'resonant' wave. The explanation given here amounts to the same thing – that the reflected wave merges with the systolic part of the pressure wave because of the long duration of ejection, and that this together with the heavy attenuation of the wave in travel through small arteries is responsible for the late systolic peak and the absence of any diastolic fluctuation.

In cold blooded animals such as the lizard and snake, the arterial pressure and flow waves show no diastolic waves, and no other evidence of wave reflection (Fig. 11.1). In these, pulse wave velocity is similar to that in mammals but because heart rate is slow, and duration of ejection long, reflected waves merge with the systolic part of the wave, as in smaller mammals. Further, as discussed on page 173, the wide range of distances to peripheral reflecting sites in snakes eliminates discrete wave reflection, even under abnormal conditions when ventricular ejection is markedly abbreviated.

VASCULAR IMPEDANCE

Vascular impedance has been determined in the

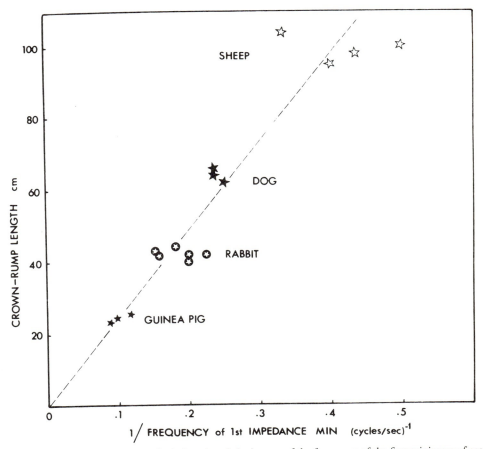

Fig. 11.6 Relationship between crown-rump body length and the inverse of the frequency of the first minimum of ascending aortic impedance in different sized animals. From data presented by Gow and O'Rourke (1970)

ascending aorta of rats (Milnor 1979), guinea pigs and rabbits (Avolio et al 1976), dogs (Patel et al 1963, O'Rourke and Taylor 1967, Noble et al 1967), sheep (Avolio 1976) and man (Mills et al 1970, Nichols et al 1977, Murgo et al 1980, O'Rourke and Avolio 1980). No studies in larger animals have yet been reported. All data are remarkably similar and can be interpreted on the same basis as arterial pressure and flow waves – on the basis of wave reflection from a single functionally discrete reflecting site in the upper part of the body, and a second functionally discrete reflecting site in the lower part of the body (p. 112). The first minimal value of impedance modulus depends on the position of the most distal lower body reflecting site. This occurs at a higher frequency in smaller animals, and at a lower frequency in the large animals (Fig. 8.17). Since this frequency depends on the distance to functionally discrete reflecting site in the lower body and on wave velocity between the heart and this site, and

since wave velocity is similar in different mammals, there is an inverse relationship between this frequency and body length (Fig. 11.6, Gow and O'Rourke 1970).

Published values of impedance modulus and characteristic impedance show large differences between different species. This is a consequence of expressing flow in volumetric terms (ml sec^{-1}), and impedance as dyne sec cm^{-5}. Volume flow is markedly different in the ascending aorta of different-sized animals, but linear flow velocity is not (p. 133). When impedance modulus is expressed in terms of linear flow velocity (i.e. as dyne sec cm^{-3}), absolute values of impedance modulus are almost identical in different species, as would be expected, since wave velocity is similar and there is an almost 1:1 relationship between the absolute value of pulse wave velocity in cms sec^{-1}, and characteristic impedance in dyne sec cm^{-3} (p. 117).

Differences in ascending aortic impedance spec-

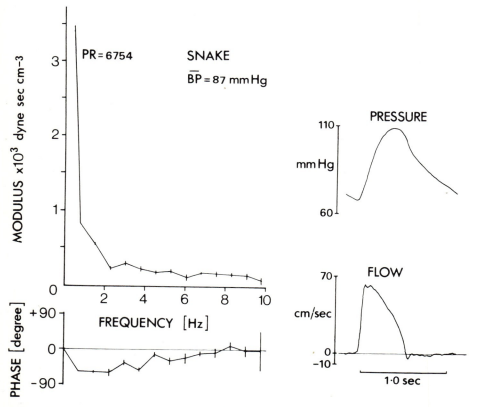

Fig. 11.7 Impedance in the proximal left aortic arch of a 2.92 metre, 5.9 kg diamond python snake. Bars represent ± 1 standard deviation (10 pulses). Data obtained in collaboration with A. Avolio, B. Bulliman, K. Mang, M. Webster

tra in man, sheep, dogs, rabbits, and guinea pigs have been explained (p. 112) on the basis of different timing and intensity of reflection from peripheral body sites. Apparent intensity of reflection (as evidenced by fluctuations of impedance modulus) depends on the degree of cancellation of wave reflection from upper and lower body sites. In dogs, the ratio of distance to upper and lower body sites is approximately 1:2 so that cancellation is maximal (since the first minimum of modulus for the upper body site corresponds to the first maximum of modulus for the lower body site (p. 105, Fig. 8.11)). One expects that cancellation of reflection should be less marked on either side of this ratio so that impedance fluctuations in other mammals may be more apparent. This appears to be the case in man (where the ratio is approximately 2:3) and is sheep and rabbits (where the ratio is approximately 1:3). One would predict that ascending aortic impedance fluctuations would also be greater in giraffes (where the ratio is approximately 1:1) and in kangaroos (where the ratio is approximately 1:5). Studies of ascending aortic impedance in giraffes have not yet been

undertaken, but kangaroos (unpublished data) do show the expected patterns.

There are no reports of impedance determinations in birds, and only limited information from lizards and snakes (Harrison 1967, Avolio et al 1980). In these reptiles, aortic pressure waves suggest that the arterial system behaves like a *Windkessel*. (Fig. 11.1) Impedance patterns (Fig. 11.7) are completely consistent with this.

BODY LENGTH AS THE DETERMINANT OF OPTIMAL HEART RATE

Favourable matching of the heart's properties to its hydraulic load is apparent throughout the mammalian kingdom (though as discussed below some qualification must be made with respect to the smallest mammals). The hydraulic load is determined by vascular properties and is expressed in terms of input impedance to the right and left ventricles. The modulus of input impedance shows a minimal value at a frequency which depends on the distance between heart and peripher-

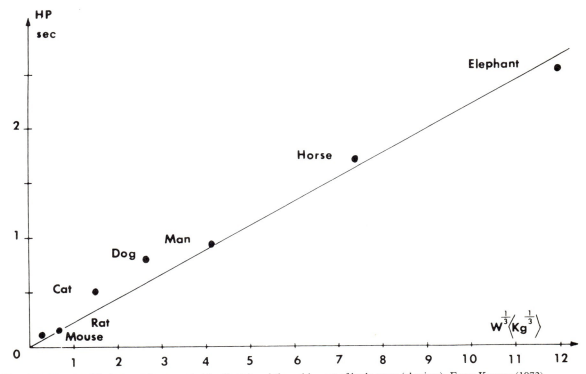

Fig. 11.8 Relationship between heart period (ordinate) and the cubic root of body mass (abscissa). From Kenner (1972).

al reflecting sites and the wave velocity over intervening arteries. Since the ratio of arterial length/wave velocity is similar for systemic and pulmonary circulations in any one animal, this minimal value occurs at approximately the same frequency in ascending aortic and pulmonary artery impedance spectra (Caro and McDonald 1961, Patel et al 1963). However this minimal value occurs at different frequencies in different animals, and this frequency for different animals is inversely related to body length (Fig. 11.6, Gow and O'Rourke 1970). But heart rate is also inversely related to body length and to the cube root of body weight (Clark 1927, Lambert and Tessier 1927, O'Rourke 1965, Dittmer and Grebe 1959, Kenner 1972, Fig. 11.8), so that there is a direct relationship in different mammals of different size between heart rate and the minimal value of impedance modulus in the ascending aorta and pulmonary artery (Taylor 1967, O'Rourke 1965, 1967, Gow and O'Rourke 1970). This is highly desirable since any mismatch between heart rate and impedance minima would increase external and total heart work, and myocardial oxygen requirement and may decrease ventricular output (Ch. 10).

A mismatch between heart and vascular system is most crucial when heart rate is inappropriately low. This can be illustrated by the following example:– If, say, the rabbit had the same heart rate as man, impedance modulus would be extremely high at the frequency of the first flow harmonic (which is invariably the largest), and the aortic pressure fluctuation generated would be inappropriately and unfavourably high, and cardiac performance would be impaired. If, on the other hand, the position was reversed, and man had the same heart rate as the rabbit, pressure fluctuations in the aorta would not be markedly altered (since impedance modulus is virtually constant at high frequencies) but the heart itself would be at considerable disadvantage because, among other things, its own oxygen requirement is dependent on heart rate as well as pressure generated (Katz and Feinberg 1958). The human heart cannot function efficiently at the basal heart rate of the rabbit. The association between heart rate and myocardial oxygen requirement does not apply between different species; the myocardium of small-

er mammals can contract more rapidly and with less energy cost than that of larger mammals (Loiselle and Gibbs 1979). Considerations such as these indicate that the lower limit of optimal heart rates is set by arterial design while the upper limit is set by cardiac limitations (O'Rourke 1967). Since an inappropriately low or high heart rate would be a disadvantage to an animal in generating and maintaining cardiac output and so chasing prey or escaping from predators, it was suggested by O'Rourke (1965), spelling out the verbally-expressed views of McDonald and Taylor, that body length determines the lower limit of optimal heart rate, and that cardiac properties have evolved in conformity with this.

The subject of the relationship between heart rate and body length is discussed elegantly by Milnor (1979) though his claim for a 'new' hypothesis* appears inappropriate. Other relevant references on this fascinating subject include Broemser (1935), Thompson (1961), Taylor (1966), Gunther (1975), Wetterer and Kenner (1968), Kenner (1972) and Iberall (1979).

The concept that body length must determine optimal heart rate is based on elementary physical, physiological and evolutionary principles, and appears to be well accepted. There are however (as always) a number of other points and qualifications that must be mentioned in this discussion.

Heart rate in any animal varies over a wide –

---

* For students of priorities, and in fairness to M.G. Taylor and the late D.A. McDonald, the following brief historical review is offered.

The relationship between impedance minimum in the pulmonary artery and heart rate was first noted by Caro and McDonald (1961), who described this as a favourable match between heart and pulmonary vascular system, and predicted that (with higher wave velocity balancing longer arterial length) the same relationship would be seen for the systemic circulation. This was confirmed by Patel et al (1963). Caro and McDonald hinted that the relationship between heart rate and impedance minimum would be preserved at lower frequencies in larger animals. This concept was confirmed by McDonald's pupil, Michael Taylor, working with his own students in Sydney during the 1960s and is referred to in his papers and many of their theses and publications (e.g. Taylor 1967, O'Rourke 1965, 1967, O'Rourke and Taylor 1967, Gow and O'Rourke 1970, Avolio 1976, Avolio et al 1976). Independently, Iberall (1973) developed the same hypothesis – that the optimal heart rate in mammals of different size is set by body length at the lower limit and by the heart itself at the upper. Independently also, Wetterer and Kenner (see Kenner 1972) had arrived at the same conclusion.

perhaps three fold – range with different levels of activity. If this be the case, how has the heart adapted – for conditions of rest or of exercise? The evolutionary theory of adaption as a survival advantage favours the latter – that the cardiovascular system is adapted for optimal performance during exercise; this is supported by the finding that in any animal the minimum of impedance modulus is normally well above basal heart rate frequency, and suggests that the arterial system pays the price of inefficiency at rest for optimal function at peak load (Taylor 1964). This may be the case, but one must also consider: (1.) that in-phase impedance is lower at low frequencies than suggested by impedance modulus alone (Fig. 10.1); and (2.) that the shape and so relative amplitude of different harmonics of the ventricular ejection (flow) wave varies with heart rate (Fig. 10.3). The first effect extends somewhat the lower limit of favourable impedance characteristics, while the latter serves to maintain energy of the ventricular ejection wave over a narrow frequency band despite changes in heart rate. Optimisation, viewed as the relationship between in-phase impedance and ventricular flow energy, appears to be preserved over a range that includes conditions of rest and activity.

A favourable relationship between heart rate and body length may be viewed usefully in terms of impedance characteristics, and so in the match between these and the harmonic content of the ventricular ejection wave. This has been done, (p. 104, 154) and it has been inferred that undesirable effects on the heart result from increase in ascending aortic and pulmonary artery systolic pressures. The same argument can be advanced through consideration of reflection in the time domain, so that the arterial system can be described as inefficient when it permits return of a major reflected wave or waves during ventricular ejection. This approach complements the former, but also permits consideration of another important factor – reduction in coronary perfusion pressure – which acts to the heart's disadvantage when echoes return inappropriately early.

In large mammals and under normal circumstances, wave reflection from lower body sites normally returns to the heart immediately after aortic valve closure, and so augments aortic pressure during early diastole. So close is the correspondence that 'incisura' (caused by aortic valve closure) and 'dicrotic notch' (caused by return of the reflected wave) are often taken to be synonomous. Aortic pressure during diastole is a major determinant of coronary blood flow (Berne and Rubio 1979). Early diastolic pressure augmentation increases coronary blood flow; (Fig. 11.9) its absence is likely to be an important limiting factor for coronary blood flow when diastolic period is reduced at rapid heart rates. Thus, early wave reflection has two adverse effects on the heart, both through increase in late systolic pressure, and cor-

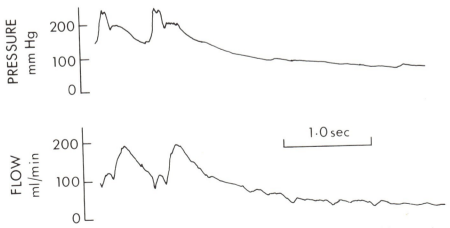

Fig. 11.9 Relationship between aortic pressure (above) and circumflex coronary artery flow (below) in a conscious dog with complete heart block. The fall in pressure and coronary flow at right occurred when the electrical pacemaker was disconnected. After Bellamy (1978) with permission American Heart Association Inc.

responding decrease in early diastolic pressure:– myocardial blood needs are increased, while concomitantly, coronary flow is jeopardised. Thus, impaired coronary flow is another disadvantage of early wave reflection from lower body sites.

ARTERIAL EFFICIENCY IN SMALL MAMMALS

Despite the general principles enunciated above, there is evidence that the arterial system in small mammals is not as efficient as in larger types. The reasons for this are unclear, but are probably related to the factors which limit the smallest size of warm blooded mammals (Thompson 1961, Iberall 1973). One expects (from previous considerations) that heart rate should be related to body length, but one also knows that total body metabolism and cardiac output is relatively high in relation to body weight in small mammals. There may be a disparity between increased heart rate, and cardiac output which is increased (relatively) to an even greater degree.

Woodbury and Hamilton (1937) in their classic studies noted that the carotid arterial pressure waves in unanesthetised mice and rats showed no diastolic pressure wave, but instead, a late systolic pressure peak and an exponential decay during diastole. They noted further that a late systolic peak was also apparent in proximal aortic and left ventricular pressure tracings, and even in the right ventricular pressure wave as well in these small animals. They also pointed out that duration of ventricular ejection is long in relation to cycle length as compared to larger mammals.

Avolio et al (1976) found similar pressure wave contour and similarly long duration of ejection in guinea pigs (Fig. 11.10). In a comparative study of arterial hemodynamics in rabbits and guinea pigs, Avolio et al showed that this pressure wave contour in guinea pigs is associated with an apparent mismatch between ascending aortic impedance spectra and energy of the ventricular ejection wave. In guinea pigs, the minimum of impedance modulus was reached at around 12 Hz whereas most of the energy of the ventricular ejection wave was in the first two harmonics at around 4 and 8 Hz (Fig. 8.18). These findings contrasted

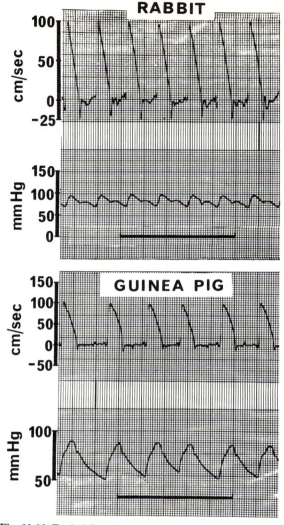

Fig. 11.10 Typical flow (above) and pressure (below) tracings in the ascending aorta of a rabbit (top) and guinea pig (bottom). From Avolio et al (1976)

to those in rabbits, studied concurrently, in which the first minimum of impedance modulus was seen at 4.25 Hz (Fig. 8.18). Heart rate and ejection duration were almost identical in the guinea pigs and rabbits.

Avolio et al (1976) attributed their findings in guinea pigs to an inappropriate match between arterial dimensions on the one hand, and heart rate and duration of ejection on the other. Duration of ventricular ejection was considered to be inappropriately long, so that wave reflection from lower body sites returned to the heart while the heart was still contracting, so adding to its pressure load. The identical pressure wave contour in mice and rats can be explained in the same way, and to be equally detrimental to cardiac function. The finding of a late systolic peak in the right ventricular trace of mice (Woodbury and Hamilton 1937) supports this view that ejection duration in these small mammals is inappropriately long in relation to all body dimensions. The hearts of these small mammals appear to suffer the disadvantages of wave reflection with none of its advantages.

The impedance mismatch in guinea pigs, and the arterial pressure wave contour in guinea pigs, rats and mice are remarkably similar to those in patients with arterial degenerative disease (O'Rourke et al 1968, p. 206). Surprisingly, these small mammals may prove to be good models for studies of the effects of arterial degeneration in man.

The reason for arterial inefficiency in small animals is not apparent. Further investigations of pressure and flow in small animals – which have languished despite technicological advances since the early work of Hamilton, Gregg and others 40 years ago – may give fresh insight into abnormal arterial function in man. The unusual findings in small animals provide yet another reason for seeking explanations of biological phenomena and mechanisms from studies of comparative physiology.

REFERENCES

Avolio AP 1976 Haemodynamic studies and modelling of the systemic arterial system. Thesis for Ph D. University of New South Wales, Sydney

Avolio AP, O'Rourke MF, Webster M 1980 Pulsatile hemodynamics in the arterial system of the snake. Proceedings, 28th International Congress of Physiological Sciences, Budapest. p. 306

Avolio AP, O'Rourke MF, Mang K, Bason PT, Gow BS 1976 A comparative study of pulsatile arterial hemodynamics in rabbits and guinea pigs. American Journal of Physiology 230: 868–875

Avolio AP, O'Rourke MF, Webster M 1980 Pulsatile hemodynamics in the arterial system of the snake. Proceedings 28th International Congress of Physiological Sciences Budapest p. 306

Baird DK 1962 Pressure pulse studies in the rabbit. Thesis for B. Sc (Med) University of Sydney

Bellamy RF 1978 Diastolic coronary artery pressure – flow relations in the dog. Circulation Research 43: 92–101

Berne RM, Rubio R 1979 Coronary circulation. In: Handbook of Physiology Section 2 The Cardiovascular System Volume 1 The Heart American Physiological Society Bethesda p. 873–952

Broemser PH 1935 Unber die optimalen Beziehungen zwischen Herztaetigkeit und physikalischen Konstanten des Gefae β systems. Zeitschrift fur Biologie 96: 1–10

Campbell KB, Rhode EA, Cox RH, Hunter WC, Noordergraaf 1981 Functional consequences of expanded aortic bulb: a model study. American Journal of Physiology 240: R200–R210

Caro CG, McDonald DA 1961 The relation of pulsatile pressure and flow in the pulmonary vascular bed. Journal of Physiology (London) 157: 426–453

Caro CG, Pedley TJ, Schroter RC, Seed WA 1978 The mechanics of the circulation. Oxford University Press, New York

Clark AJ 1927 Comparative Physiology of the heart. MacMillan New York

Dittmer D, Grebe RM, 1959 Handbook of Circulation Saunders Philadelphia

Doyle JT, Patterson JL, Warren JV, Detwiller DK 1960 Observations on the circulation of domestic cattle. Circulation Research 8: 4–15

Dujardin JP, Stone DN, Paul LT, Pieper HP 1980 Effect of acute volume loading on aortic smooth muscle activity in intact dogs. American Journal of Physiology 238: H379–H383

Dujardin JP, Stone DN, Paul LT, Pieper HP 1980 Response of systemic arterial input impedance to volume expansion and hemorrhage. American Journal of Physiology 238: H902–H908

Fisher EW, Dalton RG 1959 Cardiac output in horses. Nature 134: 2020–2021

Frank O 1905 Der Puls in den Arterien. Zeitschrift fur Biologie 46: 441–553

Goetz RH, Warren JV, Gauer OH, Patterson JL, Doyle JT, Keen EN, McGregor M 1960 Circulation of the giraffe. Circulation Research 8: 1049–1058

Gow BS, O'Rourke MF 1970 Comparison of pressure and flow in the ascending aorta of different mammals. Proceedings, Australian Physiological and Pharmacological Society 1: 68

Gross DR 1979 Animal models in cardiovascular research. In: Hwang NH, Gross DR, Patel DJ (eds) Quantitative Cardiovascular Studies University Park Baltimore Ch. 1: 3–40

Gunther B 1975 Dimensional analysis and theory of biological similarity. Physiological Reviews 55: 659–699

Hamilton WF 1944 The Patterns of the arterial pressure pulse. American Journal of Physiology 141: 235–241

Harrison M 1965 The cardiovascular system in reptiles with especial reference to the goanna, Varanus varius. Thesis for B. Sc. (Med) University of Sydney

Harvey W 1628 De motu cordis et sanguinis in animlibus. Fitzer Frankfurt Translated by Franklin KJ 1957 Blackwell Oxford

Harvey W 1649 De circulatione sanguinis. Translated by Franklin KJ 1957 Blackwell Oxford

Iberall AS 1973 On growth, form and function. A fantasia on the design of a mammal In: Regulation and Control in Physiological Systems Iberall AS and Guyton A ISA Pittsburg (eds) p. 135–139

Iberall AS 1979 Some comparative scale factors for mammals; comments on Milnor's paper concerning a feature of cardiovascular design. American Journal of Physiology 237: R7–R9

Katz LN, Feinberg H 1958 The relation of cardiac effort to myocardial oxygen consumption and coronary flow. Circulation Research 6: 656–669

Kenner T 1972 Flow and pressure in the arteries. In: Fung YC, Perrone N, Anliker M (eds) Biomechanics: Its foundations and objectives, Prentice Hill New Jersey p. 381–434

Lambert R, Tessier G 1927 Theorie de la Similitude Biologique, Annals de Physiologie 3: 212–246

Loiselle DS, Gibbs CL 1979 Species differences in cardiac energetics. American Journal of Physiology 237: H90–H98

McDonald DA 1974 Blood flow in arteries. 2nd edn Arnold London

Mc Lachlan E 1962 Studies in the arterial system of the domestic goose and turkey with a comparison with that in the rabbit. Thesis for BSc (Hons) University of Sydney

Mills CJ, Gabe IT, Gault JH, Mason DT, Ross J Jr, Braunwald E, Shillingford J 1970 Pressure-flow relationships and vascular impedance in man. Cardiovascular Research 4: 404–417

Milnor WR 1979 Aortic wavelength as a determinant of the relation between heart rate and body size in mammals. American Journal of Physiology 237: R3–R6

Morris MJ 1965 Pressure and flow in the pulmonary vasculature of the dog. Thesis for BSc (Med) University of Sydney

Murgo JP, Westerhof N, Giolma JP, Altobelli SA 1980 Aortic input impedance in normal man; relationship to pressure waveforms. Circulation 62: 105–116

Nichols WW, Conti CR, Walker WE, Milnor WR 1977 Input impedance of the systemic circulation in man. Circulation Research 40: 451–458

Noble MIM, Gabe IT, Trenchard O, Guz A 1967 Blood pressure and flow in the ascending aorta of conscious dogs. Cardiovascular Research 1: 9–20

O'Rourke MF 1965 Pressure and flow in arteries. Thesis for MD University of Sydney

O'Rourke MF 1981 Commentary on aortic wavelength as a determinant of the relationship between heart rate and body size in mammals. American Journal of Physiology 240: R393–R395.

O'Rourke MF, Taylor MG 1967 Input impedance to the systemic circulation. Circulation Research 20:365–380

O'Rourke MF 1967 Steady and pulsatile energy losses in the systemic circulation under normal conditions and in simulated arterial disease. Cardiovascular Research 1:313 326

O'Rourke MF, Avolio AP 1980 Pulsatile flow and pressure in human systemic arteries; studies in man and in a multibranched model of the human systemic arterial tree. Circulation Research 46: 363–372

O'Rourke MF, Blazek JV, Morreels CL, Krovetz LJ 1968 Pressure wave transmission along the human aorta; changes with age and in arterial degenerative disease. Circulation Research 23: 567–579

Patel DJ, deFreitas FM, Fry DL 1963 Hydraulic input impedance to aorta and pulmonary artery in dogs. Journal of Applied Physiology 18: 134–140

Patterson JL Jr. 1965 Cardiorespiratory dynamics in the ox and giraffe with comparative observations on man and other mammals. Annals New York Academy of Sciences 127: 393–413

Reeves JT, Grover RF, Will DH, Alexander AF 1962 Hemodynamics in normal cattle. Circulation Research 10: 166–171

Remington JW 1963 The physiology of the aorta and major arteries. Handbook of Physiology, American Physiological Society Washington DC Volume 2 Circulation 2 p. 799–838

Rollo DJ 1963 Pressure pulse wave transmission in the arterial system. Thesis for BSc (Med) University of Sydney

Taylor MG 1964 Wave travel in arteries and the design of the cardiovascular system. In: Pulsatile Blood Flow EO Attinger (ed) McGraw Hill New York p. 343–367

Taylor MG 1966a The input impedance to an assembly of randomly-branching elastic tubes. Biophysical Journal 6: 29–51

Taylor MG 1966b An introduction to some recent developments in arterial hemodynamics. Australasian Annals of Medicine 15: 71–86

Thompson DA 1917 On Growth and Form. Abridged edition edited by Bonner JT Cambridge University Press Cambridge

Van Citters RL, Franklin D, Vatner S, Patrick T, Warren JV 1969 Cerebral hemodynamics in the giraffe. Transactions of the Association of American Physicians 82: 293–303

Warren JV 1974 The physiology of the giraffe. Scientific American 231: 96–105

Wetterer E 1954 Flow and pressure in the arterial system, their hemodynamic relationship and the principles of the measurement. Minnesota Medicine 37: 77–86

Wetterer E, Kenner T 1968 Grundlagen der Dynamik des Arterienpulses. Springer Verlag, Berline, Heidelberg, New York

Wiggers CJ 1928 Pressure pulses in the cardiovascular system. Longmans London p. 65–90

Wolinsky H, Glagov S 1967a Lamellar unit of aortic medial structure and function in mammals. Circulation Research 20:99–111

Wolinsky H, Glagov S 1967b Nature of species differences in the medial distribution of aortic vasa vasorum in mammals. Circulation Research 20: 409–421

Wolinsky H, Glagov S 1969 Comparison of abdominal and thoracic aortic medial structure in mammals: deviation of man from the usual pattern. Circulation Research 25: 677–686

Woodbury RA, Hamilton WF 1937 Blood pressure studies in small animals. American Journal of Physiology 119: 663–674

Yates FE 1979 Comparative physiology: compared to what? American Journal of Physiology 237: 6 R1–R3

PART 4

Clinical implications of altered cushioning function

This section is directed at cushioning function of the arterial system and arterial disease:– how disturbances of cushioning function in disease alter pulsatile phenomena and adversely affect cardiac performance, and how pulsatile phenomena may initiate and aggravate arterial disease. The effects of arterial disease on the conduit function of arteries was described in Chapter 5. Disturbances in the conduit function of arteries have their principal ill effects downstream and are usually manifest as organ or tissue ischemia. Disturbances in cushioning function on the other hand, have no ill effects on tissues downstream, but alter stresses on the heart and other arteries, and their ill effects are explicable on this basis. In this section I propose to discuss individual conditions and individual diseases which affect cushioning function of arteries, and where appropriate, therapeutic strategies. Some repetition with physiological principles, discussed earlier, is inevitable.

In discussing the functional effects of arterial disease, I wish to avoid semantics, and so the arguments and differences of opinion that attend distinctions between 'arteriosclerosis' and 'atherosclerosis', and between different forms of medial degeneration, and between disease and (?) normal ageing processes. I will use the general term 'arterial degeneration' to refer to those conditions which affect predominantly the media of the aorta and major arteries and alter their distensibility, and 'atherosclerosis' to describe that disease which affects principally the intima, and has its major ill effect through obstructing blood flow.

12

Ageing and arterial function

'Only in the case of young children do we find that the elasticity of arteries is so perfectly adapted to the requirements of the organism as it is in the case of the lower animals'

CS Roy 1880

'The amount of energy expended by the heart as measured by its oxygen consumption or CO_2 output has been shown to be proportional to the pressure developed (Rohde 1910, 1914); hence the amount of energy which the heart has to expend per beat, other things being equal, varies inversely with the elasticity of the arterial system'

JC Bramwell, AV Hill 1922

The principal changes which take place in the vascular system with age are:—

1. Dilation of the aorta and major arteries
2. Increase in thickness of the walls of the aorta and major arteries
3. Decrease in distensibility of the aorta and major arteries
4. Decrease in vascularity of bodily organs and tissues

The obvious consequences of these changes are:—

1. Increase in arterial pulse wave velocity with age
2. Increase in pulse pressure with age
3. Decrease in organ blood flow and in cardiac output with age
4. Rise in peripheral resistance and in mean arterial pressure with age

The less obvious consequences result from impaired arterial distensibility and include:—

1. Alteration in contour of the arterial pressure (and flow) pulse
2. Alteration in amplification of the pressure pulse between ascending aorta and peripheral arteries
3. Alteration in input impedance to the systemic circulation
4. Mismatch between aortic impedance characteristics and energy of the left ventricular ejection wave

5. Increased pulsatile energy losses in arteries
6. Increase in mean aortic systolic pressure with —
   a Increased ventricular oxygen requirements
   b Increased afterload, hindering ventricular ejection
7. Relative decrease in mean aortic diastolic pressure and so, compromise in capacity for coronary blood flow

Roy (1880), Frank (1905, 1920, 1928), Bramwell and Hill (1922), Remington and Hamilton (1947) and many other physiologists appreciated the importance of arterial distensibility with respect to cardiac performance, and the ill effects of ageing on the heart. This information was not however applied to clinical problems. During the first part of this century, clinicians appeared preoccupied with ageing changes as they affected arterial pressure and as they applied to the classification and diagnosis of hypertension. An unduly simplistic view of the arterial system was probably responsible for the concept that systolic pressure was determined by cardiac factors and diastolic pressure by vascular factors; a high systolic pressure meant that the heart was pumping strongly and a low systolic pressure suggested cardiac weakness; a high diastolic pressure implied arteriolar constriction and 'hypertension', and a low diastolic pressure, peripheral vasodilation – even when this was due to aortic valve incompetence (Wood 1956). Clinicians had become slaves of the tool they were using – the sphygmomanometer – and came to think that the numbers they were able to obtain had as much physiological significance with respect to cardiac and vascular properties as the pulse rate, instead of the extremes of pressure fluctuation around an unknown mean value. Doubtless the approach to hypertension would have been different had an instrument been available to measure mean pressure instead of the peak and nadir of the arterial pressure wave.

There has been much conjecture on what changes in arterial pressure occur with age, whether these are abnormal or not, and what mechanism is responsible for these. These matters are well summarised in Pickering's classic (1968) monograph. Seen from the point of view espoused in this book, one seeks an explanation, not in terms of factors influencing systolic and diastolic pressure individually, but rather in terms of factors affecting mean pressure, and pulse pressure. The explanation one would advance is a simple one:– that changes in recorded systolic and diastolic pressures with age are secondary to a rise in mean pressure (which is caused by decreased bodily vascularity, and so, by increased peripheral resistance), and by decreased arterial distensibility (Fig. 12.1). Such an explanation readily explains why systolic pressure rises more with age than diastolic pressure, and also why in some instances (when change in distensibility is great) diastolic pressure may not rise at all. This simple explanation of change in arterial pressure with age is not new, having been proposed by Mackenzie nearly 80 years ago in his influental monograph (Mackenzie 1902), prepared before the sphygmomanometer had become widely used.

Over the first part of this century, and even up until the early 1970s clinicians accepted an increase in systolic pressure with age as a natural phenomenom which denoted a healthy heart and for which no treatment was possible or necessary. Elevation of systolic pressure was generally regarded as irrelevant to the diagnosis of hypertension (which was gauged on diastolic pressure alone), and not to warrant antihypertensive therapy so long as diastolic pressure was normal, even in the presence of overt heart failure.

Over the last ten years, attention of clinicians has been directed at decreased arterial distensibility as an important factor in determining left ventricular load (through elevating pressure during systole) and coronary perfusion (through concomitant reduction in pressure throughout cardiac diastole). This has followed better understanding of the factors which determine the heart's requirement for and supply of blood (p. 166), better understanding of how systolic pressure alters cardiac ejection (p. 164) and of how cardiac performance can be improved by vasodilator agents (p. 234). Over the same period, epidemiological studies have established that systolic pressure is as important (if not more so) than diastolic pressure in predicting the complications of hypertension and mortality from these (Coleandrea et al 1970, Kannel et al 1971 ab, 1972, Koch Weser 1973), and vasodilator agents have become standard therapy for cardiac failure, even in normotensive patients (Smith and Braunwald 1980).

In discussing the functional effects of ageing on arterial function, and on cardiac performance, the key is the change in physical properties of arteries, and the resultant effects of decreased arterial distensibility on the arteries themselves, and on the heart.

STRUCTURAL CHANGES IN THE AORTIC AND ARTERIAL WALL

Structure of the normal arterial wall has been described (Ch. 3). At birth (Crawford 1977) the intima comprises a single layer of cells almost direct-

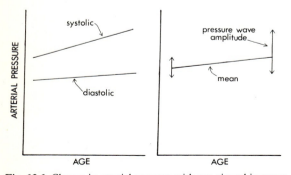

Fig. 12.1 Change in arterial pressure with age viewed in terms of systolic and diastolic pressure (left) and in terms of mean and pulse pressure (right).

ly attached to the internal elastic lamina. The media (which is mainly responsible for the physical properties of the artery) is bounded on the inside by the internal and on the outside by the external elastic laminae and comprises a mesh of elastic laminae and muscular fibres (the former predominating in the aorta and proximal arteries and the latter in more peripheral vessels), together with more loosely arranged collagen fibres and ground substance. The adventitia is made up of collagen fibres which at normal distending pressures is thought to play little part in determining distensibility of the vessel.

With the passage of time, progressive changes are seen in the arterial wall. These occur independently of such changes as may be attributed to atherosclerosis, and become more marked with the passage of time or when distending pressure is elevated (Moritz and Oldt 1937, Moschowitz 1950). These changes are not peculiar to man but have been seen to some degree or other in a variety of animals, depending on age (Fox 1933, Stehbens 1979). They are far more obvious in man, probably because of man's longer life span (Mitchell and Schwartz 1965, Stehbens 1979). They are however usually not apparent in experimental animals such as dogs or sheep which are usually investigated well under ten years of age.

Detailed studies of arterial changes in man with age have been reported by Moritz and Oldt (1937), Gray et al (1953), Milch (1965), Mitchell and Schwartz (1965) and Stehbens (1979). The most striking finding macroscopically is that at maturity, the arteries continue to 'grow', while growth of the rest of the body stops. There is progressive increase in arterial diameter and in wall thickness (Fig. 12.2). In later years, increase in length is apparent as well, being often manifest as 'uncoiling' of the aortic arch and tortuosity of the aorta and other arteries.

Histological examination of the aortic wall shows that the principal changes with age occur in the media and intima. From a physical point of view, the most important change is in the elastic fibres and laminae which are principally responsible for the vessel's distensibility. These elastic fibres and laminae lose the orderly arrangement seen in earlier life and display thinning, splitting, fraying and fragmentation. The degeneration of elastic fibres is associated with increase in collagenous fibres and in ground substance, and often with calcium deposition in degenerate elastic material. In the intima there is a steady increase in connective tissue between the endothelial cells and internal elastic lamina. Any or all of these processes may occur to an extreme, with intimal hyperplasia, cystic degeneration of the media, or extensive medial calcification (Monckeberg's sclerosis).

These changes in the arterial wall with age are accelerated in hypertension, when the process is sometimes referred to as arteriosclerosis (Moscho-

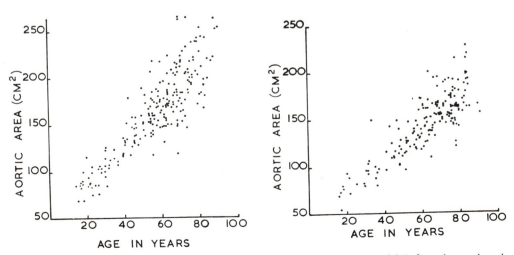

Fig. 12.2 Increase in size of the thoracic aorta with increasing age in men (left) and women (right), from the unselected necropsy sample studied by Mitchell and Schwartz (1965).

witz 1950, Gray et al 1953, Stehbens 1979). The changes seen however are exactly the same as those which accompany ageing in normotensive subjects and are usually attributed to the effects of fatigue or 'wear and tear'. An important point is that the process has to be regarded as a self-perpetuating one (Gray et al 1953, Stehbens 1979). As the artery dilates, wall tension and pulsatile stresses increase according to LaPlace's law and appear to accentuate the degeneration which has already occurred. It is hardly surprising that in this setting, with increased stresses applied to a degenerating wall, that localised problems such as aneurysmal dilation at points of weakness may occur.

Even in the absence of hypertension, or of atherosclerosis, the aortic and arterial wall of the average adult human subject is already affected by the degeneration of age. This degeneration probably begins at or before birth, becomes apparent histologically from the late teens, and leads to

steady and relentless loss of arterial distensibility, and deterioration in arterial function.

PHYSICAL PROPERTIES OF ARTERIES

Changes in elastic properties of the aorta and large arteries with age were first documented by Roy in 1880; he was also the first to point out the increased stiffness of adult human arteries as compared to those of adult experimental animals, and to comment on the onset of degeneration from childhood. Many subsequent studies have shown similar results, with increased stiffness apparent as increase in elastic modulus (Remington et al 1947, Learoyd and Taylor 1966, Gonza et al 1974), and/ or pulse wave velocity (Bramwell and Hill 1922, Schimmler 1965, Learoyd and Taylor 1966, O'Rourke et al 1968, Kenner 1972, Gonza et al 1974) (Fig. 12.3). The most marked alterations in wave velocity with age are seen in the abdominal

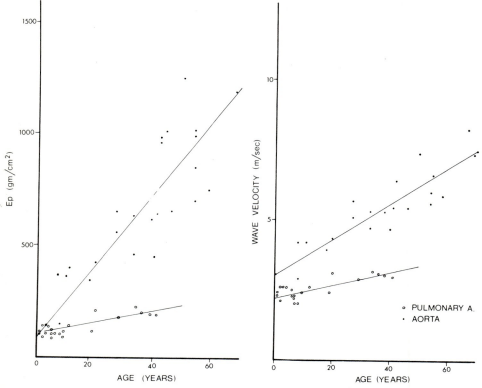

Fig. 12.3 Increase in incremental elastic modulus (Ep) (left) and calculated pulse wave velocity (right) with age in the proximal thoracic aorta and pulmonary artery of human subjects. From data published by Gonza et al (1974)

aorta and iliac arteries. These vessels are more affected by arterial degenerative changes than the thoracic aorta and upper body vessels, possibly because of the higher mean distending pressure when in the upright position. Nonetheless, changes in the thoracic aorta are also quite marked. Nichols and McDonald (1972) recorded pulse wave velocity of 4.1 metre sec^{-1} in the ascending aorta of dogs. Gonza et al calculated the same wave velocity in adolescents around 15 years of age; by 60 years, this had increased to around 6.5 metre sec^{-1}. Murgo et al (1980) measured pulse wave velocity at 6.7 metre sec^{-1} in the ascending aorta of a group of apparently normal human subjects whose average age was 34 years.

Pulse wave contour

The effects of arterial stiffening and of increased pulse wave velocity on pressure pulse contour are predictable: earlier return of reflected waves from peripheral sites merging with the initial wave generated by left ventricular ejection (Fig. 9.5). Such changes of the arterial pulse contour were described by O'Rourke et al (1968), who also noted that these are associated with disappearance of the diastolic pressure wave and decreased amplification of the pressure wave between the ascending aorta and femoral artery (Fig.

12.4). Freis et al (1967) studied the effects of ageing on the carotid pressure pulse, recorded indirectly through a transducer applied to the skin over this vessel. Freis et al noted that with advancing years, the early systolic pressure peak is replaced by a peak in late systole, and that at the same time, the diastolic pressure wave becomes inapparent. In another study of the volume pulse in the leg, Puls et al (1967) showed disappearance of the diastolic wave with age.

The most detailed and accurate studies of pressure pulse contour in the human ascending aorta have recently been reported by Murgo et al (1980). Using high fidelity Millar catheter transducers, Murgo and colleagues showed that the pressure wave recorded in the ascending aorta of human adults is quite different to that seen in experimental animals, being characterised by a notch in the mid-late part of systole, followed by a secondary wave. They identified this secondary wave as resulting from wave reflection in the lower part of the body. In young patients (average age 24 ± 2 years) the notch occurred close to the incisura and the second systolic peak was of lower amplitude than the initial peak, whereas in older patients (average age 40 ± 4 years) the notch occurred earlier and the secondary systolic wave was of large amplitude and accounted for the high peak of the pressure wave, which was apparent in

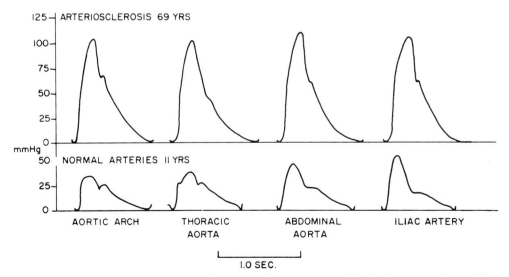

Fig. 12.4 Pressure waves recorded in the aortic arch (left), descending thoracic and abdominal aorta (middle), and iliac artery (right) of a child (below) and of an elderly subject (above)

late systole, and was responsible for substantial increase in pulse pressure (Fig. 12.5). As in the previous studies, Murgo et al (1980) showed that early return of wave reflection during systole was associated with disappearance of the diastolic pressure wave.

The typical pressure wave contour in the human adult ascending aorta is dependent on early wave reflection with normal duration of ejection. If wave reflection is delayed, as in hypotension, or if duration of ejection is shortened, as in hypovolemic shock or in heart failure or during the Valsalva manouver, the reflected wave does not merge with the initial wave generated by the heart, and is readily apparent as an obvious diastolic wave (Fig. 9.15 Kroeker and Wood, 1956; Mills et al, 1970).

There have been no reported studies on the effects of ageing on the contour of arterial flow waves. One would expect however that with earlier return of wave reflection during systole, and with inapparent diastolic pressure fluctuations, that diastolic flow oscillations would likewise be small in adult humans, so that the flow wave in the descending aorta and peripheral arteries would resemble those in the ascending aorta. This appears to be the case (Mills et al 1970, O'Rourke and Avolio 1980).

Pressure wave transmission

Increasing stiffness of arteries and increasing pulse wave velocity with age affect pressure wave contour in all systemic arteries. Since the incident and reflected waves summate in central as well as in peripheral arteries, there is a general increase in pulse pressure throughout the arterial tree so that pressure wave contour and amplitude become similar in all arteries. (Fig. 12.4), and amplification of the pressure pulse between the ascending aorta and peripheral arteries is markedly reduced. This effect of ageing is most apparent in amplification of the pressure pulse between the ascending aorta and iliac artery; in children this averages around 50 percent but only around 10 percent in humans over age 60 (Fig. 9.13).

There have been no systematic studies reported on changes in brachial pressure wave amplification with age. It is likely however that these are similar to changes in femoral wave amplification. Clinicians usually consider that the systolic and diastolic pressures they record with a sphygmomanometer pertain to pressure at the aortic valve and elsewhere throughout the arterial tree. This is erroneous because the brachial pressure wave is of higher amplitude than that in the proximal aorta. In the absence of precise data one cannot make

PRESSURE WAVEFORM CLASSIFICATION

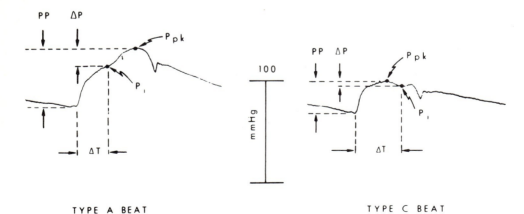

Fig. 12.5 Typical ascending aortic pressure pulses in an older adult human (type A), left, and in a younger subject (type C), right. PP, pulse pressure; P_{pk}, peak systolic pressure; P_i, inflection pressure; $P = P_{pk} - P_i$; T is the time interval between onset of systolic pressure wave form and P_i. From Murgo et al (1980) by permission American Heart Association Inc.

any definite statements on the clinical implications of changes in brachial pressure wave amplication with age. However since there is some reduction in amplification with age, one can say that increase in pulse pressure with age in the central aorta is probably greater than apparent from recordings of brachial artery pressure.

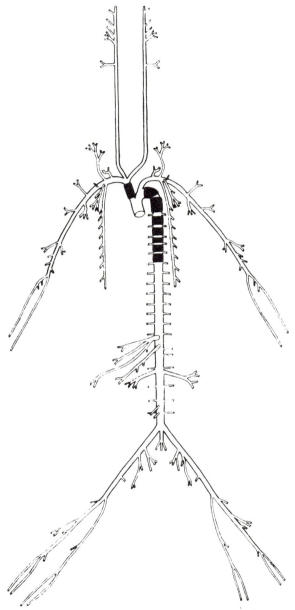

Fig. 12.6 Simulation of arterial degeneration in a dog by application of rigid lucite ferrules to the descending thoracic aorta and brachiocephalic artery

Vascular impedance

The effects of arterial stiffening on ascending aortic impedance have been simulated by application of rigid lucite ferrules to segments of the descending thoracic aorta and brachiocephalic artery (Figs. 12.6, 12.7, O'Rourke 1967). Stiffening of the proximal vessels leads to increase in characteristic impedance. When arterial stiffening is generalised, one would expect impedance curves to be shifted to the right (as they are in hypertension) so that minima of modulus occur at higher frequencies than under normal conditions. Both these effects – increase in characteristic impedance and shifting of impedance curves to the right – have the effect of increasing impedance modulus and its in-phase component (Z cosine φ) over that frequency band that normally contain most of the energy of the left ventricular ejection wave, and so causing a mismatch between ventricular ejection and impedance presented by the systemic circulation (Fig. 10.4).

There have been no studies reported on the effects of ageing on ascending aortic impedance in man. There are no data at all on ascending aortic impedance in children. Murgo et al (1980) subdivided their 18 patients – none with evidence of cardiac or arterial disease – on the basis of pressure wave contour in the ascending aorta (p. 123). Three different pressure wave patterns were seen in young (24 ± 2 years), older (33 ± 3 years), and oldest (40 ± 4 years) young adults; these different pressure wave patterns corresponded to differences in ascending aortic impedance spectra (Fig. 8.27), the youngest being similar to that seen in dogs with little fluctuation in modulus above the frequency of the first minimum, and the oldest showing considerable fluctuation consistent with the presence of a single functionally discrete reflecting site in the systemic vascular bed. These findings have been discussed, and the differences in impedance spectra have been attributed to a greater degree of degeneration in the descending aorta and lower limb vessels of the older patients (p. 125). Impedance spectra obtained for the ascending aorta of man by others (Gabe et al 1965, Patel et al 1965, Nichols et al 1977, O'Rourke and Avolio 1980) have been similar to that found by Murgo et al in their older sub-

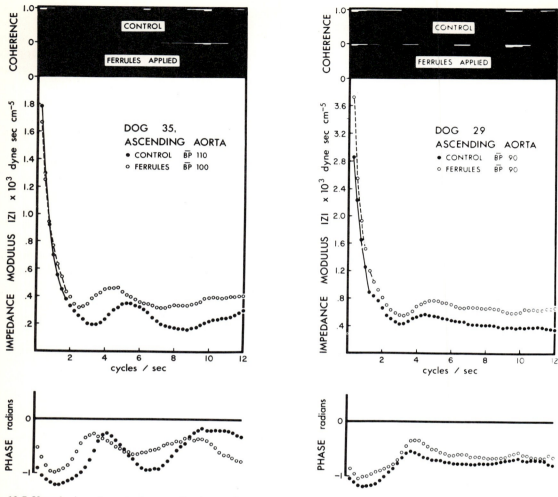

Fig. 12.7 Vascular impedance in the ascending aorta of two dogs before (solid line) and after (dotted line) application of lucite ferrules to the brachiocephalic artery and descending thoracic aorta. From O'Rourke (1967)

jects. These patterns differ from those seen in experimental animals in two other respects:– characteristic impedance appears to be greater, and minima of impedance are reached at higher frequencies than one would expect on the basis of body length. All these findings can be explained on the same basis as pulse contour and wave transmission – on the basis of arterial degeneration causing increase in characteristic impedance and in pulse wave velocity.

Impedance spectra in the human ascending aorta do not show the same favourable match with harmonic content of the ventricular ejection wave as seen in experimental animals (see Figs. 10.1,

13.11). This has been discussed on page 162). The impedance mismatch is apparent as a relative increase in the pulsatile component of external heart work – that energy generated by the heart which is lost in vascular pulsations (p. 157). In a series of dogs (O'Rourke 1967) this averaged 10 percent of total (steady plus pulsatile) external heart work, whereas in humans, reported values are higher, in the range 10–26 percent (O'Rourke 1967, Porjé 1967, Nichols et al 1977).

While detailed studies of vascular impedance with age have yet to be conducted, there is already strong evidence to support Roy's century old statement that by adult life, the human systemic arterial tree is less efficient than that of experimental animals in accepting pulsatile flow from the heart.

EFFECTS OF ARTERIAL DEGENERATION ON CARDIAC PERFORMANCE

The functional effects of arterial degeneration on the heart are apparent in the frequency domain as an increase in ascending aortic impedance modulus, a mismatch between aortic impedance and frequency content of the ventricular ejection wave, and an increase in the pulsatile component of external heart work.

In the time domain, the ill effects of arterial degeneration are manifest as a higher pulse pressure in the ascending aorta, with change in pulse wave contour, so that there is considerable increase in the pressure maintained in the ascending aorta during systole, and corresponding decrease in the pressure maintained during diastole (Fig. 12.8). Increase in systolic pressure increases myocardial oxygen requirements (as noted by Bramwell and Hill in 1922, and by Rohde in 1910, and confirmed by Sarnoff and many others subsequently) and leads to cardiac hypertrophy – with further increase in oxygen demands, and subsequent degeneration, and also tends to reduce left ventricular output – particularly when myocardial contractility is impaired (p. 164). Decrease in pressure during diastole reduces coronary perfusion pressure and contributes to a potential imbalance between demand of the ventricle for blood, and its capacity for supply through the coronary arteries during diastole (p. 166).

Studies of arterial hemodynamics in dogs and other large experimental animals have provided abundant evidence of a favourable match between cardiac and arterial properties (p. 154). This is largely due to the timing of wave reflection which under normal circumstances helps to reduce pressure during systole against which the heart must pump, while augmenting pressure during diastole and aiding coronary blood flow. Studies on adult man show the opposite – that wave reflection augments heart work and impairs coronary perfusion. Age and arterial degeneration change the timing of wave reflection so that it works to the heart's disadvantage.

The clinical implications of these considerations remain to be explored. It would seem a wise strategy where possible and appropriate, to aim through therapy to maintain the favourable match between heart and arteries with which we enter life, but begin to lose soon after.

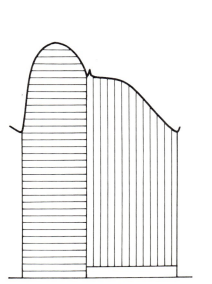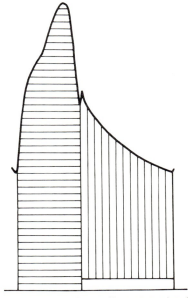

Fig. 12.8 Diagramatic representation of the effects of arterial degeneration (right) on aortic systolic pressure time index (horizontal hatched area) and aortic diastolic pressure time index (vertical hatched area)

REFERENCES

Abboud FM, Huston JH 1961 The effects of ageing and degenerative vascular disease on the measurement of arterial rigidity in man. Journal of Clinical Investigation 40: 933–939

Abramson DI, Turman CA 1961 Aging changes in blood vessels. In: Bourne GH, Wilson EMH Structural aspects of ageing Hafner New York p. 45–59

Bazett HC, Cotton FS, LaPlace LB, Scott JC 1935 The calculation of cardiac output and effective peripheral resistance from blood pressure measurements with an appendix on the size of the aorta in man. American Journal of Physiology 113: 312–334

Berry CL, Greenwald SE, Rivett JF 1975 Static mechanical properties of the developing and mature rat aorta. Cardiovascular Research 9: 669–678

Bramwell JV, Hill AV 1922 Velocity of transmission of the pulse wave and elasticity of arteries. Lancet 1: 891–892

Colandrea MA, Friedman GD, Nichaman MZ, Lynd CN 1970 Systolic hypertension in the elderly. An epidemiological assessment. Circulation 41: 239–245

Cox R 1977 Effects of age on the mechanical properties of rat carotid artery American Journal of Physiology 233: H256–263

Crawford T 1977 Blood and lymph vessels. In: Anderson WAD, Kissane JM (eds) Pathology Mosby St. Louis p. 879–927

Dittmer DS, Grebe RM 1959 Handbook of Circulation Saunders Philadelphia

Fleisch JH, Hooker CS 1976 Relationship between age and relaxation of vascular smooth muscle in rabbit and rat. Circulation Research 38: 243–249

Fowler NO 1979 Diseases of the aorta. In: Cecil Textbook of Medicine p. 1288–1298

Fowler NO 1979 Diseases of the aorta. In: Cecil Textbook of Medicine

Fox H 1933 Arteriosclerosis in lower mammals and birds; its relation to the disease in man. In Cowdrey EV (ed) Arteriosclerosis McMillan New York p. 153–194

Frank O 1905 Der Puls in den Arterien. Zeitschrift fur Biologie 46: 441–553

Frank O 1920 Die Elastizitat der Blutegefasse. Zeitschrift fur Biologie 71:255–272

Frank O 1928 Die Elastizitat der Blutegefasse 11. Zeitschrift fur Biologie 88: 105–118

Freis ED, Heath WC, Luchsinger PC, Snell RE 1966 Changes in the carotid pulse which occur with age and hypertension. American Heart Journal 71: 757–765

Gabe IT, Karnell J, Porje IG, Rudewald B 1964 The measurement of input impedance and apparent phase velocity in the human aorta. Acta Physiologica Scandinavica 61: 73–84

Goldstein S 1971 The biology of aging. New England Journal of Medicine 285: 1120–1129

Gonza EK, Marble AE, Shaw A, Holland JG 1974 Age related changes in the mechanics of the aorta and pulmonary artery of man. Journal of Applied Physiology 36: 407–411

Gray RJ, Handler FP, Blanche JO, Zuckner J, Blumenthal HT 1953 Aging process of aorta and pulmonary artery in negro and white races. Archives of Pathology 56: 238–253

Gresham GA, Howard AN, 1965 Studies on aortic atherosclerosis in the turkey. In: Comparative Atherosclerosis Harper and Row New York p. 62–65

Hallock P, Benson IC 1937 Studies on the elastic properties of human isolated aorta. Journal of Clinical Investigation 15: 595–602

Kannel WB, Gordon T, Schwartz MJ 1971 Systolic versus diastolic blood pressure and risk of coronary heart disease. American Journal of Cardiology 27: 335–345

Kannel WB, Castelli WP, McNamara PM, McKee PA, Feinleib M 1972 Role of blood pressure in the development of congestive heart failure; the Framingham study. New England Journal of Medicine 287: 781–787

Kenner T 1972 Flow and pressure in the arteries. In: Fung YC, Peronne N. Anliker M (Eds) Biomechanics: Its Foundations and Objectives New Jersey Prentice-Hill p. 381–434

Koch–Weser J 1973 The therapeutic challenge of systolic hypertension. New England Journal of Medicine 289: 481–483

Korenchevsky V 1961 Physiological and pathological ageing. Hafner New York p. 409–431

Kroeker EJ, Wood EH 1956 Beat-to-beat alterations in relationship of simultaneously recorded central and peripheral arterial pressure pulses during Valsalva manouver and prolonged expiration in man. Journal of Applied Physiology 8: 483–494

Kurtz HJ 1969 Histological features of atherogenesis and aortic rupture in turkeys. American Journal of Veterinary Research 30: 243–249

Lakatta EG 1980 Age-related alterations in the cardiovascular response to adrenergic mediated stress. Federation Proceedings 39: 3173–3177

Learoyd BM, Taylor MG 1966 Alterations with age in the viscoelastic properties of human arterial walls. Circulation Research 18: 278–292

Mackenzie J 1902 The study of the pulse. McMillan Edinburgh

Milch RA 1965 Matrix properties of the ageing arterial wall. Monographs of the Surgical Sciences 2: 261–341

Mitchell JRA, Schwartz CJ 1965 Arterial disease. Oxford Blackwell

Moritz AR, Oldt MR 1937 Arteriolar sclerosis in hypertensives and non-hypotensives. American Journal of Pathology 13: 679–728

Moschcowitz E 1949 The association of capillary sclerosis with arteriosclerosis and phlebosclerosis. Its pathogenesis and clinical significance. Annals of Internal Medicine 30: 1156–1158

Moschcowitz E 1950 Hyperplastic arteriosclerosis versus atherosclerosis. Journal of the American Medical Association 143: 861–865

Murgo JP, Westerhof N, Giolma JP, Altobelli SA 1980 Aortic input impedance in normal man; relationship to pressure waveshapes. Circulation 62: 105–116

Nakashima T, Tanikawa J 1971 A study of human aortic distensibility with relation to atherosclerosis and aging. Angiology 22: 477–490

Newman D, Lallemand R 1978 The effect of age on the distensibility of the abdominal aorta of man. Surgery Gynecology and Obstetrics 147: 211–214

Nichols WW, Conti CR, Walker WW, Milnor WR 1977 Input impedance of the systemic circulation in man. Circulation Research 40: 451–458

O'Rourke MF 1967 Steady and pulsatile energy losses in the

systemic circulation under normal conditions and in simulated arterial disease. Cardiovascular Research 1: 313–326

O'Rourke MF, Avolio AP 1980 Pulsatile flow and pressure in human systemic arteries; studies in man and in a multi–branched model of the human systemic arterial tree. Circulation Research 46: 363–372

Pagani M, Mirsky I, Baig H, Manders P, Kerkhof P, Vatner SF 1979 Effects of age on aortic pressure-diameter and elastic stiffness-stress relationships in unanesthetised sheep. Circulation Research 44: 420–429

Page IH 1974 Arterial hypertension in retrospect. Circulation Research 34: 133–142

Patel DJ, Greenfield JC, Austen WG, Morrow AG, Fry DL 1965 Pressure–flow relationships in the ascending aorta and femoral artery of man. Journal of Applied Physiology 20: 459–463

Pickering GW 1968 High blood pressure. Churchill London

Porjé IG 1967 The energy design of the human circulatory system. Proceedings, Seventh International Conference on Medical and Biological Engineering Stockholm p. 153

Puls RJ, Heizer KW 1967 Pulse wave changes with aging. Journal of the American Geriatrics Society 15: 153–165

Remington JW, Noback CR, Hamilton WF, Gold JJ 1948 Volume–elasticity characteristics of the human aorta and prediction of the stroke volume from the pressure pulse. American Journal of Physiology 153: 298–308

Rohde E 1910 Zeitschrift fur Physiologische Chemie 68: 181 (quoted by Bramwell and Hill, 1922)

Roy CS 1880 The elastic properties of the arterial wall. Journal of Physiology (London) 3: 125–159

Schimmler W 1965 Untersuchungen zum Elastizitaetsproblem der Aorta (Statistische Korrelation der Pulswellengeschwindigkeit zu Alter, Geschlecht und Blutdruck). Archiv KreislForsch 47: 189–233

Schwartz CJ, Wethessen NT, Wolf S. 1980 Structure and function of the Circulation. New York Plenum

Sen S, Tarazi RC, Bumpus M 1981 Reversal of cardiac hypertrophy in renal hypertensive rats: medical vs surgical therapy. American Journal of Physiology 240: H408–H412

Simon AC, Safar ME, Levenson JA, Kheder AM, Levy BI 1979 Systolic hypertension; hemodynamic mechanism and choice of antihypertensive treatment. American Journal of Cardiology 44: 505–511

Smith TW, Braunwald E 1980 The management of heart failure. In: Heart Disease Braunwald E (ed.) Philadelphia Saunders p. 509–570

Stehbens WE 1979 Hemodynamics and the blood vessel wall. Thomas Springfield

Templeton GH, Platt MR, Willerson JT, Weisfeldt ML 1979 Influence of aging on left ventricular hemodynamics and stiffness in beagles. Circulation Research 44: 189–194

Weisfeldt M 1980 Aging of the cardiovascular system. New England Journal of Medicine 303: 1172–1174

Weisfeldt ML 1980 Research on aging in Weisfeldt ML (Ed) The Aging Heart New York Raven

White PD 1952 The heart and great vessels in old age. In: Cowdrey's Problems of ageing. Williams and Wilkins Baltimore p. 277–289

Wood P 1968 Diseases of the heart and circulation. London Dyre and Spottiswoode p. 71

Yin F 1980 The aging vasculature and its effects on the heart in Weisfeldt ML (Ed) The Aging Heart. Its function and response to stress. New York Raven

Yin F, Milnor WR, Weisfeldt ML 1981 Role of aortic input impedance in the decreased cardiovascular response to exercise with aging in dogs. Journal of Clinical Investigation 68: 28–38

13

Disease of major arteries

AORTIC COARCTATION

In simple post ductal aortic coarctation, the descending thoracic aorta is narrowed or occluded immediately beyond the origin of the left subclavian artery and blood flow is channelled through large collateral branches of the subclavian and intercostal arteries into the aorta beyond this obstruction. Though most obviously an obstructive lesion, the clinical features of aortic coarctation are primarily a consequence of altered arterial hemodynamics in the upper part of the body, not of reduced blood flow to the lower part. It has been standard practice in the past to relate these hemodynamic abnormalities in the upper part of the body to 'hypertension', though it is recognised that this condition is more sinister in its prognosis than essential hypertension of equal severity (Pickering 1968, Wood 1968, Campbell 1970).

Aortic coarctation is best considered in terms of its effects on conduit and cushioning function of the arterial system, through separate consideration of steady pressure and flow phenomena, and of pulsatile pressure and flow phenomena. When this is done, a relatively simple picture emerges that explains changes in arterial pressure on each side of the coarctation, and that provides a logical view of mechanisms determining complications, and principles of optimal management.

Hemodynamic alterations

Figure 13.1 shows changes in arterial pressure in the ascending aorta and femoral artery when, under acute conditions, the proximal descending aorta is progressively narrowed. These data, taken from Gupta and Wiggers (1951) are similar to

those in Chapter 5 and show a fall in mean pressure and in pulse pressure beyond the obstruction when the aorta is progressively narrowed. This is not a good simulation however, of the clinical condition, because in this, blood flow to the lower part of the body is maintained at near normal levels (Lewis 1933, Patterson et al 1957, Taylor and Donald 1960) – at rest and during exercise – through many large dilated collateral vessels. Because of the presence of these collateral vessels,

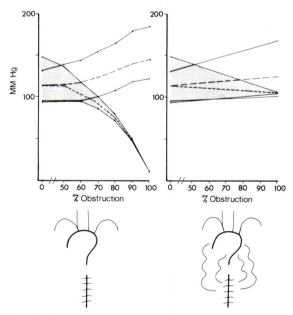

Fig. 13.1 The effects of graded occlusion of the descending thoracic aorta on systolic, diastolic and mean pressure immediately above and immediately below the obstruction. Dashed line indicates mean pressure above, and dotted line mean pressure below the obstruction. The shaded area indicates pulse pressure immediately below the coarctation. Left panel: No collateral vessels. Right panel: Plentiful collaterals

mean pressure below the coarctation (even when the aorta is totally obstructed) is far greater than that seen under acute conditions, and is usually within normal limits (Bing et al 1948, Fuller et al 1952, Pickering 1968, Fig. 13.2). While mean arterial pressure is maintained at or near normal, pulse pressure is markedly reduced beyond the coarctation, as a result of attenuation of the pulse in travel through the long, tortuous and narrow collateral vessels (p. 135). The influence of abundant collateral vessels in aortic coarctation on mean pressure and on pulse pressure is illustrated diagrammatically in the right panel of Figure 13.1. The presence of collateral vessels causes mean pressure to fall only slightly in arteries below the coarctation, and to rise only slightly in the arteries above. The collaterals however have a great effect on pulsatile phenomena so that pulsatile pressure is markedly attenuated below the coarctation (in the same way as when this is induced acutely) and augmented above. In terms of conduit and cushioning function of the arterial system, one can say that the collateral vessels provide almost complete compensation for abnormal conduit function, but little or no compensation for altered cushioning function.

Figure 13.1 illustrates the changes in mean and pulsatile pressure that would be expected in the presence of abundant collateral vessels. Figure 13.3 shows the pressure waves one would expect to record above and below the coarctation in patients with different degrees of collateral development. The adequacy of collaterals determines the extent of fall in mean pressure while the presence of coarctation and of collateral vessels appears to reduce pulse pressure to much the same extent in all. Such an explanation accounts easily for the change in mean level and amplitude of the pressure wave below the coarctation, and so for the systolic and diastolic pressures. The explanation is not so obvious when one considers systolic and diastolic pressures only, and seeks to account separately for differences in systolic pressure above and below the coarctation and of diastolic pressure above and below. It is clear that in the presence of abundant collaterals, diastolic pressure may be higher below the coarctation than above (Fig. 13.3). In the past, this occasional finding has been a source of confusion to clinicians, shackled as they are (or were) to the sphygmomanometer and to the notion that diastolic pressure is the sole indicator of arterial hypertension. The finding of a higher than normal diastolic pressure below the coarctation in many patients was the source of the theory that there is generalised arteriolar vasocon-

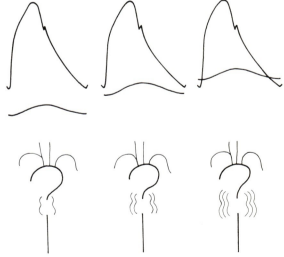

Fig. 13.3 Diagramatic representation of different degrees of collateral development on arterial pressure waves above and below an obstruction in the descending thoracic aorta. When collaterals are poorly developed, both systolic and diastolic pressures are lower beyond the obstruction. When collaterals are well developed, diastolic pressure may be higher beyond the obstruction

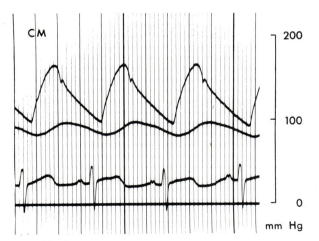

Fig. 13.2 Pressure waves recorded simultaneously in the aortic arch (above) and lower thoracic aorta (below) in a 9 year old boy with uncomplicated postductal aortic coarctation. From O'Rourke and Cartmill (1971) with permission, American Heart Association Inc.

striction in aortic coarctation (Steele 1941), and is still frequently quoted to support the theory that a renal mechanism is partly responsible for hypertension in this condition (Goldblatt and Kahn 1933, Habib and Nanson 1968, Pickering 1968).

While there is some evidence that hypertension in coarctation is partly based on a renal mechanism, and that such a mechanism may be responsible for the frequency of unexplained residual hypertension (around 15 percent according to Nanton and Olley 1976) following surgical correction, this has been disputed (Bing et al 1948, Patterson et al 1957, Pickering 1968) and in any case is not the major issue in determining complications of coarctation. Preoccupation with diastolic pressure, hypertension, and rival theories of hypertension in aortic coarctation (Goldblatt and Kahn 1938, Steele 1941, Bing et al 1948, Gupta and Wiggers 1951, Habib and Nanson 1968, Pickering 1968) appears to have diverted attention from the real problem – that only one third of the whole arterial system is able to act as the cushion to intermittent left ventricular ejection (Taylor and Donald 1960, O'Rourke and Cartmill 1971, Fig. 13.4).

Pressure pulse contour

When the proximal descending aorta is acutely occluded, the contour of the ascending aortic pressure pulse is considerably altered, with increase in pressure during the latter part of systole and disappearance of the diastolic pressure wave (p. 106, Gupta and Wiggers 1951). The pressure wave in acute aortic obstruction resembles that seen in hypertension (p. 215) and arterial degeneration (p. 137) and can be explained on the same basis – early return of wave reflection summating with pressure during systole and so augmenting the systolic peak. In contrast to hypertension and arterial degeneration however, early wave reflection arises from an abnormal site (the coarctation itself) close to the heart whereas in the other two conditions reflected waves return early from normally placed sites (the peripheral arterioles) because of increased pulse wave velocity (Fig. 13.4)

Because of the absence of collateral vessels, acute aortic obstruction is not strictly comparable with the clinical condition of aortic coarctation. Nonetheless the proximal aortic pressure wave in chronic experimental coarctation

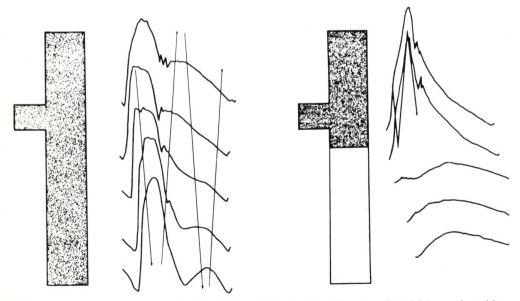

Fig. 13.4 Model of the normal arterial system (left) and the arterial system in aortic coarctation (right), together with pressure waves recorded in a normal dog (left) and in a dog with aortic coarctation (right) at points corresponding to their position in the respective model. Superimposed on the waves are lines with arrows, which show the impulse generated by ventricular ejection passing back and forth over the arterial system at the velocity of the pulse (approximately 6 m sec^{-1}). It is shown that contour of the waves is attributable to summation of incident and reflected components. From O'Rourke and Cartmill (1971) with permission American Heart Association Inc.

(Fig. 13.5), and in patients with coarctation (Fig. 13.2) is exactly the same as in acute aortic constriction. The only difference is that mean pressure is lower than when the aorta is acutely obstructed. These findings support the view that collateral vessels restore steady flow and so maintain adequate conduit function, while the coarctation itself is responsible for alterations in pulsatile phenomena in upper body arteries.

The pressure wave in Figure 13.2 is typical of the pressure waves recorded in the ascending aorta of patients (even children) with aortic coarctation. O'Rourke and Cartmill (1971) found evidence of a diastolic wave in only one of 27 young patients with aortic coarctation. Children and young adults almost always exhibit a diastolic wave in the proximal aorta (p. 144, O'Rourke et al 1968). Absence of a diastolic pressure wave in the ascending aorta or in peripheral arteries of children and young adults is quite abnormal and is suggestive of coarctation, hypertension, or premature arterial degeneration.

Change in contour of the arterial pressure wave in aortic coarctation can be explained on the basis of early return of wave reflection, with summation of primary and subsequent echos with the incident wave (Fig. 13.4). Alternatively one can look at these phenomena in terms of smaller volume-distensibility of the arterial system (p. 211), and by likening this to a *Windkessel* of reduced dimensions. The two explanations amount to the same thing.

Vascular impedance

Figure 13.6 shows ascending aortic impedance in three control dogs (left) and in three litter mates in whom aortic coarctation had been induced three months previously. The first minimum of impedance modulus has been attributed to wave reflection from the lower part of the body (p. 106, O'Rourke and Taylor 1967). This minimum is, predictably, lost in the dogs with coarctation, so that impedance modulus is considerably higher up

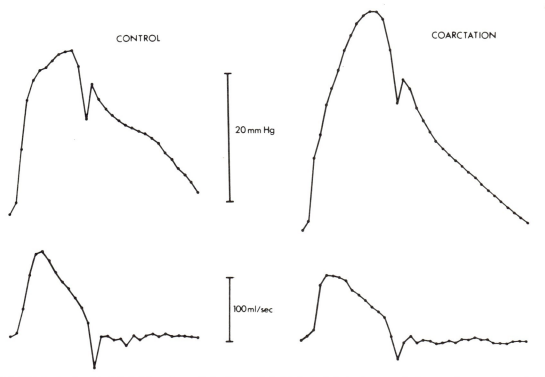

Fig. 13.5 Pressure waves (above) and flow waves (below) recorded simultaneously in the ascending aorta of a normal dog (left) and in a litter mate with surgically induced aortic coarctation (right). From O'Rourke and Cartmill (1971) with permission American Heart Association Inc.

to 8 Hz than under normal conditions. Alteration of impedance spectra in coarctation is responsible for the higher amplitude and altered contour of the ascending aortic pressure wave, and for mismatch between aortic impedance and ventricular ejection. Figure 13.7 shows impedance spectra in two of these dogs together with moduli of the first 5–6 harmonics of the ventricular ejection wave.

The favourable relationship between impedance minima and harmonic content of the left ventricular ejection wave (p. 154) is lost in the dogs with aortic coarctation. No data on ascending aortic impedance in patients with aortic coarctation are presently available, but the ventricular ejection wave and ascending aortic pressure wave are known to be similar to those in dogs with chronically induced aortic coarctation (Porjé 1967, O'Rourke and Cartmill 1971). One would expect ascending aortic impedance spectra in humans with coarctation to show the same features as dogs.

Pulsatile external heart work

The mismatch between heart and vascular system in aortic coarctation is apparent as an increase in the pulsatile component of external left ventricular work. This (p. 157) represents energy lost in vascular pulsations – principally in the large arteries and in coarctation, within the long tortuous collateral vessels as well. In the young dogs with experimentally induced chronic coarctation reported by O'Rourke and Cartmill (1971), the ratio of pulsatile to total (steady plus pulsatile) external left ventricular work increased to 7.3 percent from 4.1 percent in control litter mates. The change was not as great as one might have predicted on the basis of impedance modulus alone, since the accompanying alteration in impedance phase led to a lesser increase in the in-phase component of impedance (which determines the magnitude of pulsatile external heart work (p. 154)) than the impedance modulus itself. As described elsewhere

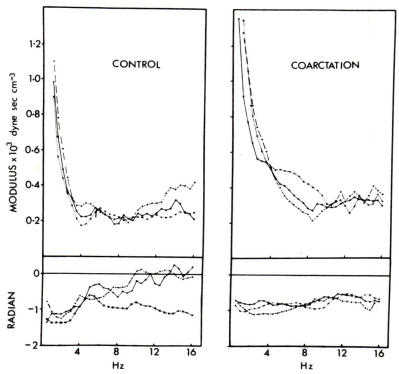

Fig. 13.6 Input impedance to the systemic circulation in three normal dogs (left) and in three litter mates with aortic coarctation (right). From O'Rourke and Cartmill (1971) with permission American Heart Association Inc.

(p. 162) however, the impedance modulus is a better guide than in-phase impedance of the amplitude of aortic systolic pressure, and so of total heart work and left ventricular load and oxygen requirement.

Porjé (1967) measured the steady and pulsatile components of external left ventricular work in two patients with aortic coarctation, and found that the ratio of pulsatile to total work was considerably higher (24 and 37 percent) than in patients with normal arterial systems where the value was 10–17, mean 14 percent.

Changes of arterial pressure with exercise

Murgo et al (1980) have studied the effects of exercise on arterial hemodynamics in the ascending aorta of patients with apparently normal vascular trees. They have shown that mild supine exercise causes no significant alteration in the frequency dependent components of impedance even though it leads to reduction in the resistive term. There is no reason to believe that ascending aortic impedance in aortic coarctation behaves differently. Murgo et al found that the first five harmonics of the ventricular ejection wave are approximately doubled in mild supine exercise when cardiac output is doubled, and that this leads to a similar increase in aortic pressure moduli, and so, near doubling of the aortic pressure pulse. If one applies the same considerations to the nine year old boy whose pressure wave is shown in Figure 13.2

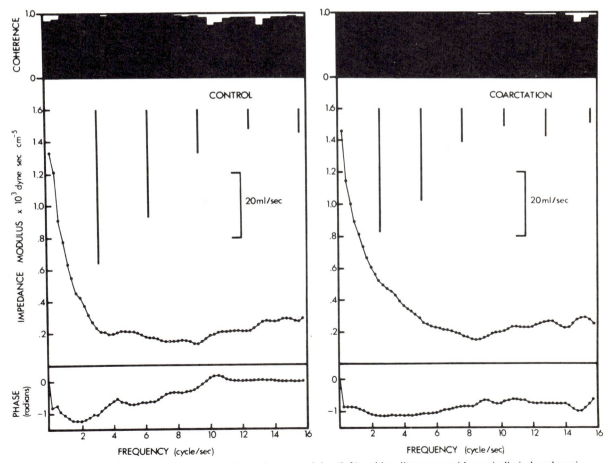

Fig. 13.7 Input impedance to the systemic circulation in a normal dog (left) and in a litter mate with surgically induced aortic coarctation (right). Bars indicate amplitude of the first five to six harmonics of the flow wave in the ascending aorta. From O'Rourke and Cartmill (1971) with permission American Heart Association Inc.

and if one allows the same increase in mean pressure as found by Murgo et al in normal subjects – around 14 mm Hg – (which probably underestimates the rise in coarctation) one can calculate that with mild supine exercise, this child would generate a pressure wave of amplitude 135 mm Hg and a peak systolic pressure of over 230 mm Hg in the ascending aorta. Strenuous exercise would be expected to cause correspondingly greater pressure fluctuations and peaks.

Taylor and Donald (1960) drew attention to the dramatic increases in brachial artery pressure that occur during exercise in patients with aortic coarctation, and showed that these are far greater than seen in patients with severe essential hypertension who would be considered to require urgent medical therapy and restriction of activity (Fig. 13.8). These authors also pointed out that such changes in pressure usually occur without symptoms (although they can induce cardiac failure), with moderate exertion only and in patients otherwise asymptomatic, and who usually have had no advice to reduce their activities. These pressure increases are precisely what one would expect from reduction in cushioning capacity of the arterial system. Their potential damaging effects on the heart and arteries were stressed by Taylor and Donald, and by others (O'Rourke and Cartmill 1971, Maron et al 1973, Nanton and Olley 1976), and will be discussed further below.

Pathophysiology

In aortic coarctation, conduit function of the arterial system is preserved, while cushioning function is markedly disturbed, with unusually high pressure fluctuations being generated in the proximal aorta and upper body arteries by normal left ventricular ejection. The most apparent pathological features of this condition (apart from the coarctation itself) are cardiac hypertrophy and pronounced degenerative changes in the proximal aorta and upper body arteries. These degenerative changes include thinning, splitting, and fragmentation of elastic fibres and laminae, mucoid degeneration of the aortic media and development of aneurysms in the Circle of Willis and within the brain substance itself. These pathological features are similar to those seen with ageing, and in hypertension, (Glynn 1940, Davis and Fisher

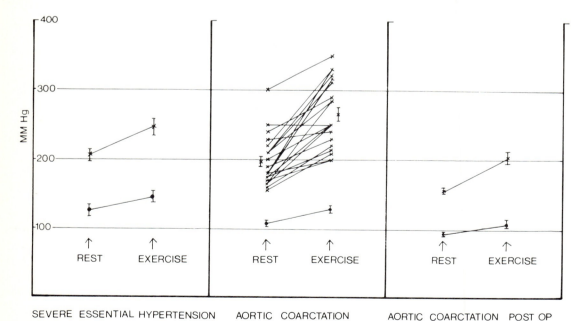

Fig. 13.8 Systolic and diastolic pressures in the brachial artery at rest and during exercise of similar intensity in a group of patients with severe essential hypertension (left), patients with aortic coarctation (centre), and patients with surgically corrected aortic coarctation (right). Individual values are shown for systolic pressure in all patients with coarctation. Other values are mean ± 1 SEM. Figure prepared from data published by Taylor and Donald (1960)

1943, Refenstein et al 1947, Blumenthal et al 1954, Pickering 1968, Stehbens 1979), but occur at a much earlier age, and are attributable (as are those of ageing (p. 188) and hypertension (p. 216) to fatigue and damage of structural components of the arterial wall as a result of repeated high pulsatile stresses over a long period of time. These pathological changes in the heart and arteries are the basis of the lethal complications of aortic coarctation – subarachnoid hemorrhage, cerebral hemorrhage, aortic rupture and cardiac failure; abnormally high stresses on the (often bicuspid) aortic valves and at the coarctation itself probably also contribute to the development of endocarditis and endarteritis at these sites. These complications of aortic coarctation are the most common causes of death, which usually in 'simple' aortic coarctation occurs before age 40 (Wood 1968, Campbell 1970, Fig. 13.9). Onset of these complications is often abrupt, in a patient previously asymptomatic, but autopsy almost invariably shows the presence of gross arterial degeneration and of cardiac hypertrophy (Pickering 1968, Stehbens 1979).

Aortic coarctation is a sinister condition with an ominous prognosis. Patients usually appear quite normal until disaster strikes, and the main manifestation of the disorder is elevation of blood pressure in the upper part of the body. Since, in the past, the ill effects of coarctation were deemed to result from 'hypertension', and 'hypertension'

was gauged on the basis of diastolic blood pressure level (which is less altered in aortic coarctation than systolic or pulse pressure), operation was often deferred while the arterial system was literally being 'ripped to pieces'. Misunderstanding of the pathophysiology of this condition is evident in textbooks published as recently as 1968 when Paul Wood stated that 'Surgical repair should only be advised when the blood pressure is at least moderately elevated' (a moderate elevation being defined by Wood as diastolic pressure 110–125 or systolic pressure 180–230) 'since nothing is gained by restoring the course of the blood flow *ipso facto*'. The presence of aortic coarctation is now generally agreed as an indication for surgery (Hartman et al 1977, Keith 1978, Kirklin and Pacifico 1978), and the only point of contention seems to be how early in childhood this should be performed (Maron et al 1973, Nanton and Olley 1976). Improvement in operative mortality, and appreciation that degenerative arterial lesions are a consequence of longstanding high arterial stresses have led to progressive decrease in the recommended age at which the defect is to be repaired. In addition it is now appreciated that the residual hypertension after surgical repair and the late complications after surgery depend on the age at which this is performed (Maron et al 1973, Nanton and Olley 1976, Keith 1978). From the pathophysiological viewpoint alone, one would

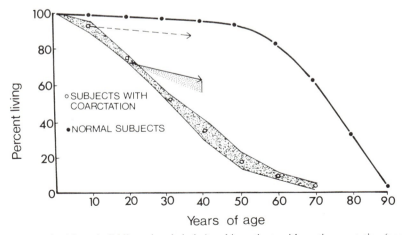

Fig. 13.9 Life tables in normal subjects (solid line, closed circles) and in patients with aortic coarctation (open circles, with steppled area), after Campbell (1970). The solid line with arrow indicates improvement in survival after surgical correction of coarctation, as described by Maron et al (1973). The shaded area below this line indicates the possible lower survival if patients lost to follow-up in this survey had died. The dashed line with arrow indicates the hopefully better prognosis in patients operated on electively at an earlier age

think that the earlier corrective surgery is performed, the better. The arguments presented here support Keith's recommendation that elective surgery be undertaken at 4–7 years.

Effects of surgery in aortic coarctation

Repair of aortic coarctation involves resection and end-to-end anastomosis or resection with patch or conduit grafting. The operation carries an appreciable risk, even now, because of the abundant collateral vessels in the chest wall and about the anastomosis site, and because of the friable nature of the degenerate aorta when the condition has persisted into adolescence. The post-operative course of this condition is sometimes characterised by two interesting complications. The first of these is reactive hypertension which is probably due to altered baroreceptor activity (March 1960, Keith 1978), and frequently requires hypotensive therapy for several days. The second, rarely seen now that blood pressure is well controlled post operatively is acute arterial and arteriolar damage and necrosis which are attributable to excessive stresses on and fracture of elastic fibres, laminae, and muscle fibres in atrophic lower body arteries and arterioles (Benson and Sealy 1956, Pickering 1968, Keith 1978). The relationship of this condition to fibrinoid necrosis in malignant hypertension is discussed on page 217. Like the arterial degeneration in upper body arteries, this condition is attributable to excessive and damaging stresses on the arterial wall, but in this case, applied acutely, and in vessels structurally weak, and so, more easily damaged, even by normal or only slightly elevated pressures.

Repair of aortic coarctation is usually curative, with reduction of arterial pressure in the upper body (Fig. 13.10), return of normal femoral pulses, regression of collateral vessels, and decrease or disappearance of electrocardiographic evidence of left ventricular hypertrophy (Wright et al 1956, Taylor and Donald 1960, Simon and Zloto 1974, Maron et al 1973, Keith 1978). However, residual problems often remain, especially in patients undergoing surgery after childhood. These problems are attributable to aortic narrowing at the site of the original coarctation –

due to problems at surgery or to growth of the child with non-growth of the anastomosis – and to persistence of degenerative changes caused by the coarctation before operative repair. Systemic hypertension (systolic rather than diastolic) is more common than in the normal population, and was found by Nanton and Olley (1976) in 24 percent of patients operated on at the Toronto Hospital for Sick Children, and by Maron et al (1973) in approximately 40 percent of patients undergoing surgery (usually at an older age) at the Johns Hopkins Hospital. An unusually high increase in systolic pressure during exercise was noted by Taylor and Donald (1960) (see also Fig. 13.8), and by James and Kaplan (1974), even in patients whose resting arterial pressures were normal. In their detailed long term follow up, Maron et al (1973) noted a very high incidence of premature cardiovascular disease and cardiovascular death in patients who had undergone aortic coarctectomy.

It is likely that with improved surgical techniques, early diagnosis and surgery, and with reoperation where necessary, that there will be further improvement in the results of corrective surgery for aortic coarctation. Since changes in the attitudes to surgery have only come about in the last 10–15 years, such long term benefits – if present – may not become evident for some years to come.

Clinical implications in management of aortic coarctation

Attention has been directed here to the abnormal cushioning function of the arterial system in aortic coarctation as the cause of asymptomatic arterial degeneration and cardiac hypertrophy, and of early death from the effects of these. It has been pointed out that abnormal cushioning function may accompany quite modest gradients (less than 10 mm Hg) of mean pressure between proximal and distal aorta, and that diastolic pressure in upper body arteries is a poor guide to the significance of coarctation. The importance of assessing pressure change during exercise has been stressed, as has the importance of restricting exertion when pressure changes are great. Early operative correction of aortic coarctation has been advised (even if reoperation has to be undertaken during adolescence) in order to prevent the relentless progression of arterial degeneration which is the basis of early death in this condition, and of late complications, even after corrective surgery.

ATHEROSCLEROSIS

The effects of atherosclerosis on conduit function of arteries was discussed in Chapter 5. Concern

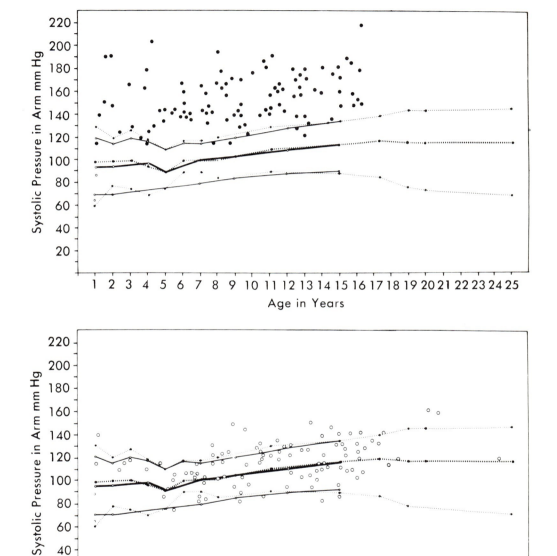

Fig. 13.10 Systolic pressures in the arm before surgery (top) and at the last follow up (bottom) in 95 young patients after correction of aortic coarctation. The mean ± standard deviation lines represent values from a normal population. Eighty percent of patients after operation have pressures within the normal limits (from Keith, 1978 in: Heart Disease in Infancy and Childhood, Macmillan.)

with conduit function, and with effects on organs and tissues downstream from an obstructive lesion has dominated thinking in studies of arterial hemodynamics. There have been no systematic studies performed on the effects of atherosclerosis on cushioning function of arteries. However, studies of pulsatile arterial hemodynamics in man have included patients with known atherosclerosis in the coronary arteries and elsewhere (O'Rourke et al 1968, Nichols et al 1977); patients considered 'normal' in other studies have undoubtedly included many with asymptomatic atherosclerosis affecting the aorta and major arteries.

Although no specific data are available, the effects of atherosclerosis on cushioning function of the arterial system are predictable, and would be expected to affect the arteries and heart in the same way as the medial degeneration of aging (discussed in Ch. 12) and (though to a lesser degree) aortic coarctation. In atherosclerosis (p. 225) there is patchy thickening of the aortic and arterial intima, associated with focal degeneration of elastic tissue and deposition of fibrous tissue and sometimes calcium as well. Affected segments of artery

lose their distensibility and usually impinge on the lumen as well. The decrease in distensibility and thickening of the wall lead to an increase in pulse wave velocity (p. 41) and an impedance mismatch with adjoining segments of normal artery (p. 88). The net effects of atherosclerosis are increase in overall pulse wave velocity in the systemic arterial tree, and creation of new reflecting sites closer to the heart than the peripheral arterioles which normally are responsible for reflection of the arterial pulse. Patients with atherosclerosis predictably show evidence of early return to wave reflection, with increase in the frequency of ascending aortic impedance minima (Nichols et al 1977, Fig. 13.11), and presence of a late systolic peak with absence of diastolic fluctuation in the proximal aortic pressure wave (O'Rourke et al 1968). With decreased distensibility of the proximal aorta and major arteries, characteristic impedance in the proximal aorta is also increased (Fig. 13.11, Nichols et al 1977).

Through its effects on wave velocity and wave reflection, atherosclerosis affects the arteries and heart in the same way as medial degeneration and

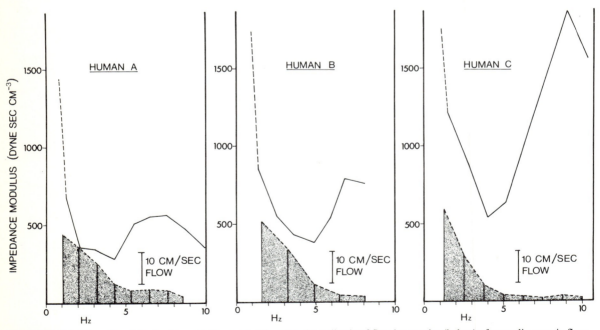

Fig. 13.11 Impedance modulus in the ascending aorta (above) and amplitude of flow harmonics (below) of ascending aortic flow waves in three groups of human subjects – A, no known cardiac or vascular disease, B. subjects with known atherosclerosis and C, subjects with hypertension and known atherosclerosis. Modulus plotted in terms of linear flow velocity. Rearranged from data of Nichols et al (1977). Contrast with Fig. 10.1.

aortic coarctation. Since, however, a vessel as large as the descending aorta is never occluded by atherosclerosis, the detrimental effects of new reflecting sites would never be as pronounced as in aortic coarctation.

Atherosclerosis thus adversely affects the heart by increasing systolic pressure – so increasing myocardial blood need (p. 166), and tending to reduce ventricular ejection (p. 164), and by reducing aortic pressure during cardiac diastole (so reducing coronary perfusion pressure and facilitating development of myocardial ischemia) (p. 166). Atherosclerosis adversely affects the arteries themselves by increasing the peak and pulse pressure, so increasing stresses in the aortic wall and hastening further damage and degeneration (p. 216).

PATENT DUCTUS ARTERIOSUS AND ARTERIOVENOUS FISTULA

There have been no studies reported on the effects of patent ductus arteriosus on pulsatile arterial hemodynamics in the proximal aorta of humans. In the presence of such shunts, left ventricular output and stroke volume are increased, perhaps up to three times normal, and pulse pressure is increased to a similar degree as stroke volume. The contour of the aortic pressure wave in this condition has no specific features, and a diastolic wave appears to be present with the same frequency as in normal subjects. There are no specific arterial complications that can be attributed to altered arterial dynamics (although one might expect that with high pulse pressure, arterial degeneration would be hastened), and, in patients surviving infancy without problems, left ventricular function is usually well preserved. The heart can tolerate a volume load far better than a pressure load (Wood 1968).

Mang (1976) and Mang et al (1976) attempted to simulate the clinical condition of patent ductus arteriosus in dogs by creating an acute shunt between the aortic arch and right atrium. When the shunt was opened, peripheral resistance fell, and stroke volume, peak left ventricular ejection velocity, and pulse pressure all increased to a similar degree (Fig. 13.12) but there was no alteration in contour of the left ventricular ejection wave or of the aortic pressure wave, and no consistent change at all in ascending aortic impedance (Fig. 13.13).

The impedance spectra and pressure wave patterns in dogs with arterio-venous shunts are quite different to those seen when cardiac output is increased and peripheral resistance reduced by peripheral vasodilation. During vasodilation (p. 108, Fig. 8.16, O'Rourke and Taylor 1966, 1967, O'Rourke and Avolio 1981) there is decrease in oscillation of impedance modulus and phase, and decrease in amplitude of the diastolic pressure wave in the ascending aorta. These changes with vasodilation are attributable to decrease in

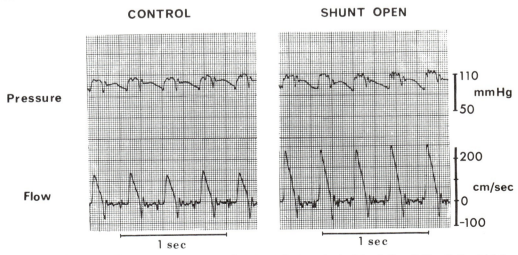

Fig. 13.12 Pressure (above) and flow (below) in the ascending aorta of an anesthetised dog before (left) and after (right) opening a shunt between aortic arch and right atrium. From Mang (1976)

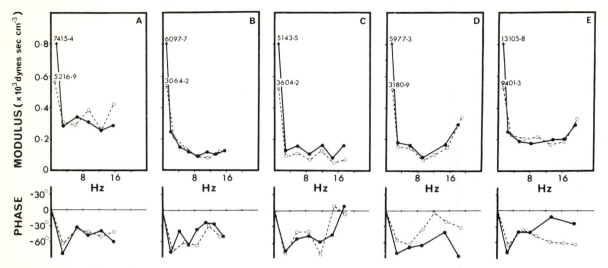

Fig. 13.13 Ascending aortic impedance in five dogs before (closed circles, solid lines) and after (open circles, dashed lines) opening a shunt between aortic arch and right atrium. From Mang (1976)

peripheral reflection coefficient, and so to lesser influence of wave reflection on impedance spectra and pressure wave patterns in the proximal aorta. In arteriovenous shunt, peripheral reflection is unchanged, but a new abnormal 'open end' reflecting site is created close to the heart. It appears that abnormal wave reflection at this site occurs too early to be apparent in the aortic pressure wave, and at too high a frequency to be apparent in impedance spectra.

The trivial effects of simulated patent ductus arteriosus on arterial cushioning function contrast with the gross effects of altered arterial distensibility and of aortic obstruction.

Clearly, the types of study described here are in their infancy, but data already available suggest that this approach may provide satisfactory explanations for, and new insights into, the differing effects of major arterial disease on arterial function and cardiac performance. Extension of the techniques applied by Mills et al (1970), Nichols et al (1977), and Murgo et al (1980, 1981) to these clinical problems is awaited with interest.

REFERENCES

Abbott M 1928 Statistical study and historical retrospect of 200 recorded cases with autopsy, of stenosis or obliteration of the descending arch. American Heart Journal 3: 392–421; 574–618

Benson WR, Sealy WC 1956 Arterial necrosis following resection of coarctation of the aorta. Laboratory Investigation 5: 359–376

Bing RJ, Handelsman JC, Campbell JA, Griswold HE, Blalock A 1948 The surgical treatment and pathophysiology of coarctation of the aorta. Annals of Surgery 128: 803–824

Blumenthal HT, Handler FP, Blache JO 1954 The histogenesis of arteriosclerosis of the larger cerebral arteries with an analysis of the importance of mechanical factors. American Journal of Medicine 17: 337–347

Campbell M 1968 Natural history of persistent ductus arteriosus. British Heart Journal 30: 4–13

Campbell M 1970 Natural history of coarctation of the aorta. British Heart Journal 32: 633–640

Davies JNP, Fisher JA 1943 Coarctation of the aorta, double mitral AV orifice, and leaking cerebral aneurysm. British Heart Journal 5: 197–204

Eliakim M, Sapoznikov D, Weinman J 1971 Pulse wave velocity in healthy subjects and in patients with various disease states. American Heart Journal 82: 448–457

Farrar DJ, Green HD, Gene Bond MG, Wagner WD, Gobbee RA 1978 Aortic pulse wave velocity, elasticity, and composition in a nonhuman primate model of atherosclerosis. Circulation Research 43: 52–62

Farrar DJ, Green HD, Wagner WD, Bond MG 1980 Reduction in pulse wave velocity and improvement in aortic distensibility accompanying regression of atherosclerosis in the rhesus monkey. Circulation Research 47: 425–432

Fuller J. Taylor BE, Clagett OT, Wood EH 1952 Blood pressure in the aorta during resection and repair of coarctation of the aorta. Journal of Laboratory and Clinical Medicine 39: 10–25

Glynn LE 1940 Medial defects in circle of Willis and their relation to aneurysm formation. Journal of Pathology and Bacteriology 51: 213–222

Goldblatt H, Kahn JR 1938 Experimental hypertension: Constriction of the aorta at various levels. Journal of the American Medical Association 110: p. 686

Gross RE 1950 Coarctation of the aorta; surgical treatment of one hundred cases. Circulation 1: 41–55

Gunn GC, Dobson HL, Gray J, Geddes LA, Vallbona C 1965 Studies of pulse wave velocity in potential diabetic subjects. Diabetes 14: 489–492

Gupta TC, Wiggers CJ 1951 Basic hemodynamic changes produced by aortic coarctation of different degrees. Circulation 3: 17–31

Habib WK, Nanson EM 1968 The causes of hypertension in coarctation of the aorta. Annals of Surgery 168: 771–778

Hamilton WF, Abbott ME 1928 Coarctation of the aorta of the adult type. American Heart Journal: 4: 381–392

Hartmann AF, Goldring D, Strauss AW, Hernandez A, McKnight RC, Weldon CS 1977 Coarctation of the aorta. In: Moss AJ, Adams FH, Emmanouilides GC (eds) Heart Disease in Infancy, Childhood and Adolescence Williams and Wilkins Baltimore p. 199–209

Heath D, Edwards JE 1959 Configuration of elastic tissue of aortic media in aortic coarctation. American Heart Journal 57: 29–35

James FW, Kaplan S 1974 Systolic hypertension during submaximal exercise after correction of coarctation of the aorta. Circulation 50 (Supplement 2): 27–34

Keith JD 1978 Coarctation of the aorta. In: Keith JD, Rowe RD, Vlad P (eds) Heart Disease in Infancy and Childhood New York McMillan p. 736–760.

Kirklin JW, Pacifico AD 1978 Surgical treatment of congenital heart disease. In: Hurst JW (ed) The Heart, Arteries and Veins McGraw New York p. 901–946

Magarey FR, Stehbens WE, Sharp A 1959 Effects of experimental coarctation of the aorta on the blood pressure of sheep. Circulation Research 7: 147–151

Malinow MR 1980 Atherosclerosis. Regression in non human primates. Circulation Research 46: 311–320

Mang K 1976 Impedance studies in the arterial system with arterio-venous shunt. Thesis for BSc (Hons) New South Wales Institute of Technology Sydney

Mang K, O'Rourke MF 1976 Input impedance to the systemic circulation in the presence of arteriovenous shunt. Proceedings of the Australian Physiological and Pharmacological Society 7: p. 44

March HW, Hultgren HW, Gerbode F 1960 Immediate and remote effects of resection on the hypertension in coarctation of the aorta. British Heart Journal 22: 361–373

Maron BJ, Humphries JO, Rowe RD, Mellitis ED 1973 Prognosis of surgically corrected coarctation of the aorta; a 20 year post operative appraisal. Circulation 47: 119–126

Mills CJ, Gabe IT, Gault JH, Mason DT, Ross J Jr., Braunwald E, Shillingford JP 1970 Pressure-flow relationships and vascular impedance in man. Cardiovascular Research 4: 405–417

Murgo JP, Westerhof N, Giolma JP, Altobelli SA 1980 Aortic input impedance in normal man; relationship to pressure waveshapes. Circulation 62: 105–116

Murgo JP, Westerhof N, Giolma JP, Altobelli SA 1980 Effects of exercise on aortic input impedance and pressure waveshapes in normal man. Circulation Research 48: 334–343

Nanton MA, Olley PA 1976 Residual hypertension after coarctectomy in children. American Journal of Cardiology 37: 769–772

Nichols WW, Conti CR, Walker WW, Milnor WR 1977 Input impedance of the systemic circulation in man. Circulation Research 40: 451–458

O'Rourke MF, Blazek JV, Morreels CL, Krovetz LJ 1968 Pressure wave transmission along the human aorta; changes with age and in arterial degenerative disease. Circulation Research 23: 567–579

O'Rourke MF, Cartmill TB 1971 Influence of aortic coarctation on pulsatile hemodynamics in the proximal aorta. Circulation 44: 281–292

O'Rourke MF, Avolio AP 1980 Ascending aortic impedance as the load presented to the left ventricle; effects of change in mean pressure, arterial compliance and peripheral resistance. (In press)

O'Rourke MF, Taylor MG 1966 Vascular impedance of the femoral bed. Circulation Research 18: 126–139

O'Rourke MF, Taylor MG 1967 Input impedance of the systemic circulation. Circulation Research 20: 365–380

Patterson GC, Shepherd JT, Whelan RF 1957 The resistance to blood flow in the upper and lower limb vessels in patients with coarctation of the aorta. Clinical Science 16: 627–632

Pickering GW 1968 High blood pressure. Churchill London p. 582–591

Porjé IG 1967 The energy design of the human circulatory system. Cardiologia 51: 293–306

Reifenstein JE, Levine SA, Gross RE 1947 Coarctation of the aorta; a review of 104 autopsied cases of the 'adult' type 2 years of age or older. American Heart Journal 33: 146–168

Shearer WT, Rutman JY, Weinberg WA, Goldring D 1970 Coarctation of the aorta and cerebrovascular accident. A proposal for early corrective surgery. Journal of Pediatrics 77: 1004–1009

Simon AB, Zloto AE 1974 Coarctation of the aorta; longitudinal assessment of operated patients. Circulation 50: 456–464

Stehbens WE 1962 Cerebral aneurysms and congenital abnormalities. Australasian Annals of Medicine 11: 102–112

Stehbens WE 1975 The role of hemodynamics in the pathogenesis of atherosclerosis. Progress in Cardiovascular Diseases 18: 89–103

Stehbens WE 1979 Hemodynamics and the blood vessel wall. Thomas Springfield

Taylor SH, Donald KW 1960 Circulatory studies at rest and during exercise in coarctation of the aorta before and after operation. British Heart Journal 22: 117–139

Wood P 1968 Diseases of the heart and circulation. Eyre and Spottiswoode London p. 71

Woolam GL, Schnur PL, Vallbona C, Hoff HE 1962 The pulse wave velocity as an early indicator of atherosclerosis in diabetic subjects. Circulation 25: 533–539

Wright JL, Burchell HB, Wood EH, Hines EA Jr, Clagett OT 1956 Hemodynamic and clinical appraisal of coarctation four to seven years after resection and end-to-end anastomosis of the aorta. Circulation 24: 806–814

Wright JL, Wood EH 1958 The value of aortic and radial pressure pulses in the diagnosis of cardiovascular disorders. American Heart Journal 56: p. 64

14

Hypertension

INTRODUCTION

Arterial hypertension is generally regarded as a disease, characterised by abnormally high arterial pressure, in which there is accelerated degeneration of arteries and an increased load on the heart, increased risk of vascular damage to brain, heart and kidneys, and of heart failure, and reduction in life expectancy. This is conventional teaching: this is the simple story.

The closer one looks at arterial hypertension, the less comfortable one becomes, and the more one has to agree with Pickering (1968) that hypertension is a sign, not a disease. The problems in viewing hypertension as a disease include:–

1. The arbitrary definition of hypertension; – is it to be defined in terms of a particular value of diastolic and/or systolic pressure irrespective of age or is it to be defined in terms of normal values at a particular age?

2. Arterial pressure increases progressively with age; – is this a normal process or do more people develop hypertension as age advances?

3. None of the complications of hypertension are specific to this condition. All but one (fibrinoid necrosis) occur with increasing frequency as age advances, even in the presence of normal arterial pressure, and fibrinoid necrosis can occur with normal arterial pressure in a weak or diseased arteriole (p. 204). Are the complications those of age, of hypertension or of some common factor?

4. Hypertension is associated with decreased life expectancy, but the relationship between arterial pressure and life expectancy continues into the normal range of arterial pressure. Is hypertension a disease with different mortality risk at different levels of severity, or is arterial pressure simply one

factor with a graded effect on life expectancy?

5. Drugs used successfully in the treatment of hypertensive heart failure are now used with equal benefit in treatment of normotensive heart failure (Ch. 16). Is heart failure due to hypertension or is arterial pressure simply one factor which aggravates heart failure under different conditions?

6. Drug treatment of hypertension has proved effective in lowering mortality from cardiovascular disease, even in groups of subjects who by some definitions would be considered to be within the normal range for arterial pressure. Is the benefit that of converting hypertension to normotension or simply the lowering of arterial pressure. If the latter, at what level does the benefit end?

Consideration of these points and of the vast amount of epidemiological, clinical, and research data that has accumulated over the twelve years since publication of Pickering's book serves to emphasise further his view that hypertension is not a disease, but that *High Blood Pressure* (the title of his book) is a sign. Perhaps it would be better still to identify the real problem as 'higher blood pressure' and the solution as 'lower blood pressure', so eliminating the need for a definition and stressing the graded increase in risk of cardiovascular complications with rising blood pressure, and the graded benefit of therapy as blood pressure is lowered.

The approach to be taken in this chapter will be application of the concepts presented in earlier chapters to the problem of 'hypertension' (Though uncomfortable with the term 'hypertension', I must acquiesce to the majority view – as did Pickering whose simpler text (Pickering 1968b) is titled 'Hypertension'). The concept of arteries as conduit and cushion helps in the understanding of

blood pressure changes with ageing, and the interpretation of hypertension according to levels of
systolic and diastolic pressure. While hypertension
is caused by increase in peripheral resistance, most
of its complications can be attributed to pulsatile
phenomena and so to altered cushioning function
of the arterial system.

Increased peripheral resistance as the cause of hypertension

It is generally agreed that the fundamental defect
in hypertension is an increase in peripheral resistance (Platt 1960, Pickering 1968, Frolich et al
1969). This was first demonstrated by Pickering
(1936) and by Prinzmetal and Wilson (1936), who
showed that forearm blood flow is within normal
limits (for age) despite elevated arterial pressure.
Since viscosity was shown to be normal in
hypertensive patients, increased resistance was
attributed to vasoconstriction. Normal subjects
show quite marked vasoconstriction in peripheral
arterioles. Hypertensive subjects show a little
more. The search for the cause of this 'little bit
more' was pursued by Pickering for 40 years only
to be described by him in 1968 as the 'Holy Grail'.
The search for this 'Holy Grail' has cost countless
millions of dollars and has been discussed in countless thousands of scientific papers. The nature of
the problem – a fractional increase in normal
arteriolar tone – suggests that for essential hypertension, the Holy Grail will not be found as a specific pathophysiological process. The fundamental
problem in essential hypertension is probably a
statistical one, with some subjects having a little
more, and some a little less, than others.

Effects of increased peripheral resistance on mean, systolic, and diastolic pressure

The level of mean arterial pressure depends on
cardiac output and peripheral resistance. The systolic and diastolic pressures however depend not
only on mean pressure but on the distensibility of
the arterial system. This is illustrated in Figure
14.1 where arterial distensibility is represented by
a *Windkessel*, and peripheral resistance by the
calibre of the output nozzle. With normally high
arterial distensibility, pressure fluctuations are

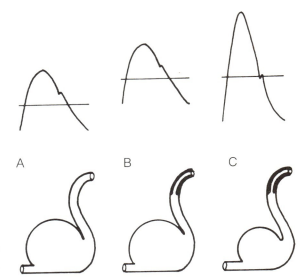

Fig. 14.1 Effects of increased resistance and decreased
compliance on arterial pressure waves (top) in three
'*Windkessel*' models of the arterial system (bottom).
A: Normal compliance, normal resistance
B: Normal compliance, increased resistance
C: Reduced compliance, increased resistance
Mean arterial pressure is represented by the solid line

small. When resistance is increased, but distensibility is unchanged, mean pressure will rise and
wave shape will be identical, so that peak (systolic)
and lowest (diastolic) pressures will be increased
to the same degree as mean pressure. When increased mean pressure is accompanied by decreased arterial distensibility, the pressure wave
will have a higher amplitude, so that systolic
pressure will be higher, and diastolic pressure,
lower than before. Indeed, diastolic pressure may
be the same as before peripheral resistance and
mean pressure were raised.

This simple model illustrates an important
point. Diastolic pressure is not a satisfactory guide
to mean pressure or peripheral resistance when
arterial distensibility is altered. Some who assess
the degree of hypertension according to the level
of diastolic pressure, would have hypertension
more severe in Case B than in Case C. Yet Case C
has the same increase in peripheral resistance and
mean pressure – but with signs of impaired
cushioning function caused by arterial degeneration as well.

In the past, little attention was given to 'systolic

hypertension', partly because it showed greater variation with emotional state of a patient, and partly because it was considered to be irrelevant to the etiology of hypertension and to incidence of complications (Wood 1968, Page 1974, 1979). Fundamental mechanistic and physiological considerations of arterial hemodynamics (as discussed above and elsewhere – p. 164, p. 216) argue that systolic pressure should be more important than diastolic pressure. Surprisingly, the importance of 'systolic hypertension' has only been generally recognised over the past ten years (Colandrea et al 1970, Kannel et al 1971, 1972, Koch–Weser 1973, Simon et al 1979).

Arterial hypertension and change in arterial pressure with age

This has been considered in Chapter 12 (Fig. 14.2). There has been a great deal of debate in the past on the changes in arterial pressure with age, the cause of these changes, and their relationship to arterial hypertension. Much of this conflict has arisen from consideration separately of systolic pressure and of diastolic pressure, as though these had separate and special significance in terms of cardiac and arteriolar properties (Platt 1960, Wood 1968) instead of representing the extremes of the arterial pressure wave. Peripheral re-

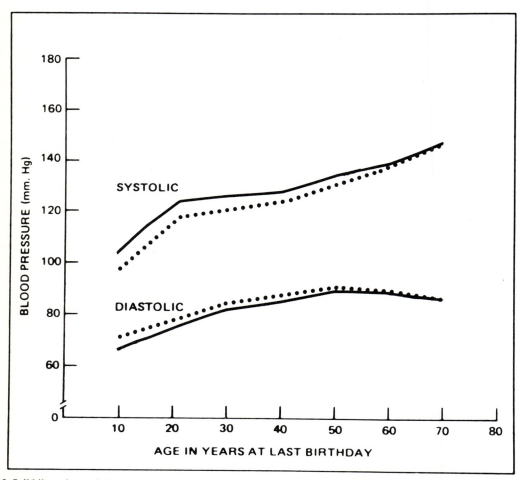

Fig. 14.2 Solid line: change in brachial systolic and diastolic pressures with age in American males. From the U.S. National Center for Health Statistics National Survey, 1977. Dotted line indicates expected change in ascending aortic systolic and diastolic pressures with age, assuming decreased amplification with increasing age

sistance is known to increase progressively with age (Pickering 1936, Dittmer and Grebe 1959); arterial distensibility is known to decrease progressively with age (p. 188, Bramwell and Hill 1922, Kenner 1972). The changes in arterial pressure with ageing are attributable to these two factors – with increasing resistance leading to increase in mean pressure, and decreasing distensibility to increasing pulse pressure (Fig. 14. 2). Changes in ascending aortic pressure with age are doubtless greater than determined indirectly with a sphygmomanometer over the brachial artery. In young subjects, there is considerable amplification of the pressure pulse between central and peripheral arteries, but with advancing years, amplification declines (p. 190, O'Rourke et al 1968). Figure 14. 2 shows (with dotted lines) the changes one might expect to see in ascending aortic systolic and diastolic pressures with advancing years.

In population studies such as those conducted by the U.S. Government National Center for Health Statistics, hypertension is defined in terms of absolute values of systolic and/or diastolic pressure. For the 1977 survey, definite hypertension was defined as either systolic pressure greater than 160 mm Hg or diastolic pressure greater than 95 mm Hg. It is obvious (Fig. 14.3), that with increasing blood pressure with age, this definition will include many older subjects (some 25 percent of the survey population over age 50) while excluding the upper 5 percent of this population under age 25. Perhaps one would be better considering the upper 10 percent of the population at any age to be hypertensive. Were one to do this however, one would have to regard a 20 year old male with diastolic blood pressure of 85 mm Hg to be definitely hypertensive, but not a 50 year old man with diastolic pressure 102 mm Hg (Fig. 14.3).

These considerations of ageing and of hypertension are germane to the problems faced commonly by physicians in assessing individual patients. The answers to the problems however are easier than the problems' specific definitions. Some are available from actuarial tables compiled by Life Insurance Companies. Some have been answered

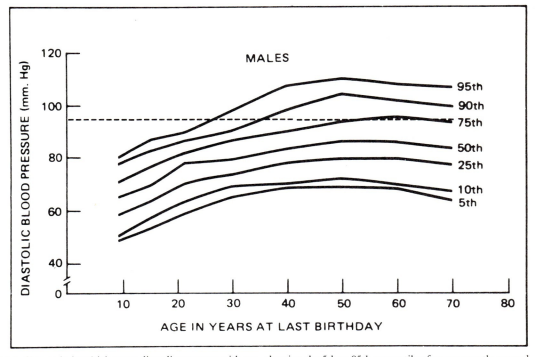

Fig. 14.3 Change in brachial artery diastolic pressure with age, showing the 5th to 95th percentile of an apparently normal population of American males. The generally accepted upper limit of normal pressure – 95 mm Hg – includes approximately 25% of this population over age 50. From the National Survey, US National Center for Health Statistics, 1977

by reports from the Veterans Administration Cooperative Study Group on Anti-Hypertensive Agents (1967, 1970), and some by the more recent reports from the Hypertension Detection and Follow-up Program Cooperative Group (1979a,b). At all ages, life expectancy is related to arterial pressure; the higher the pressure (even within the normal range) the lower the life expectancy. Actuarial tables provide other information, in graded form. The lower the age for a given level of raised arterial pressure, the greater is the reduction in life expectancy. The Co-operative studies on anti-hypertensive therapy have shown definite reduction in mortality for patients aged 30–69 years with diastolic pressure greater than 90 mm Hg, when the arterial pressure was lowered by drug therapy under close medical supervision.

Effects of increased arterial pressure on pulsatile arterial hemodynamics

When arterial pressure is raised, the aorta and major arteries dilate, and wall stress is borne to a greater degree by the collagenous components of the wall (p. 29). Thus, with rise in arterial pressure, elastic modulus of the arterial wall is increased, and so in consequence are pulse wave velocity and aortic characteristic impedance (p. 42). In acute hypertension, the increase in wave velocity and characteristic impedance are caused by distension of the wall alone. In chronic hypertension, degenerative changes in the wall potentiate these effects by increasing Young's modulus and increasing wall thickness (p. 187).

Alterations in pulsatile arterial hemodynamics in hypertension are thus attributable to three factors: – *increased peripheral resistance, increased characteristic impedance*, and *increased pulse wave velocity*. These three effects are apparent in ascending aortic impedance spectra (Fig. 14.4 O'Rourke and Taylor 1967, O'Rourke 1970, Nichols et al 1977, Merillon et al 1980) and in the aortic pressure wave (Broadbent 1890 Freis et al 1966, O'Rourke 1970).

Figure 14.4 shows diagrammatically ascending aortic impedance spectra in a normal and a hypertensive subject. (Impedance spectra in dogs with acute hypertension and humans with chronic

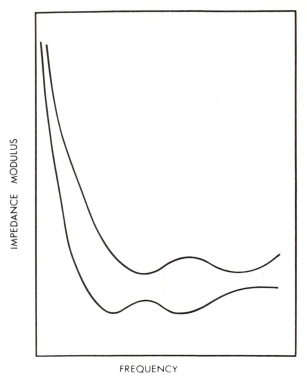

Fig. 14.4 Diagrammatic representation of the effects of hypertension on impedance modulus in the ascending aorta. Upper curve – hypertensive subject; lower curve – normal subject. Differences are 1. Increased impedance modulus at zero frequency, 2. Increased characteristic impedance, and 3. Shift of impedance curve to the right

hypertension are shown in Figures 8.15 and 13.11 respectively.) Increased peripheral resistance increases the zero frequency component of impedance modulus. Increased characteristic impedance raises the general level of impedance modulus (p. 191), while increased pulse wave velocity shifts the curve to the right as a result of earlier return of wave reflection (p. 109). These impedance changes are responsible for the typical changes in contour of the aortic pressure wave (Fig. 14.5). Increased resistance increases mean pressure. Increased characteristic impedance causes pressure to rise further (and at a faster rate i.e. a higher dp/dt) up to the first shoulder which corresponds to the peak of ventricular ejection (p. 77, Murgo et al 1980). Faster wave velocity causes wave reflection to return early, during systole, where it merges with the late systolic part of the wave, causing the late systolic pressure peak, and disappearance of the diastolic wave (p. 78).

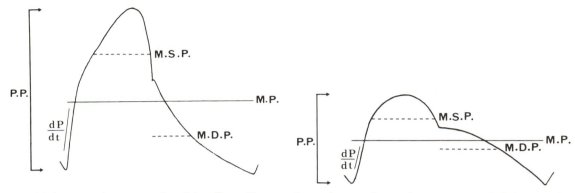

Fig. 14.5 Diagrammatic representation of the effects of hypertension on the ascending aortic pressure wave. Left: hypertensive subject, right: normotensive subject. P.P. Pulse pressure, MSP. mean systolic pressure, MDP. mean diastolic pressure, MP. Mean pressure throughout the whole cardiac cycle, dP/dT. Maximum rate of rise of pressure. In hypertension, MP is increased as a result of increased peripheral resistance, dP/dT is increased as a result of increased characteristic impedance, and PP is increased as a result of this and early return of wave reflection during late systole

Effects of altered pulsatile arterial dynamics on the heart and arteries

The ill effects of hypertension on the heart and arteries are similar to those of ageing (p. 193), aortic coarctation (p. 200), and atherosclerosis (p. 206) and are explicable on the same basis of increased impedance at those frequencies which contain most of the energy of the ventricular ejection wave. Impedance mismatch between left ventricle and systemic arterial system in hypertension leads to greater pulsatile energy losses within the arterial tree (Porjé 1967, Nichols et al 1977). Increased pressure during systole increases total heart work and myocardial oxygen consumption (p. 166), impairs ventricular ejection (p. 164), and induces ventricular hypertrophy. From consideration of physiological mechanisms related to heart work (p. 166), myocardial blood requirement (p. 166), and ventricular ejection (p. 164), it is apparent that 'systolic hypertension' is less favourable than diastolic hypertension. How it could ever have been thought otherwise (Wood 1968, Page 1979) remains an enigma. Vascular complications of hypertension are attributable to higher systolic pressure, and greater rate and extent of pressure fluctuation – that is to altered cushioning function of the arterial system. In hypertension, altered cushioning function is a consequence both of increased wall stretch – an acute and immediately reversible effect, and to arterial degeneration – a chronic and irreversible phenomenon. Both acute

and chronic effects increase peak pressure, pulsatile pressure, and rate of change of pressure, and it appears both accelerate the process of degeneration, as described below.

The ill effects of hypertension on blood vessels (apart from acute fibrinoid necrosis) appear not to be specific for hypertension, but to be a consequence of the amplitude of arterial pressure and of time (Moritz and Oldt 1937, Moschcowitz 1950, Pickering 1968). Given enough time, they occur in all subjects; in a shorter time they occur only in those whose blood pressure is high – i.e. in hypertensive patients. There appears to be a continuous gradation with (age × arterial pressure) being directly related to the frequency of vascular complications. Pickering (1968) has described hypertensive chronic vascular disease as an accelerated form of ageing.

Vascular complications of hypertension are explicable on the basis of alteration in arterial hemodynamics consequent on impaired cushioning function of the arterial system. The following account extends the approach of Pickering (1968), and of Byrom (1954, 1969, 1974) in explaining complications of hypertension in terms of increased vascular stresses, and discusses logical approaches to therapy.

Mechanical factors in complications of hypertension

The incidence of chronic hypertensive complications is related to the level of arterial pressure, being appreciable in the normal population, increased according to degree of pressure increase in hypertensive subjects, and decreased when pressure is reduced by drug therapy (Corcoran et al 1956, Pickering 1968, Veterans Administration Co-operative Study Group on Anti-Hypertensive Agents 1967, 1970, Hypertension Detection and Follow-up Program Co-operative Group 1979ab, Relman 1980). Complications of acute hypertension (fibrinoid necrosis of arterioles with hypertensive encephalopathy, acute renal failure, and acute left ventricular failure) are likewise related to the height of arterial pressure increase, no matter how this is brought about (Pickering 1968, Byrom 1954, 1969, 1974), and are relieved completely by reduction in arterial pressure. Since increase in arterial pressure is a common factor in etiology of these complications, and its reduction in their relief, it is only logical that one should seek an explanation for these complications in terms of mechanical stresses within the arterial and arteriolar wall. This has been done with considerable success (Byrom 1969, 1974, Wolinsky 1970, 1971, 1972, Roach 1977), but most texts and reviews still emphasise the influence of humoral factors as of the greatest importance in hypertensive complications and relegate mechanical factors to a subsidiary role such as causing rupture in an already weakened artery (Page 1974, Gavras et al 1974).

The role of mechanical factors in vascular complications of hypertension may be understood by seeking analogies with physical systems (Sandor 1972, Gent 1972, O'Rourke 1976). With physical materials, acute damage is manifest as fracture or rupture and is caused by a stress that the material cannot withstand. The load that needs be applied depends on the physical material and on its thickness. The nature of the applied load also is important:— a steadily applied stress is less likely to cause fracture than one with a pulsatile component, especially when this is changing rapidly. Rate of change of stress is especially important in elastomers such as the materials that make up the arterial wall (Gent 1972). These principles are familiar to all in simple everyday operations. When we wish to tear a page or rip a branch from a tree, we do best by tugging quickly, not by pulling steadily.

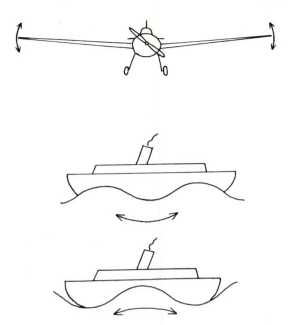

Fig. 14.6 Cyclic stresses causing fatigue and ultimately fracture in physical materials. After Sandor, 1972

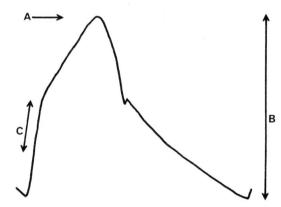

Fig. 14.7 Stresses in the arterial wall. A: Peak stress, B: Cyclic stress, C: Maximal rate of change of stress

While acute damage is manifest as an acute fracture or tear, chronic damage to materials is caused by fatigue, which involves rearrangement of molecular structure, and leads ultimately to fracture at a lower level of stress than needed to cause acute fracture. Fatigue is the important factor determining durability of physical materials in aircraft, bridges, ships, and other man—made objects. As with acute stress, the oscillating component is more important than the steadily-applied component of stress (Sandor 1972). It is the extent and rapidity with which an aircraft's wings are bent, or the span of a bridge is loaded that determine fatigue and fracture (Fig. 14. 6). In the arterial system, the important factors appear to be peak stress (*i.e.* systolic pressure), the amplitude of pulsatile stress (which is related to pulse pressure), and the rate of application of stress (related to maximal dp/dt). All these (Fig. 14. 7) are increased in hypertension.

These mechanical concepts of acute fracture and chronic fatigue have found little application to date in biological phenomena (O'Rourke 1976, Stehbens 1979). Certainly the arterial wall is a non-homogeneous structure, and is made up of living material which may not respond in the same way as an inert physical material. Nonetheless stresses in the arterial wall are borne by non-living components – elastin and collagen – which would be expected to behave in the same way as steel or rubber. While one must be cautious in applying such principles to the arterial wall, one also cannot neglect them and view non-living components of the arterial wall as behaving quite differently than other physical materials.

In what follows, acute arterial and arteriolar damage will be described in terms of acute fracture of components in the vessel wall, and chronic arterial damage related to chronic stresses in, and fatigue, then fracture of arterial wall components. Humoral factors, though important in modifying effects of mechanical stresses, are emphasised elsewhere and will not be considered here.

Acute damage to arterioles and small arteries – fibrinoidnecrosis

Fibrinoid necrosis is the characteristic lesion of malignant hypertension. In malignant hypertension, arterial pressure is markedly elevated, and there is usually evidence of renal insufficiency and retinal damage, and often hypertensive encephalopathy and acute left ventricular failure as well. Untreated, malignant hypertension has a grave prognosis. When treated, evidence of cerebral, renal and cardiac malfunction regresses, sometimes within hours, usually within days, and the optic fundi and apparently other organs as well can return completely to normal (Pickering 1968).

Malignant hypertension with fibrinoid necrosis can occur in any form of hypertension; all that seems necessary is a pressure high enough to cause arteriolar damage (Pickering 1968, Byrom 1969).

Search for the cause of fibrinoid necrosis has generated a lively controversy which continues to the present. While it is doubtful that any one mechanism can explain fibrinoid necrosis of arterioles and small arteries under all conditions, there is compelling evidence that high mechanical stress is the major factor (Byrom 1969, 1974). Despite this, influence of the renin – angiotensin system and auto-immune concepts appear to overshadow interest in mechanical factors (Goldby and Beilin 1972ab, Olsen 1969, Geise 1973, Heptinstall 1974, Gavras et al 1974, Brunner and Gavras 1975, Lynch and Edwards 1978). In their galenic love of mystery and of complexity, many physicians seem reluctant to consider seriously that fibrinoid necrosis may be simply an incomplete arteriolar tear.

The pathogical features of fibrinoid necrosis are well known. There are signs of acute damage to and necrosis of endothelial and medial smooth muscle cells, with separation of endothelial cell junctions and accumulation of acid-Schiff staining material within the arteriolar wall. These changes are accompanied by fragmentation and rupture of the internal and external elastic laminae, and may be associated with extravasation of blood into the wall, aneurysmal dilation of the vessel or by frank rupture of the vessel. Perivascular oedema is usually present, and unless the process is acute, a perivascular inflammatory response is usually seen (Byrom 1954, 1969, 1974, Aikawa and Koletsky 1970, Heptinstall 1974).

The concept that fibrinoid necrosis may represent an incomplete tear of arteriole or small artery was developed by Byrom in a series of articles over many years, which have been summarised in a brief monograph, which is in some ways a modern day version of 'De Motu Cordis.....'. Byrom showed that a variety of interventions can cause fibrinoid necrosis, but that all have a common mechanism:– very high arterial pressure in a previously normal arteriole or small artery, or (in vessels downstream after removal of a Goldblatt clamp or correction of aortic coarctation), application of a moderately high arterial pressure to a structurally weak arterial wall.

Although his interpretations have been challenged, Byrom's observations of vascular changes of malignant hypertension in experimental animals have been repeatedly confirmed. When arterial pressure is extremely high, either following application of a Goldblatt clamp or during infusion of angiotensin II or norepinephrine or methoxamine, or even when arterial pressure is suddenly increased by forceful intra-arterial injection of saline, arterioles and small arteries (i.e. those in the region of $100\ \mu$ diameter) show focal areas of constriction and dilation. Constriction has been attributed to abnormal reactivity or spasm of smooth muscle. Histological lesions of fibrinoid necrosis are not seen however at these sites of constriction, but in the regions where the vessels are dilated. In life, abnormal permeability of these dilated segments has been demonstrated, with accumulation of fluorescent macromolecules and colloidal carbon particles in the wall after their intravenous infusion (Giese 1973, Goldby and Beilen 1972).

These changes in the wall of dilated arterioles and small arteries have been attributed (Giese 1973, Garvas et al 1974, Bruner and Garvas 1975) to stretching of the endothelium and retraction of endothelial cells under the influence of angiotensin II, with resulting increase of endothelial permeability, entrance of plasma proteins into the vessel wall with resultant necrosis of the media and the characteristic histological changes. Byrom (1969) considered this hypothesis, and was inclined to reject it, pointing out that for it to hold, there must always be plasma protein in the vessel wall, there must be evidence that plasma proteins are toxic to smooth muscle cells, and there must be evidence that exudation of plasma proteins always precedes medial necrosis. These conditions have not been satisfied. The available evidence supports the view that the initial event at the points of dilation is overstretching and fragmentation of elastic laminae, followed by stretching and tearing of smooth muscle cells, then secondary entrance of plasma protein into the vessel wall through defects in the overstretched intima, and filtration of fluid into the perivascular space. The inflammatory response with infiltration of granulocytes probably represents the process of repair. Byrom's mechanical hypothesis is completely consistent with histological appearances and other findings and explains the further progression of the lesions into aneurysmal dilation or frank rupture of the vessel. The explanation also accounts for fibrinoid necrosis in atrophic arteries at only moderately elevated pressures (Byrom 1969, Benson and Sealy 1956), and the appearance of pathological changes only where vessels are dilated where wall tension is higher (according to LaPlace's law) than in vessels of normal calibre. One would expect (though no direct measurements are currently available) that pulsatile pressure fluctuations are greatest in dilated small arteries and arterioles immediately proximal to the abnormally constricted vessel, where the pulse wave is reflected and incident and reflected waves summate (p. 8). Dilation of arteries upstream under the influence of elevated pressure, is likely to reduce attenuation of the pulse and increase its amplitude in very small vessels.

Byrom's hypothesis gives a logical explanation for the therapeutic approach to malignant hypertension with fibrinoid necrosis. If the problem is caused by excessive stretch of the vessel wall, the solution is to reduce stretch by lowering arterial pressure. If this is done before arteriolar rupture occurs or irreversible ischemic damage has occurred downstream, the condition, it seems, can be completely cured (Pickering 1968). The accepted therapy certainly is mechanical – reduction of arterial pressure. The converse – abnormally high arterial pressure, may well be the only cause.

Chronic damage to the aorta and large arteries

Arteriosclerosis

Arteriosclerosis is a condition characterised by generalised dilation and tortuosity of systemic arteries, associated with thickening and sclerosis of the wall. Arteriosclerosis is commonly identified in hypertension, but the changes seen are similar to, though more extensive then, those seen with ageing, and described under the general heading of 'medial degeneration' (p. 186). The mechanism of medial degeneration appears to be the same and is related to pulsatile stresses in the arterial wall over long periods of time (Pickering 1968, Moritz and Oldt 1937, Moschcowitz 1950, Wolinsky 1972)

Wolinsky (1970, 1971, 1972) studied the effects of hypertension on the arterial wall structure, and on arterial wall stresses in rats. He showed that the wall response was biphasic, characterised early (at 10 weeks) by hypertrophy and hyperplasia of smooth muscle cells in the arterial wall, and late (16 months) by striking increase in collagen and elastin within the wall, leading to substantial increase in wall thickness. Wolinsky showed that with chronic hypertension, the number of elastic laminae in the wall remained constant, even though elastin and collagen content of the wall increased substantially. The end result was that wall stress (wall tension per unit wall thickness) was not increased compared to controls, but that tension per lamellar unit was considerably elevated. Wolinsky (1972) studied arterial wall changes with hypertension only up to 16 months. Beyond this time there appears to be a third phase, with hypertension being associated with degenerative changes in the vessel wall characterised by fraying, splitting, and fragmentation of elastic fibres with accumulation of intercellular substance having the staining characteristics of elastin, and deposition of calcium within this degenerate material (Pickering 1968, Aikawa and Kolitsky 1970, Stehbens 1979). The same changes are seen with ageing (p. 187). The common factors in ageing and hypertension are repeated high pulsatile stresses in the arterial wall over long periods of time. Whether degenerative changes in structural components of the wall are caused by stress fatigue or from cellular components in the wall outgrowing their blood supply is not known. That the greatest change is seen in non-living material (the elastic fibres) argues for the former.

These considerations seem to explain the progression of medial degeneration at an ever increasing pace. In young healthy animals, and in man, there is a constant relationship between aortic wall stress and the number of elastic lamellar units within the aortic wall, such that throughout the mammalian kingdom, the tension per lamellar unit is relatively constant at around 2000 dynes/unit (Wolinsky and Glagov 1967, Fig. 11.2). There is every reason to believe that this arrangement is desirable for optimal arterial function. With chronic hypertension, tension per lamellar unit is increased, and as lamellae degenerate and fragment, more tension still is exerted on remaining lamellae. The newly deposited elastic tissue and collagen fibres are not arranged in the orderly structural fashion seen in youth, and obviously are less efficient in bearing arterial stresses. The degenerative process appears to be a vicious cycle with high stresses on the wall causing degeneration, and degeneration increasing stresses on the remaining normal constituents in the wall.

Arteriosclerosis affects cushioning function of arteries, and is the principal cause of increased impedance and pulse wave velocity in hypertension. Its ill effects are felt by the heart as increased afterload (p. 164) and relatively decreased coronary perfusion pressure (p. 166), and by the arteries themselves as increased pulsatile pressure – an important factor in the vicious circle of degeneration (p. 188).

Cystic medial degeneration (Medionecrosis)

Clinical complication: dissecting aortic aneurysm. Cystic medial degeneration of the aorta appears to be an extreme example of medial degeneration, where elastic fibres degenerate and fragment, and the aorta contains multiple cystic areas containing homogeneous material between the elastic laminae. This is seen commonly in patients with Marfan's syndrome, where there is an inherited defect in elastic tissue, but is also seen (at a later age) in patients with long standing hypertension, and even in some elderly patients without known hypertension. The medial degeneration in these cases is attributable to high stresses on elastic components of the wall, and their degeneration into homogeneous mucoid material. Cystic medial degeneration is the antecedent of dissecting aortic aneurysm.

In dissecting aortic aneurysm, there is partial rupture of the aortic wall, (Roberts 1981) and the media is stripped by blood over a long distance, even down to and into the iliac and femoral arteries. Death from dissecting aneurysm is caused by adventitial breakdown and complete aortic rupture, compression and occlusion of a vital artery, or by unseating of the aortic valve attachment. No therapy is known for medionecrosis, but in experimental animals, dissecting aneurysm can be prevented by therapy aimed to reduce stresses in the arterial wall (Ringer 1960, Palmer and Wheat, 1967). In humans, medical therapy is the basis for treatment of dissecting aneurysm (Palmer and Wheat 1967, McFarland et al 1972, Lynch and Edwards 1968), with additional surgery usually reserved for aneurysms involving the ascending aorta.

In most cases, dissecting aortic aneurysm is a complication of hypertension. The underlying lesion (cystic medial necrosis) can be attributed to chronically increased stresses in the aortic wall. The intimal tear can be attributed to an acute stress in the wall, while progression of the dissection can be attributed to continuation of these high stresses, accentuated by obstruction of the aorta or major arteries, and sometimes by renal ischemia as well.

The aim of medical therapy in aortic dissection is to reduce disruptive stresses in the aortic wall, so that the dissection will not progress, and the intimal tear will heal. Therapy must be prompt, and aggressive, and must be continued indefinitely so that dissection will not recur. In medical treatment, one aims to reduce systolic pressure, and the rate of rise of pressure. This is accomplished by vasodilator agents which reduce arteriolar tone, venous tone, and venous return, in combination with beta blocking drugs which reduce myocardial contractility, and so stroke volume and rate of aortic pressure rise (dp/dt). Such therapy is perfectly logical, and has proved extremely effective, but has only been in general use since 1967. Prior to this time the role of high aortic stresses in aortic dissection appears to have been largely ignored, and the condition was regarded as a surgical one, with results that were generally catastrophic (Palmer and Wheat 1967).

Arterial aneurysms

Clinical complications: subarachnoid and cerebral hemorrhage Aneurysms of the larger cerebral arteries, especially around the Circle of Willis are usually considered to result from a congenital defect of smooth muscle (Forbus 1930) or of the elastic laminae (Ross-Russell 1963, Walker and Allegre 1954) at points of bifurcation. They are common however, and more frequently rupture, in patients with increased stresses in the arterial wall, as a result of hypertension or aortic coarctation (Pickering 1968). It is generally agreed that a combination of wall weakness and wall stress is necessary for their development (Stehbens 1962, 1979). The initial anatomical defect is doubtless a small bulge in the arterial wall at a point of weakness. Once a bulge has developed, physical factors would hasten the process of expansion, since on the one hand, tension would be increased with increased diameter according to LaPlace's law, and on the other, the stretched wall would become progressively thinner. A relentless progression of expansion and ultimate rupture would be expected unless thrombus formed in the aneurysmal sac or reparative processes led to strengthening of the wall. Abnormally high stresses in the aneurysmal wall undoubtedly are responsible for expansion and ultimate rupture. Rupture causes hemorrhage into the subarachnoid space, and sometimes into the brain substance as well.

In hypertension, cerebral hemorrhage usually results from rupture of a small artery within the substance of the brain. It is now clear (Pickering 1968) that arteries rupture at points of weakness where tiny aneurysms (first recognised by Charchot and Bouchard in 1868 and now called after them) give way. These aneurysms appear to develop with advancing years, but at any age are more common in patients with hypertension (Pickering 1968), and are very common in elderly hypertensive subjects. The localised medial weakness in Charcot Bouchard aneurysm appears to be acquired as a result of arterial degeneration, (not from a congenital defect as with aneurysms in larger cerebral arteries), but to expand and progress to aneurysmal dilation and rupture under the influence of the same vicious circle as these.

Atherosclerosis

Clinical complications: Myocardial Ischemia, myocardial infarction, cerebral infarction, leg ischemia and gangrene, aortic aneurysm and rupture. Atherosclerosis is accelerated in hypertension, presumably because of increased stresses in the arterial wall (Ch. 15). Atherosclerosis causes organ ischemia as a result of arterial narrowing (Ch. 5), but its most frequent lethal complications result from superadded arterial thrombosis. Some lethal complications however, including rupture of abdominal aortic aneurysm are attributable to continuation of high stresses in the aortic wall, with bulging at localised points of weakness, and to the same vicious cycle as described for aneurysms of cerebral arteries.

Cardiac hypertrophy

Clinical complication heart failure. The earliest response to increased ventricular load is hypertrophy of myocardial cells. Hyperplasia does not occur. At an early stage hypertrophy is completely reversible, and the process is referred to as 'Physiological' (Wikman–Coffelt et al 1979). At a later stage however, the process becomes 'Pathological' and hypertrophied muscle fibres degenerate, with early disarray of myofilaments, increase in width of Z band and of intercalated discs, and later necrosis and replacement of muscle cells by fibrous tissue. In 'Pathological' hypertrophy, myocardial structure is quite abnormal and disorganised. It is not known what converts 'Physiological' into 'Pathological' hypertrophy. Hypertrophic myocardial changes in hypertension are in some ways similar to those which occur in the medial smooth muscle within the arterial wall, with early hypertrophy, and later degeneration. In both sites, degeneration has been attributed to hypertrophied cells outgrowing nutrient supply (Wikman–Coffelt et al 1979). Recent studies (Adomian et al 1975) using new methods for preparation and staining, have shown another process that has

been noted in severe hypertension:– tearing of myocardial filaments and rupture of myocardial cells when acute outflow obstruction was produced experimentally. Rupture of skeletal muscle fibres, and of tendons, are common sporting injuries, but the fact that the same process can occur in the heart is not generally known. The end results of myocardial cell rupture are not known. Damaged cells may die, or the healing process may be responsible for fibrosis or for the disorganisation of myocardial filaments and cells that are seen in severe myocardial hypertrophy, and to an extreme degree in obstructive cardiomyopathy (Bulkley et al 1977).

SUMMARY:– ROLE OF MECHANICAL FACTORS IN COMPLICATIONS OF HYPERTENSION

Table 14. 1 summarises the effects of mechanical factors in complications of hypertension. With the exception of fibrinoid necrosis, all these complications can be regarded as having a predisposing and precipitating cause. Increased arterial pressure is of variable importance in predisposition to and precipitation of these complications. In myocardial infarction for instance, hypertension appears to play no role in precipitation, wheras in hypertensive encephalopathy or acute renal failure, hypertension appears to play a major, and perhaps the only, role. One would expect that control of arterial pressure would be most effective and most obvious in reducing incidence of hypertensive complications which are precipitated by hypertension,

Table 14.1 Role of increased arterial pressure in clinical complications of hypertension

Complication	Predisposition	Precipitation	Response to hypotensive therapy	Prevention by hypotensive therapy
Left ventricular failure	+++	++++	√√√	√√√
Malignant phase				
(Hypertensive encephalopathy)	0	++++	√√√	√√√√
(Acute renal failure)	0	++++	√√√	√√√√
Cerebral hemorrhage	+++	+++	–	√√√
Subarachnoid hemorrhage	++	++	–	√√
Dissecting aneurysm	+++	+++	√√	√√√
Abdominal aortic aneurysm with rupture	++	+++	–	√√
Myocardial infarction	++	0	√	√

while being less effective, less obvious, and slower in reducing other complications where increased arterial pressure plays no role in precipitation. This appears to be the case. Control of arterial pressure has virtually abolished hypertensive encephalopathy and acute renal failure as complications of hypertension (Pickering 1968), and has markedly reduced the incidence of hemorrhagic stroke (Veterans Administration Co-operative Study Group on Anti–Hypertensive Agents (1967, 1970). Benefit of arterial pressure control in reduction of incidence of myocardial infarction has been less apparent but has recently been documented (Hypertension Detection and Follow–Up Program Cooperative Group 1979ab). On the basis of different roles of hypertension in predisposition and precipitation, these points have a ready explanation.

PULMONARY HYPERTENSION

Increase in pulmonary artery pressure causes the same increase in pulmonary vascular impedance as seen in the ascending aorta, with increase in characteristic impedance and shift to the right of impedance curves, as a result of increased pulse wave velocity (Bergel and Milnor 1965, Milnor et al 1969, Elkins et al 1974). In some experimental work, failure of characteristic impedance to increase at high pressure has been attributed to restriction of arterial expansion by a cuff–type flow transducer (p. 115).

Milnor et al (1969) showed that in pulmonary hypertension in man, increased characteristic impedance and pulse wave velocity are associated with increased pulmonary arterial pressure fluctuations, increased right ventricular work, and increased pulsatile energy losses within the pulmonary circulation; these approached and sometimes exceeded energy losses in maintaining steady flow. They stressed that altered elasticity of the pulmonary arterial tree in pulmonary hypertension is as important as the state of the arterioles and capillaries in determining right ventricular work. As with systemic hypertension, altered distensibility of the pulmonary arterial tree may result from increased pressure *per se* or from secondary arterial degeneration.

There has been less interest in the mechanical complications of pulmonary than of systemic hypertension, presumably because these are less frequently lethal, and also because it is often difficult to distinguish cause of pulmonary hypertension from its effects, especially in the smaller vessels. It is known that pulmonary hypertension is associated with medial hypertrophic and degenerative changes, as in systemic hypertension, and that pulmonary hypertension, when chronic, may be associated with atherosclerosis as well (Stehbens 1979).

REFERENCES

Adomian GE, Laks MM, Swan HJC 1975 Fragmentation of the actin filaments by acute pressure overload to the right ventricle of the conscious dog. 33rd Annual Proceedings of the Electron Microscopy Society of America GW Bailey (ed) p542

Aikawa M, Koletsky S 1970 Arteriosclerosis of the mesenteric arteries of rats with renal hypertension. American Journal of Pathology 61: 293–322

Benson WR, Sealy WC 1956 Arterial necrosis following resection of coarctation of the aorta. Laboratory Investigation 5: 359–376

Bergel DH, Milnor WR 1965 Pulmonary vascular impedance in the dog. Circulation Research 16: 401–415

Broadbent W 1890 The pulse. Lea Philadelphia

Brunner HR, Gavras H 1975 Vascular damage in hypertension. Hospital Practice 103: 97–108

Bulkley BH, Weisfelt ML, Hutchins GM 1977 Asymmetrical septal hypertrophy and myocardial fibre disarray: features of normal developing and malformed hearts. Circulation 56: 292–298

Byrom F. 1954 The pathogenesis of hypertensive encephalopathy and its relation to the malignant phase of hypertension. Lancet 2: 201–211

Byrom F 1969 The hypertensive vascular crisis – an experimental study. Heinemann London

Byrom F 1974 The evolution of acute hypertensive arterial disease. Progress in Cardiovascular Diseases 17: 31–37

Castleman B, Smithwick RH 1948 The relation of vascular disease to the hypertensive state 11 The adequacy of renal biopsy as determined from a study of 500 patients. New England Journal of Medicine 239: 729–732

Charcot JM, Bouchard 1868 Nouvelles Recherches sur la pathogenie du l'hemorrhagie cerebrale. Archives de Physiologie 1: 110, 643 and 725

Colandrea MA, Friedman GD, Nichaman MZ, Lynd CN 1970 Systolic hypertension in the elderly. An epidemiological assessment. Circulation 41: 239–245

Corcoran AC, Lewis LA, Dunstan HP, Page IH 1956 Atherosclerotic complications in hypertensive disease. Annals New York Academy of Sciences 64: 620–629

Cox RH 1979 Comparison of arterial wall mechanics in normotensive and spontaneously hypertensive rats. American Journal of Physiology 237: H159–H167

Dittmer DS, Grebe RM 1959 Handbook of circulation. Saunders Philadelphia

Elkins RC, Peyton MD, Greenfield LJ 1974 Pulmonary vascular impedance in chronic pulmonary hypertension. Surgery 76: 57–64

Folkow B 1978 Cardiovascular structural adaptation; its role in the initiation and maintenance of primary hypertension. Clinical Science and Molecular Medicine 55 (Suppl 4) 3s–22s

Forbus W 1930 On the origin of miliary aneurysms of the superficial cerebral arteries. Bulletin Johns Hopkins Hospital 47: 239–284

Freis ED, Heath WC, Luchsinger PC, Snell RE 1966 Changes in the carotid pulse which occur with age and hypertension. American Heart Journal 71: 757–765

Frohlich ED, Tarazi RC, Dunstan HP 1969 Re-examination of the hemodynamics of hypertension. American Journal of Medical Science 257: 9–23

Gavras H, Brunner HR, Laragh 1974 Renin and aldosterone and the pathogenesis of hypertensive vascular damage. Progress in Cardiovascular Diseases 17: 39–49

Geddes LA, Whistler SJ 1978 The error in indirect blood pressure measurement with the incorrect size of cuff. American Heart Journal 96: 4–8

Gent AN 1972 Fracture of elastomers. In:Fracture H Liebowitz (ed) Academic Press New York

Giese J 1973 Renin, angiotensin and hypertensive vascular damage–A review. American Journal of Medicine 55: 315–332

Goldby FS, Beilin LJ 1972 Relationship between arterial pressure and the permeability of arterioles to carbon particles in acute hypertension in the rat. Cardiovascular Research 6: 384–390

Goldby FS, Beilin LJ 1972 How an acute rise in arterial pressure damages arterioles. Electron microscopic changes during angiotensin infusion. Cardiovascular Research 6: 569–584

Gribbin B 1974 A study of baroreceptor function and arterial distensibility in normal and hypertensive man. MD Thesis University of Dundee

Gribbin B, Steptoe A, Sleight P 1976 Pulse wave velocity as a measure of blood pressure change. Psychophysiology 13: 86–90

Guyton A 1980 Circulatory Physiology 3: Arterial Pressure and Hypertension. Saunders Philadelphia.

Heptinstall RH 1974 Relation of hypertension to changes in the arteries. Progress in Cardiovascular Diseases 17: 25–30

Hinghofer-Szalkay H, Pascale K, Kenner T 1976 Experimental measurement of arterial pulse wave propagation and the influence of arterial blood pressure. Pflugers Archives 362: R6

Hirst EA Jr, Johns VJ Jr 1962 Experimental dissection of media of aorta by pressure; its relation to spontaneous dissecting aneurysm. Circulation Research 10: 897–903

Hypertension Detection and Follow up Program Co operative Group 1979a Five year findings of the hypertension detection and follow up program
1. Reduction in mortality of persons with high blood pressure including mild hypertension. Journal of the American Medical Association 242: 2562–2571

Hypertension Detection and Follow up Program Cooperative Group 1979b Five year findings of the hypertension detection and follow-up program

11. Mortality by race, sex and age. Journal of the American Medical Association 242: 2572–2577

Kannel WB, Gordon T, Schwartz MJ 1971 Systolic versus diastolic blood pressure and risk of coronary heart disease. American Journal of Cardiology 27: 335–345

Kannel WB, Castelli WP, McNamara PM, McKee PA, Feinleib M 1972 Role of blood pressure in the development of congestive heart failure. The Framingham study. New England Journal of Medicine 287: 781–787

Koch–Weser J 1973 The therapeutic challenge of systolic hypertension. New England Journal of Medicine 289: 481–483

Lynch RP, Edwards JE 1978 Pathology of systemic hypertension including background and complications. In: Hurst JW, Logue RB, Schlant RC, Wenger N (eds) The Heart, Arteries and veins 4th edition McGraw New York p. 1380–1390

Mackenzie J 1902 The Study of the pulse. MacMillan Edinburgh

McFarland J, Willerson JT, Dinsmore RE, Austen WG, Buckley MJ, Sanders CA, De Sanctis RW 1972 The medical treatment of dissecting aortic aneurysms. New England Journal of Medicine 286: 116–119

Management Committee 1980 The Australian Therapeutic Trial in Mild Hypertension. Lancet 1: 1262–1267

Merillon JP, Fontenier G, Chastre J, Lerallut JF, Jaffrin MY, Gourgon R 1980 Etude du spectre d'impedance chez l'homme normal et hypertendu. Effects de l'accroissement de frequence cardiaque et des crogues vasomotrices. Archives Des Maladies De Coeur 73: 83–90

Milnor WR, Conti CR, Lewis KB, O'Rourke MF 1969 Pulmonary arterial pulse wave velocity and impedance in man. Circulation Research 25: 637–649

Mitchell JRA, Schwartz CJ 1965 Arterial disease. Oxford Blackwell

Moritz AR, Oldt MR 1937 Arteriolar sclerosis in hypertensives and non hypertensives. American Journal of Pathology 13: 679–728

Moschcowitz E 1950 Hyperplastic arteriosclerosis versus atherosclerosis. Journal of the American Medical Association 143: 861–865

Niarchos AP, Laragh JH 1980 Hypertension in the elderly. Modern concepts of cardiovascular disease 49: 49–54

Nichols WW, Conti CR, Walker WW, Milnor WR 1977 Input impedance of the systemic circulation in man. Circulation Research 40: 451–458

Olsen F 1969 Arteriolar permeability and destruction of elastic membrane in hypertension. Acta Pathologica Microbiologica Scandinavica 75: 527–536

O'Rourke MF 1967 Steady and pulsatile energy losses in the systemic circulation under normal conditions and in simulated arterial disease.. Cardiovascular Research 1: 313–326

O'Rourke MF 1970 Arterial hemodynamics in hypertension. Circulation Research 26 Supplement 2: 123–133

O'Rourke MF 1976 Pulsatile arterial hemodynamics in hypertension. Australian and New Zealand Journal of Medicine 6 Supplement 2: 40–48

O'Rourke MF, Taylor MG 1967 Input impedance of the systemic circulation. Circulation Research 20: 365–380

O'Rourke MF, Blazek JV, Morreels CL, Krovetz LJ 1968 Pressure wave transmission along the human aorta; changes with age and in arterial degenerative diseases. Circulation Research 23: 567–579

Page IH 1974 Arterial hypertension in retrospect. Circulation Research 34: 133–142

Page IH 1979 Two cheers for hypertension. Journal of the American Medical Association 242: 2559–2561

Palmer RF, Wheat MW 1967 Treatment of dissecting aneurysms of the aorta. Annals of Thoracic Surgery 4: 38–52

Pickering GW 1936 The peripheral resistance in persistent arterial hypertension. Clinical Science 2: 209–235

Pickering GW 1968a Hypertension. Churchill London

Pickering GW 1968b High blood pressure. Churchill London

Platt R 1960 The nature of essential hypertension. In:Bock KD, Cottier PT(eds) Essential Hypertension; an international symposium Springer Berlin p. 39–52

Porjé IG 1967 The energy design of the human circulatory system. Cardiologia 51: 293–306

Prinzmetal M, Wilson C 1936 Nature of the peripheral resistance in arterial hypertension with special reference to the vasomotor system. Journal of Clinical Investigation 15: 63–83

Relman AS 1980 Mild hypertension: no more benign neglect. New England Journal of Medicine 302: 293–294

Reuben SR 1970 Wave transmission in the pulmonary arterial system in disease in man. Circulation Research 27: 523–529

Ringer RK 1960 Aortic rupture, plasma cholesterol and arteriosclerosis following serpasil administration in turkeys. In: The second conference on the use of reserpine in poultry production Summit New Jersey CIBA p. 32–39

Roach MR 1977 – Biophysical analysis of blood vessel walls and blood flow. Annual Review of Physiology 39: 51–71

Roberts W 1981 Aortic dissection: anatomy, consequences and causes. American Heart Journal 101: 195–214

Ross-Russell RW 1963 Observations on intracranial aneurysms. Brain: 86, 425–442

Ross-Russell RW 1976 Cerebral arterial disease. Churchill Edinburgh

Sandor B 1972 Fundamentals of cyclic stress and strain. University of Wisconsin Madison p. 3

Safar M 1980 Management of hypertension in the elderly. New England Journal of Medicine 303: 1234

Safar ME, Peronneau PA, Levenson JA, Toto-Moukoud JA, Simon A 1981 Pulsed doppler: Diameter, blood flow velocity and volumic flow of the brachial artery in sustained essential hypertension. Circulation 63: 393–400

Scott DL 1980 The dynamic arterial pressure/flow relationship and total arterial compliance as a function of pressure in the normotensive and spontaneously hypertensive rat. MSC Thesis Ohio State University

Simon AC, Safar ME, Levenson JA, Kheder AM, Levy BI 1979 Systolic hypertension; hemodynamic mechanism and choice of antihypertensive treatment. American Journal of Cardiology 44: 505–511

Simon AC, Safar ME, Levenson JA, London GM, Levy BI, Chau NP 1979 An evaluation of large arteries compliance in man. American Journal of Physiology 237: H550–554

Spence JD, Sibbard WJ, Cape RD 1978 Pseudohypertension in the elderly. Clinical Science and Molecular Medicine 55: 3995–4025

Stehbens WE 1962 Cerebral aneurysms and congenital abnormalities. Australasian Annals of Medicine 11: 102–112

Stehbens WE 1979 Hemodynamics and the blood vessel wall. Thomas Springfield

Trippodo NC, Frohlich ED 1981 Similarities of genetic (spontaneous) hypertension: man and rat. Circulation Research 48: 309–319

U·S· Government National Center for Health Statistics J· Roberts (ed) 1977 Blood pressure levels of persons 6–74 years, United States 1971–1974. DHEW Publication No (HRA) 78–1648

Veterans Administration Cooperative Study Group on Anti–hypertensive Agents 1967 Effects of treatment on morbidity in hypertension; results in patients with diastolic blood pressures averaging 115 through 129 mm Hg. Journal of the American Medical Association 202: 1028–1034

Veterans Administration Cooperative Study Group on Anti-hypertensive Agents 1970 Effects of treatment on morbidity in hypertension 11. Results in patients with diastolic pressure averaging 90 through 114 mm Hg. Journal of the American Medical Association 213: 1143–1152

Veterans Administration Cooperative Study Group on Anti-hypertensive Agents 1972 Effects of treatment on morbidity in hypertension 111 Influence of age, diastolic pressure and prior cardiovascular disease; further analysis of side effects. Circulation 45: 991–1004

Walker AE, Allegre GW 1954 The pathology and pathogenesis of cerebral aneurysms. Journal of Neuropathology and Experimental Neurology 13: 248–259

Wikman-Coffelt J, Parmley WW, Mason DT 1979 The cardiac hypertrophy process: analysis of factors determining pathological vs physiological development. Circulation Research 45: 697–707

Wolfgarten M, Magarey FR 1959 Vascular fibrinoid necrosis in hypertension. Journal of Pathology and Bacteriology 77: 597–603

Wolinsky H 1970 Response of the rat aortic media to hypertension. Morphological and chemical studies. Circulation Research 26: 507–522.

Wolinsky H 1971 Effects of hypertension and its reversal on the thoracic aorta of male and female rats. Circulation Research 28: 622–637

Wolinsky H 1972 Long-term effects of hypertension on rat aortic wall and their relation to concurrent ageing changes. Morphological and chemical studies. Circulation Research 30: 301–309

Wolinsky H 1973 Comparative effects of castration and antiandrogen treatment on aortas of hypertensive and normotensive male rats. Circulation Research 32: 183–189

Wolinsky H, Glagov S 1967 Alamellar unit of aortic medial structure and function in mammals. Circulation Research 20: 99–111

Wood P 1968 Diseases of the Heart and Circulation Eyre and Spottiswoode London p. 71

15

Mechanical factors in atherogenesis

Atherosclerosis is the most common cause of death and disability in the western world. Atherosclerosis at just one site – in the coronary arteries of the heart – is responsible for approximately one third of all deaths in the U.S.A., Australia, and other countries with similar diet and lifestyle (Reader 1979, Levy 1979). Despite an enormous amount of research there is no agreement on how an atherosclerotic plaque first develops, nor precisely how it enlarges. The three main theories of etiology invoke totally different mechanisms – the first that the lesion results from infiltration of lipoproteins out of blood into the endothelium (Virchow 1862, Anitschkow 1933, Digirolamo and Schlant 1978, Wolinsky 1979), the second that it is due to thrombus formation on damaged endothelium with subsequent muscle cell proliferation, organisation and reendothelialisation (Duguid 1946, 1948, Pickering 1964, Mitchell and Schwartz 1965, Mustard 1974, Mustard and Packham 1975), and the third that it involves a type of neoplastic process involving smooth muscle cells (Ross and Glomset 1976, Bendit 1977). Variations of these theories and other totally different theories have also been proposed and debated (Stehbens 1975, 1979, Gessner 1973, Ross and Glomset 1976, Marzilli et al 1980, Lown and de-Silva 1980).

Although basic research on mechanisms has generated considerable controversy about initiation and subsequent growth of atheromatous plaques, epidemiological studies of the clinical manifestations of atherosclerosis have clearly identified certain risk factors which are related to these complications and presumably to the development of the atherosclerosis itself – the three most important of these being high blood pressure, high blood cholesterol, and cigarette smoking (Wolinsky 1979, Levy 1979). Awareness of these factors and widespread attempts to identify and modify them have been associated with a decline in age-specific mortality from coronary artery disease of around 25 percent in American males over the past ten years following a progressive rise up until the early 1950s (Statistical Bulletin, Metropolitan Life Insurance Co 1979, Levy 1979). A similar fall has been seen in Australia but not in most European countries (Reader 1979). Better treatment of established disease – coronary artery bypass surgery and coronary care units – may have contributed to this, but the general impression is that benefit has resulted from application of preventive measures — identification and control of high blood pressure and high blood lipids and reduction in smoking by older males, together with development of less toxic cigarettes (Levy 1979). We do not know the cause of this disease, we do not know how it progresses, we do not know why incidence of its clinical complications is now falling. The situation is somewhat like 'hypertension': clinical progress is being made despite laboratory consternation. Doubtless, however, clinical efforts would be more successful still, and certainly more satisfying if more were known about the genesis of atherosclerosis.

While many factors are involved in etiology of atherosclerosis, it is apparent that mechanical factors are very important in initiation and progression of the disease itself and for the clinical expression of established disease. Mechanical and hydraulic principles concerned in expression of established disease were discussed in Chapter 5. Here it was pointed out how (and why) atherosclerosis is usually clinically silent until an artery is narrowed to 30 percent or less of its original diameter (or to 10 percent or less of its original cross sectional area), and that with further progression of the disease, symptoms are likely to progress rapidly.

Arterial changes with ageing and hypertension were attributed to arterial stresses acting over long periods of time – to arterial 'wear and tear'. It is likely that similar factors are involved in atherogenesis. The influence of time is apparent in stu-

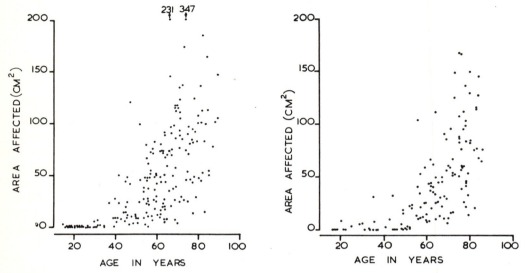

Fig. 15.1 Increasing severity of atherosclerosis with advancing years. Area of the thoracic aorta affected by complicated raised fibrous and sudanophilic plaques in the autopsy series of men (left) and women (right), reported by Mitchell and Schwartz (1965)

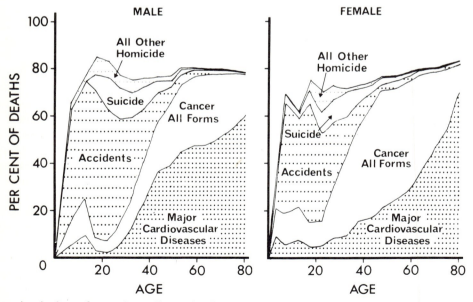

Fig. 15.2 Increasing death rate from major cardiovascular diseases with increasing age. From data published for 1978 in the Statistical Bulletin, Metropolitan Life Insurance Co. 60: p. 16, 1980. (Figure shows relative death rate from different causes. Absolute death rate from cardiovascular disease increases with age to an even greater degree because of higher total mortality with increasing age)

dies of atherosclerosis itself (Fig. 15.1) and of mortality from cardiovascular disease, most of which in later life is due to the complications of atherosclerosis (Fig. 15.2).

Evidence that mechanical factors are important in atherogenesis include (after Stehbens 1979):–

1. Atherosclerosis is virtually confined to the systemic arteries where arterial pressure and pulsatile stresses are high, and is only seen in the pulmonary arterial system and in systemic veins when stresses are abnormally high.

2. Atherosclerosis is accelerated in patients with systemic hypertension in association with increase in mean and pulsatile pressure (Ch. 14)

3. In aortic coarctation, atherosclerosis is accelerated in upper body arteries where mean pressure is high, and pulsatile pressure variations are extreme; atherosclerosis is decreased in severity in lower body arteries where mean pressure is lower, and pulsatile fluctuations are small.

4. Atherosclerosis is usually more severe in the abdominal than in the thoracic aorta, and in the lower limb compared to upper limb arteries. In the erect position, mean and pulsatile pressures are greater in the lower body as a result of gravitational forces (other factors including different medial elastin composition and vasa vasorum in the abdominal aorta may also play a role (Wolinsky & Glagov 1967, 1969).

5. Atherosclerosis is usually more severe in larger than in smaller arteries of the same organ (Blumenthal et al 1954, Young et al 1960). In the carotid artery, atherosclerosis is usually most severe in and about the dilated carotid sinus. According to LaPlace's law, wall stress is greater in larger than in smaller vessels.

6. Atherosclerosis appears to progress slowly in patients with aortic stenosis in whom mean and pulsatile arterial pressures tend to be low.

7. Atherosclerosis is most severe about the origin of branches, at bifurcations, and in the proximal segments of resulting daughter vessels; at these sites there are large and variable changes in wall stress and in blood shear (see below).

8. Atherosclerosis tends to be most severe in poorly supported arteries, and least severe in vessels with additional external support. In the heart, coronary atherosclerosis occurs only in the epicardial arteries and not in vessels surrounded by myocardium. In the vertebral arteries, atherosclerosis usually spares those segments of artery within the intervertebral foramena, while in the carotid artery, atherosclerosis usually spares that segment of vessel within the petrous temporal bone.

9. Atherosclerosis is usually most severe in arteries subjected to repeated bending or tugging – as at the base of the cardiac ventricles, or over a joint.

10. Atherosclerosis develops in systemic veins when exposed to systemic arterial pressure (and high blood flow) in an arteriovenous aneurysm or in a surgically induced shunt.

11. Atherosclerosis develops in the pulmonary arterial system only when pulmonary arterial pressure is sustained at very high levels over long periods of time.

These points establish beyond question the importance of mechanical factors in development of atherosclerosis, However, how these mechanical factors operate in atherogenesis is still uncertain. A number of recent reviews address this question (Patel et al 1974, 1979, Roach 1977, Lutz et al 1977, 1979, Caro 1979) as did a Ciba symposium in 1972 (see Adams 1973, Fry 1973, Caro 1973), and another conference in Ohio during 1974 (see Bergel et al 1976).

Mechanical factors may operate by altering stresses either in the vessel wall ('normal hemodynamic stresses') or at the vascular interface ('shearing stresses') (Fry 1969, Patel et al 1974). The 'normal' stresses counterbalance intravascular pressure and tethering and comprise tensile stresses in the circumferential and longitudinal direction, and a compressional stress in the radial direction. The radial stress is always non-uniform (i.e. it varies with distance from inner to outer surface) whereas the circumferential and longitudinal stresses are relatively uniform except at bends and about branches and in regions where disease or degeneration have has already occurred and caused structural thinning, weakness, or dilation (Patel et al 1974). 'Normal' stresses are increased when arterial pressure is elevated, and are not related directly to blood flow.

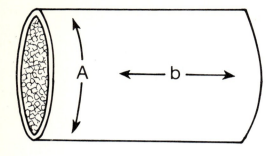

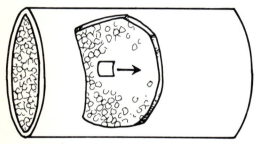

Fig. 15.3 *Top*: Circumferential (A) and longitudinal (B) stresses in the arterial wall
Bottom: Shearing stress at the vascular interface

In contrast to 'normal' stresses, shearing stresses at the vascular wall are related to blood flow, not to arterial pressure. Shearing stress at the vascular wall (Fig. 15.3) represents the viscous drag on endothelial cells, and so the forces tending to damage or dislodge them. Shearing stresses are absent when blood is not flowing, even when arterial pressure is high (as in the ascending aorta during cardiac diastole). When blood is flowing, shear stresses at the vessel wall are least when a parabolic velocity profile has been established, and greater when the velocity profile is flattened, either because of pulsatility of flow or because of disturbed (non laminar) or turbulent flow (p. 35, McDonald 1974).

Studies of mechanical factors in atherogenesis have been directed at measuring tensile stresses within the vascular wall, and shearing stresses at the vascular interface, and the effects of altered stresses on intimal properties. Although wall stress has been measured from arterial pressure and diameter in arterial segments and intact vessels by

many workers over may years, (see Chs. 2–4), the techniques applied have not proved suitable for determining differences in wall stress at those regions which are preferentially affected by atherosclerosis i.e. about bends, branches or bifurcations. More success has been achieved in measuring shearing stresses at such sites with ingenious though still relatively gross techniques (Ling et al 1968, Peronneau et al 1974, Nerem 1974, Lutz et al 1977). Much information has been obtained on differences in shearing stress at different parts of the arterial system and the effects of these on endothelial permeability, endothelial damage, and intimal proliferation (Fry 1969, Flaherty et al 1972, Fry 1973, 1976, Lutz et al 1977, 1979). These studies have been supplemented by other work on vascular models showing the alterations in flow patterns and profiles that result at bifurcations and branches under different conditions (Gutstein et al 1968, Lutz et al 1977, Malcolm and Roach 1980). This work offers explanations for initiation and progression of atherosclerosis in and about arterial branches and bifurcations.

Fry and coworkers at the National Institutes of Health in Bethesda have concentrated on shearing stresses at the vascular wall, the effects of altered shearing stresses on endothelial cells and on endothelial permeability, and on the arterial intima. Fry and colleagues have shown a general relationship between high wall shearing stress, increased permeability to plasma protein and lipoprotein, and the sites of predilection for atherosclerosis in experimental animals. They have shown that flux of protein and lipoprotein into the endothelium is related to shearing stress, and that flux is increased without evidence of damage to endothelial cells. Whether increased flux occurs through the cell wall by pinocytosis or between endothelial cells is still not established. They have also shown that when shearing stress is very high – around 400 dyne cm^{-2}, endothelial cells yield so that local denudation of endothelium occurs; this is followed by adherence of platelets to the wall with subsequent proliferation of smooth muscle cells in the intima, intimal fibrosis, and eventual reendothelialisation. In the original work on this subject (Fry 1969, Caro 1973), certain apparent contradictions existed which made it difficult to explain experimental atherosclerosis on the basis

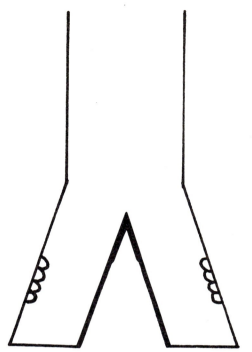

Fig. 15.4 Diagrammatic representation of an arterial bifurcation. Shear stresses are greatest but have constant orientation at the flow divider. This area is usually spared of atheroma. Shear stresses are most variable at the lateral wall of daughter branches. This area is usually most severely affected by atheroma

of increased shearing stress at the vascular wall. At bifurcations, the leading edge of flow dividers (Fig. 15.4) was usually spared, even though shearing stresses here were greatest, wheras increased endothelial permeability and greatest disease was usually apparent on the outer lateral side of the flow divider and in the daughter vessel away from the flow divider where stresses were expected to be much less. These problems now appear to have been resolved on the basis of unidirectional shear at the leading edge of the flow divider and variable shear at its lateral margin and in the daughter vessel (Fry 1973, Lutz et al 1977, 1979, Malcolm and Roach 1980). It appears that high shearing stress over the leading edge of the flow divider leads to orientation of cells and of sub endothelial collagen in the direction of continuous flow, and that such endothelium is less permeable to protein and less susceptible to desquamation – and so more resistant to atherosclerosis. On the outer side of the flow divider, and in the daughter vessel, on the

other hand, shearing stresses are both high and variable, with swirling of blood in different directions under different conditions, so preventing alignment of endothelial cells and of collagen, and so leaving this region more susceptible to denudation, and more permeable to proteins and lipoproteins.

Fry's work, which is being continued and extended, provides a logical explanation for atherogenesis at and about branching points on the basis of altered shearing stresses at the vascular interface, either through transudation of lipoprotein into the vascular wall or through endothelial damage and platelet aggregation i.e. on the basis of the two·principal theories. Although important results have already become apparent, this work is still at a relatively embryonic stage. Further studies will involve more accurate mapping of shearing stresses at more sites, and in more sophisticated vascular models, together with examination of the effects of pulsatile flow, of vessel expansion, and of different degress of tethering on shearing stresses, endothelial change, and experimental atherosclerosis.

Although shearing stresses are important, and perhaps decisive in development of atherosclerosis at branches and bifurcations, stresses within the wall – tensile or compressive – are obviously also of great importance in atherogenesis. A person whose arterial pressure is high has the same arterial anatomy and the same cardiac output as a person whose blood pressure is normal (and so presumably the same shearing stresses around bends, branches and bifurcations), yet he develops atherosclerosis much more quickly. In the pulmonary circulation, blood flow is the same as in the systemic circulation and arteries branch and bifurcate in similar fashion, yet atherosclerosis does not occur unless pulmonary artery pressure is elevated (and so wall stresses are increased) for long periods of time. It is not known how increased wall stress predisposes to atherosclerosis. Stretch of the arterial wall increases permeability of the endothelium and entry of lipoproteins (Duncan et al 1965, Glagov 1972, deForest and Hollis 1978), but it seems unlikely that this is the only (or even the principal) mechanism; if it were, one would expect that when the plaque had developed and the endothelium was splinted by underlying fibrous tissue, permeability would return to normal, and growth of the plaque would cease. Plaques tend to remain localised and to grow progressively. It is possible that there are at branches, bends and discontinuities, large differences in circumferential and longitudinal stress in contiguous parts of the vessel wall throughout the cardiac cycle, and that these are increased when blood pressure is elevated, sufficient to shear and damage components of the vessel wall, and in this way to initiate the atherosclerotic process. Fry (1973) and Lutz et al (1977, 1979) emphasised the importance in atherogenesis of transient variations in shearing stress at the vascular interface; transient variations in shear within the wall may have similar importance. Such shearing stresses within the arterial wall (if they exist) will be extremely difficult to demonstrate.

Mechanical factors – shearing stress at the vascular interface, tensile and compressional stresses within the wall – obviously play an important role in atherogenesis, but there are clearly other factors as well. Mechanisms described could explain entry of lipoproteins into the intima, muscle cell proliferation and fibrosis or accumulation of debris from thrombosis in the intima. Other factors include low phagocytic activity in the intima (Adams 1973, Stebhens 1979), poor blood supply from the adventitia, even when thickened (Stehbens 1979), and its sluggish lymphatic drainage (Courtice and Garlick 1962). The intima of arteries is very inert and is cleared very slowly of foreign substances.

While it has been accepted for many years that mechanical factors are important in atherogenesis, little specific information on arterial stresses have been previously available. Progress in this field has come from measurement of stresses and application of standard physical and engineering principles to this problem, in association with conventional histological and histochemical techniques – from the same type of interdisciplinary collaboration which led to the modern approach to pulsatile blood flow. Further important advances can be anticipated.

REFERENCES

Adams CWM 1972 Tissue changes and lipid entry in developing atheroma In: Ciba Foundation Symposium No. 12 Atherosclerosis: initiating factors. Associated Scientific Publishers Amsterdam p. 5–37

Anitschkow N 1933 Experimental arteriosclerosis in animals. In: Cowdry EV (ed) Arteriosclerosis McMillan New York p. 304–306

Atabek HB, Ling SC, Patel DJ 1975 Analysis of coronary flow fields in thoracotomised dogs Circulation Research 37: 752–761

Benditt P 1977 The origin of atherosclerosis Scientific American 236: 75–85

Bergel DH, Nerem RM, Schwartz CJ 1976 Fluid dynamic aspects of arterial disease. Atherosclerosis 23: 253–261

Blumenthal HT, Handler FP, Blache JO 1954 The histogenesis of arteriosclerosis of the larger cerebral arteries, with an analysis of the importance of mechanical factors. American Journal of Medicine 17: 337–347

Bruns DL 1959 A general theory of the causes of murmurs in the cardiovascular system. American Journal of Medicine 27: 360–374

Bruns DL, Connolly JE, Holman E, Stofer RC 1959 Experimental observations on post-stenotic dilatation. Journal of Thoracic Surgery 38: 662–669

Caro CG 1973 Transport of material between blood and wall in arteries. In: Ciba Foundation Symposium No. 12 Atherosclerosis Initiating Factors Associated Scientific Publishers Amsterdam p. 127–164

Caro C 1977 Mechanical Factors in Atherogenesis. In: Hwang NH, Norman NA (eds) Cardiovascular flow dynamics and measurements University Park Baltimore

Courtice FC, Garlick DG 1962 The permeability of the capillary wall to the different plasma lipoproteins of the hypercholesterolemic rabbit in relation to size. Quarterly Journal of Experimental Physiology 47: 221–227

DeForrest JM, Hollis TM 1978 Shear stress and aortic histamine synthesis. American Journal of Physiology 234: 701–705

DePalma RG 1979 Atherosclerosis in vascular grafts. In: Atherosclerosis Reviews Vol 6 Gotto AM, Paoletti R (eds) Raven New York

DiGirolamo M, Schlant RC 1978 Etiology of coronary atherosclerosis. In: Hurst JW, Logue RB, Schlant RC, Wenger NK (eds) The Heart, Arteries and Veins p. 1103–1121

Duguid 1946 Thrombosis as a factor in the pathogenesis of coronary atherosclerosis. Journal of Pathology and Bacteriology 58: 207–212

Duguid 1948 Thrombosis as a factor in the pathogenesis of aortic atherosclerosis. Journal of Pathology and Bacteriology 60: 57–61

Duncan JE, Buch K, Lynch A 1965 The effect of pressure and stretching on the passage of labelled albumen into canine aortic wall. Journal of Atherosclerosis Research 5: 69–78

Flaherty JT, Ferrans VJ, Pierce JE, Carew TE, Fry DL 1972 Localising factors in experimental atherosclerosis. In: Likoff W, Segal BL, Insull W Jr, Mayer JH (eds) Atherosclerosis and coronary heart disease. Grune and Stratton New York p. 40–83

Fry DL 1969a Certain histological and chemical responses of

the vascular interface to acutely induced mechanical stress in the aorta of the dog. Circulation Research 24: 93–108

Fry DL 1969b Certain chemorheologic considerations regarding the blood vascular interface with particular reference to coronary artery disease. Circulation 39, 40: Supplement 4 38–59

Fry DL 1972 Localising factors in arteriosclerosis. In: Atherosclerosis and coronary heart disease. Grune and Stratton New York p 85–104

Fry DL 1973 Responses of the arterial wall to certain physical factors. Ciba Foundation Symposium no 12 Atherogenesis initiating factors Associated Scientific Publishers Amsterdam p. 93–125

Fry DL 1976 Hemodynamic forces in atherogenesis. In: Steinberg P (ed) Cerebrovascular disease. Raven New York p. 77–95

Ganz W 1981 Coronary spasm in myocardial infarction: fact or fiction. Circulation 63: 487–488

Gazetopoulos N, Ioannidis PJ, Marselos A, Kelekis D, Lolas C, Augoustakis D, Tountas G 1976 Length of main left coronary artery in relation to atherosclerosis of its branches A coronary arteriographic study. British Heart Journal 38: 180–185

Gertz S, Uretsky G, Wajnberg R, Navot N, Gotsman M 1981 Endothelial cell damage and thrombus formation after partial arterial constriction: relevance to the role of coronary artery spasm in the pathogenesis of myocardial infarction. Circulation 63: 476–486

Gessner F. 1973 Hemodynamic theories of atherogenesis. Circulation Research 33: 259–266

Glagov S. 1972 Hemodynamic risk factors; mechanical stress, mural architecture, medial nutrition and vulnerability of arteries to atherosclerosis. In: Wissler RW, Geer JC (eds) The pathogenesis of atherosclerosis Williams and Wilkins Baltimore p. 164–168.

Gresham GA, Howard AN 1965 Studies on aortic atherosclerosis in the turkey. In: Comparative atherosclerosis. Harper and Row New York p. 62–65

Gross HL 1977 Atherosclerosis Scope Upjohn Kalamazoo

Gutstein WH, Schneck DJ, Marks JO 1968 In vitro studies of local blood flow disturbances in a region of separation. Journal of Atherosclerosis Research 8: 381–388

Kurtz HJ 1969 Histological features of atherogenesis and aortic rupture in turkeys. American Journal of Veterinary Research 30: 243–249

Levy RI 1979 Prevalence and epidemiology of cardiovascular disease. In: Cecil Textbook of Medicine Beeson PB, McDermott W, Wyngaarden JB (eds) Saunders Philadelphia

Ling SC, Atabek HB, Fry DL, Patel DJ, Janicki JS 1968 Application of heated-film velocity and shear probes to hemodynamic studies. Circulation Research 23: 789–801

Lown B, DeSilva RA 1980 Is coronary artery spasm a risk factor for coronary atherosclerosis? American Journal of Cardiology 45: 901–903

Lutz RJ, Cannon JN, Bischoff KB, Dedrick RL, Stiles RK, Fry DL 1977 Wall shear stress distribution in a model canine artery during steady flow. Circulation Research 41: 391–399

Lutz RJ, Cannon JN, Bischoff KB, Dedrick RL, Stiles RK, Fry DL 1979 Shear stress patterns in a model canine artery: their relationship to atherosclerosis. In: Hwang NH, Gross DR, Patel DJ (eds) Quantitative Cardiovascular Studies University Park Baltimore Chapter 5 233–237

McDonald DA 1974 Blood flow in arteries. 2nd edition Arnold London

McGill HC (ed) 1968 The geographic pathology of atherosclerosis. Laboratory Investigation 18: 465–653

Malcolm A, Roach M 1979 Flow disturbances at the apex and lateral angles of a variety of bifurcation models and their role in development and manifestations of arterial disease. Stroke 10: 335–343

Malinow MR 1980 Atherosclerosis: Regression in non-human primates. Circulation Research 46: 331–320

Marzilli M, Goldstein S, Trivella MG, Palumbo C, Maseri A 1980 Some clinical considerations regarding the relation of coronary vasospasm to coronary atherosclerosis: a hypothetical pathogenesis. American Journal of Cardiology 45: 882–886

Mitchell JRA, Schwartz CJ 1965 Arterial disease. Oxford Blackwell

Montenegro MR, Eggen DA 1968 Topography of atherosclerosis in the coronary arteries. Laboratory Investigation 18: 126–133

Mustard JF 1974 Platelets and thrombosis. In: Braunwald E (ed) The Myocardium, failure and infarction. HP Publishing New York p. 117–190

Mustard JF, Packham MA 1975 The role of blood and platelets in atherosclerosis and the complications of atherosclerosis. Thromb Diath Haemorr 33: 444–456

Nerem RM, Rumberger JA, Gross DR, Hamlin RL, Geiger GL 1974 Hot film anemometer velocity measurements of arterial blood flow in horses. Circulation Research 34: 193–203

Nerem RM, Rumberger JA Jr, Gross DR, Hamlin RL, Geiger GL 1974 Hot film measurements of coronary blood flow in horses. In: Nerem RM (ed) Fluid dynamic aspects of arterial diseases Pt 1: 137–160

Nerem RM, Cornhill JF 1980 Hemodynamics and Atherogenesis Atherosclerosis 36: 151–157

Patek PR, deMignaro VA, Bernick S 1968 Changes in structure of coronary arteries. Susceptability to arteriosclerosis in old rats. Archives of Pathology 85: 388–396

Patel DJ, Vaishnav RN, Gow BS, Kot PA 1974 Hemodynamics. Annual Review of Physiology 36: 125–154

Patel DJ, Vaishnav RN, Atabek HB 1979 Local mechanical properties of the vascular intima and adjacent flow fields. In: Hwang NH, Gross DR, Patel DJ (eds) Quantitative cardiovascular studies university Park Baltimore Ch 5 p. 215–231

Peronneau PA, Hinglais JR, Xhaard M, Delouche P, Philippo J 1974 The effects of curvature and stenosis on pulsatile flow in vivo and in vitro. In: Reneman RS (ed) Cardiovascular applications of ultrasound. Elsevier New York p. 203–215

Peronneau P, Bournat JP, Bugnon A, Barbet A, Xhaard M 1974 Theoretical and practical aspects of pulsed Doppler flowmetry: real time application to the measurement of instantaneous velocity profiles in vitro and in vivo. In: Reneman RS (ed) Cardiovascular applications of ultrasound North Holland Amsterdam p. 66–84

Pickering GW 1964 Pathogenesis of myocardial and cerebral infarction: nodular arteriosclerosis. British Medical Journal 1: 517–529

Reader R 1979 Heart disease in Australia 1960–1980 and the National Heart Foundation. Medical Journal of Australia 1: 323–328

Roach MR 1977 Biophysical analyses of blood vessel walls and blood flow. Annual Review of Physiology 39: 51–71

Ross R, Glomset JA 1976 The pathogenesis of atherosclerosis. New England Journal of Medicine 295: 369–377

Saltissi S, Webb-Peploe MM, Coltart DJ 1977 Effect of
  variation in coronary artery anatomy on distribution of
  stenotic lesions. British Heart Journal 42: 186–191
Statistical Bulletin Metropolitan Life Insurance Co 1979 60:00
Stehbens WE 1975 The role of hemodynamics in the
  pathogenesis of atherosclerosis. Progress in Cardiovascular
  Diseases 18: 89–103
Stehbens WE 1979 Hemodynamics and the blood vessel wall.
  Thomas Springfield
Virchow RLK 1862 Cellular pathology as based on
  physiological and pathological histology. (translated from the
  second German edition by Chance F) 1971 New York Dover
  p. 230–245
Wissler RW, Vesselinovitch D, Getz GS 1976 Abnormalities of
  the arterial wall and its metabolism in atherogenesis.
  Progress in Cardiovascular Diseases 18: 341–369

Wolinsky H 1973 Mesenchymal response of the blood vessel
  wall. A potential avenue for understanding and treating
  atherosclerosis. Circulation Research 32: 543–549
Wolinsky H 1979 Atherosclerosis. In: Beeson PB, McDermott
  W, Wyngaarden JB (eds) Cecil, Texbook of Medicine.
  Saunders Philadelphia p. 1218–1222
Wolinsky H, Glagov S 1967 Nature of species differences in
  the medial distribution of aortic vasa vasorum in mammals.
  Circulation Research 20: 409–421
Wolinsky H, Glagov S 1969 Comparison of abdominal and
  thoracic aorta medial structure in mammals. Deviation of
  man from the usual pattern. Circulation Research
  25: 677–686
Young W, Gofman JW, Tandy R, Malamud N, Waters ESG
  1960 The quantitation of atherosclerosis 1. Relationship to
  artery size. American Journal of Cardiology 6: 288–293

16

Afterload reduction and cardiac performance

BACKGROUND

One of the most fundamental properties of isolated skeletal and heart muscle preparations is that during contraction, their extent of shortening is inversely related to the afterload applied (Fig. 16.1, Hill 1938, Sonnenblick 1966). In the intact heart, the same principle holds, and left ventricular stroke volume increases when aortic systolic pressure is reduced, (Sonnenblick and Dowling 1963), and decreases when aortic systolic pressure is increased (Ross et al 1966, Wilcken et al 1964, Braunwald et al 1967, Fig. 16.2)

Clinical application of these principles was slow, and it is only in the last eight years that deliberate, controlled reduction in aortic pressure during systole (left ventricular afterload) has been practiced widely in treatment of acute normotensive heart failure, chronic normotensive heart failure, and in management of acute myocardial infarction (Chatterjee and Parmley 1977, Chatterjee et al 1976, Awan et al 1977, Chatterjee and Swan 1974). See also Cohn (1980) for key selected references.

Although reduction in left ventricular afterload has been practiced only recently in normotensive patients, it has been known for three decades that reduction in arterial pressure is an important goal in management of acute and chronic hypertensive left ventricular failure (Smirk and Alstad 1951, Pickering 1968). The relevant physiological principles are the same in normotensive and hypertensive patients – increase in cardiac output as a result of decrease in left ventricular afterload. The old notion of hypertension as a disease – challenged so effectively by Pickering (see p. 210) – was apparently responsible for this therapy being reserved for patients whose heart failure was

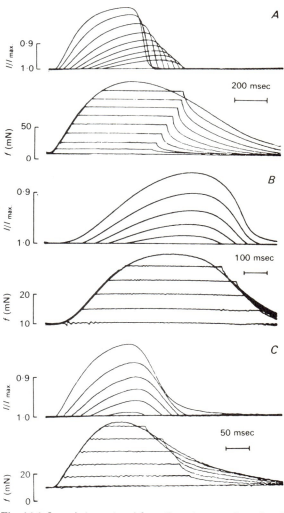

Fig. 16.1 Length (upper) and force (lower) traces of a series of afterloaded isotomic contractions against various loads in cat papillary muscle A; frog ventricular strip B; and rat papillary muscle C. Relaxation properties are different, but in all there is an inverse relationship for each contraction between degree of shortening and afterload. From Brutsaert et al (1978)

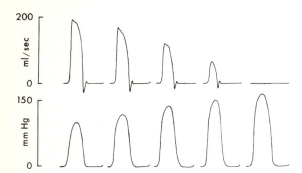

Fig. 16.2 Change in left ventricular ejection caused by stepwise increase in aortic (and so, left ventricular) pressure, with constant contractility and end-diastolic length. Redrawn from data published by Ross et al (1966)

associated with elevated arterial pressure. Benefit was ascribed to control of a disease (hypertension) and no benefit was expected in a patient already 'normotensive' in whom any degree of hypotension was considered to be undesirable. This was conventional wisdom up until the early 1970s.

The practice of left ventricular afterload reduction is thus soundly based, both on fundamental physiological properties of cardiac muscle, and on accepted treatment of patients with hypertension. The problems with drug therapy for afterload reduction are predictable, and explicable on the basis of decrease in mean pressure (fainting from transient cerebral ischemia when erect), and from decrease in pressure during diastole (possible myocardial ischemia from reduction in coronary flow). These are the same problems encountered with anti-hypertensive therapy, and have not proved to be a major hazard when modern therapy is carefully controlled.

Mechanism

The concept of left ventricular afterload as aortic or left ventricular pressure during systole was discussed in Chapter 10. The mechanisms whereby this afterload may be decreased are:- (Fig. 16.3)
1. Reduction of mean arterial pressure with drugs that reduce arteriolar tone
2. Reduction of arterial compliance, either indirectly through reduction of mean arterial pressure (p. 29), or directly through reduction in tone of smooth muscle in the wall of large arteries (p. 30).
3. Reduction in and delay of wave reflection when this is a factor in raising aortic systolic pressure (p. 145), through vasodilation and through reduction in pulse wave velocity
4. Reduction of systolic pressure preferentially with arterial counterpulsation
5. Reduction in cardiac output.

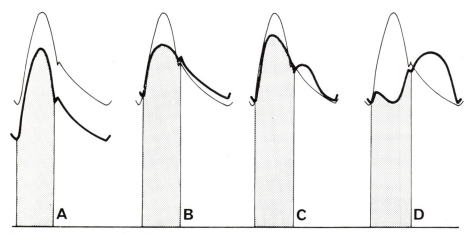

Fig 16.3 Reduction in aortic systolic pressure and in left ventricular pressure-time index (stippled area) as induced by a variety of mechanisms; from left to right
A Reduction in mean pressure without change in arterial distensibility
B Increase in arterial distensibility without change in mean pressure
C Delay in wave reflection
D Arterial counterpulsation
Superimposed in each case is the ascending aortic pressure wave as recorded in a human adult.

All but number 5 are therapeutically useful. The common factor is reduction in aortic and so left ventricular pressure during systole, be this through reduction in mean pressure (no. 1), pulse pressure (nos. 2 and 3), or through generation of a negative pressure wave in the aorta during systole (no. 4). One type of therapy may act through more than one mechanism i.e. vasodilator agents reduce mean pressure, increase arterial compliance indirectly (and perhaps directly as well – *vide infra*), and reduce and delay wave reflection.

Use of aortic pressure during systole as left ventricular afterload is a clinical convenience. One must bear in mind that the real afterload is the tension developed by the (more or less) circumferentially arranged myocardial fibres. Aortic pressure during systole will parallel changes in myocardial tension provided that (a) the period of isometric contraction and relaxation is not altered, and (b) end diastolic ventricular dimensions do not change. Another *caveat* in interpreting left ventricular afterload from arterial pressure is that one consider changes in amplification of the pulse to the brachial artery under different conditions (see p. 146); one cannot consider aortic systolic pressure to be the same as brachial artery pressure.

The beneficial action of agents which reduce ventricular afterload can readily be explained on the basis of myocardial mechanics (Figs 16.1, 16.2). The heart, when contracting against a lower pressure, can eject a greater volume. But increase in stroke volume with reduction in aortic systolic pressure is most apparent in patients with obvious cardiac failure and least obvious in patients without failure (Gold et al 1972, Chatterjee et al 1973, Cohn and Franciosa 1977). This same phenomenom is also seen in experimental animals (Reichel and Bauman 1978) and in isolated heart preparations (Elzinga and Westerhof 1974, 1978, 1979, Fig. 10.8) where greater relative increases in stroke volume are seen with decrease in afterload for lower degrees of myocardial contractility. The strongly contracting heart has been likened to a flow source (i.e. capable of ejecting the same volume against a wide range of pressures) and the weakened heart to a pressure source (i.e. capable of generating a moderate pressure only, and with volume ejection totally dependent on pressure de-

veloped) (Elzinga and Westerhof 1974, Reichel and Bauman 1978, Fig. 16.4). These findings can be explained readily on the basis of differences in ventricular function curves and pressure/volume loops as displayed by Sagawa, Suga and colleagues (Sagawa 1978, Suga et al 1980, p. 165).

Figure 16.5 shows diagramatically how differences in the slope of Frank/Starling ventricular function curves in the normal and failing heart can explain different responsiveness to afterload reduction. As the ventricle contracts, pressure rises

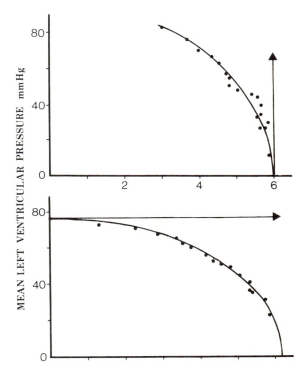

Fig. 16.4 Pump function curves redrawn from Elzinga and Westerhof (1979) with higher (top) and lower (bottom) ventricular contractility. Data points are fitted readily by ellipses with formulae

$$\frac{X^2}{6.0^2} + \frac{Y^2}{95.0^2} = 1 \text{ (top)}$$

$$\text{and } \frac{X^2}{6.2^2} + \frac{Y^2}{76.6^2} = 1 \text{ (bottom)}$$

The tangent to the ellipse at the intersection of pressure Y and flow X axes is 90°, signifying that the ventricle behaves as a pure flow source when pressure is zero and as a pure pressure source when flow is zero. When output is low the ventricle can be closely approximated to a pressure source. This could occur at normal pressure when ventricular contractility is depressed. Data prepared with Dr. A. Avolio

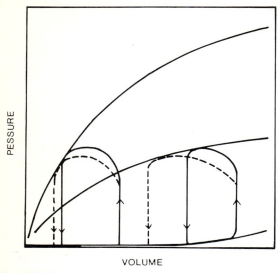

Fig. 16.5 Diagrammatic ventricular pressure-volume loops with normal and depressed ventricular contractility, illustrating the greater effect of arterial pressure reduction (dashed line) on volume ejection in the presence of impaired contractility

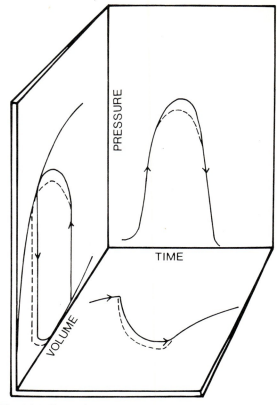

Fig. 16.6 Change in ventricular pressure (Y axis) and volume (Z axis) with time (X axis) through one cardiac cycle. The effect of reducing ventricular systolic pressure (afterload) is illustrated with a dashed line. See text.

without change in volume until aortic pressure is exceeded and the aortic valve opens. Pressure then rises slowly (in relation to volume), and ventricular volume falls. When the pressure – volume loop reaches the ventricular function curve, contraction ceases, the aortic valve shuts, and ventricular pressure falls. The dotted line shows the pressure-volume loop when afterload is reduced. With afterload reduction, ventricular ejection begins at a lower pressure, and the pressure – volume loop arches up to the ventricular function curve. Since with normal contractility, the slope of this curve is steep, the pressure – volume loop reaches the ventricular function curve at only a slightly lower volume than at the higher afterload, so only slightly more blood is ejected. When on the other hand, myocardial contractility is impaired, and the slope of the ventricular function curve is less steep, the pressure volume loop arches across further before meeting this curve at a greatly decreased systolic volume. Considerably more blood is ejected than at the higher systolic pressure. Difference in slope of the Frank/Starling curves with normal and impaired myocardial contractility thus explains the greater clinical benefit of afterload reduction in the presence of impaired myocardial contractility, the altered slope of pump function curves displayed

by Elzinga and Westerhof (1978, 1979), and the apparent change of the ventricle from flow source to pressure source when contractility is depressed (Elzinga and Westerhof 1974, Reichel and Baumann 1978).

It is fortuitous indeed that the failing ventricle responds so well to afterload reduction. A substantial rise in stroke volume can be achieved with a very small fall in aortic systolic pressure. When pressure is measured in the brachial or other peripheral artery, this change in aortic systolic pressure may not be apparent at all, because of altered pressure wave transmission (*vide infra*).

Figure 16.5 might be taken to imply that ventricular ejection is markedly prolonged when afterload is reduced. This is not the case. The ventricular pressure – volume loop takes no account of time. This can be added on a third axis (Fig. 16.6), so that the point relating pressure, volume,

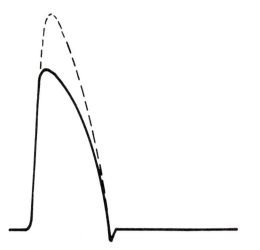

Fig. 16.7 Diagrammatic illustration of the effects of vasodilation (dashed line) on the left ventricular ejection wave. The major effect is increase in systolic flow; duration of systole is little altered

and time through the cardiac cycle can be taken to move through space in three dimensions, tracing a pressure – volume loop on the YZ axis, a ventricular pressure curve on the XY axis, and a volume – time curve (like a cardiometer curve as originally obtained by Henderson (1906) and used in the older textbooks (e.g. Wiggers 1950)) on the XZ axis. It is clear from this that when afterload is decreased, and stroke volume increased, ejection period is only slightly prolonged. The ventricular volume – time (or cardiometer) curve during systole is the integral of the ventricular volume flow ejection curve, and so may be differentiated to obtain this. Ventricular ejection curves measured during vasodilator therapy in heart failure do show the predicted pattern – an increase in peak and

mean flow with little change in ejection duration (Pepine et al 1977, Fig. 16.7).

Change in contour of the ventricular ejection wave may explain clinical benefit of vasodilator therapy in the absence of any appreciable change in brachial systolic pressure (Chatterjee and Parmley 1977, Cohn and Franciosa 1977). One cannot logically account for any beneficial effect from this therapy without reduction in ventricular afterload (reduced ventricular pressure during systole) (Braunwald 1974). However one can readily explain a difference in amplification of the aortic pressure wave to the brachial artery, such that aortic systolic pressure is reduced while brachial systolic pressure is unchanged. Amplification of the pressure pulse in transit to the brachial artery is discussed on page 146. The higher harmonics of the pressure wave between 2.5–5 Hz undergo most amplification, so that aortic pressure pulses with more energy in these components increase more in amplitude (O'Rourke 1970). The change in ascending aortic flow contour during vasodilator therapy (increase in peak flow with little change in ejection duration) is such as to increase these harmonics in the aortic pressure wave, and so cause more amplification. Possible effects of afterload reduction on aortic and brachial pressure waves are shown in Figure 16.8. No specific data on this subject are presently available so that the foregoing discussion is necessarily speculative. It is included however to emphasise the problems of inferring changes in central aortic and left ventricular systolic pressure from pressures recorded (even directly) in a peripheral artery. Indirect (sphygmomanometric) measurement of pressure introduces even more potential error (p. 148).

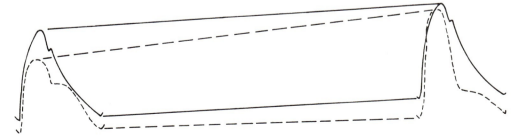

Fig. 16.8 Diagrammatic representation of pressure wave amplification between the ascending aorta (left) and brachial artery (right) under different conditions. Aortic systolic pressure may be decreased considerably without perceptible reduction in brachial systolic pressure

Vasodilator therapy of cardiac failure

Vasodilator drugs exert their therapeutic effect by reducing smooth muscle tone in blood vessels on the arterial and venous side of the circulation. All vasodilator drugs, currently available, alter arteriolar and venous tone, but relative intensity of effect varies. Phentolamine and hydralazine have their greatest influence on arteriolar tone with little effect on venous tone (Cohn and Franciosa 1977, Mehta et al 1978, Franciosa and Cohn 1978, Opie 1980).

Reduction in venous tone is beneficial in cardiac failure, since this increases venous distensibility, and so reduces venous pressure, venous return, and cardiac preload. Further discussion on change in preload with these drugs is outside the scope of this book. However it must be said that since vasodilator drugs are not specific, some decrease in preload must be expected with decrease in afterload. Usually this is a desirable therapeutic goal, but care must be exercised to ensure that this is not excessive.

Afterload reduction is achieved with vasodilator drugs primarily through reduction in peripheral resistance and so in mean arterial pressure. This is accompanied by a fall in pressure during systole (Fig. 16.3). Reduction in mean pressure has two other beneficial effects – increase in arterial distensibility (through reduction of arterial elastic modulus at lower distending pressure – p. 29) and delay of wave reflection from peripheral sites (through decrease in pulse wave velocity at lower distending pressure – p. 145). These effects are shown individually in Figure 16.3. Figure 16.9

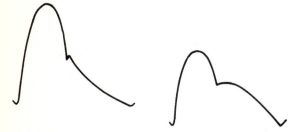

Fig. 16.9 Diagrammatic representation of the human ascending aortic pressure wave under control conditions (left) and during vasodilator therapy (right). Reduction in systolic pressure is attributable to fall in mean pressure, fall in pulsatile pressure, and delay of wave reflection

summarises the effects of vasodilator agents on aortic pressure.

Reduction in mean arterial pressure is a consequence of peripheral arteriolar vasodilation. The therapeutic effect of afterload reduction is an increase in cardiac output. Without this, mean pressure would fall to the same degree as peripheral resistance. Clearly, the fall in peripheral resistance is greater than the fall in mean pressure; however some reduction in mean pressure is necessary for continued therapeutic benefit i.e. mean pressure must remain lower than before for mean flow (cardiac output) to remain higher. This concept seems fundamental but is not unanimously accepted (see Chatterjee and Parmley 1977). Fall in mean pressure with vasodilator therapy is the basis of possible adverse effects – fainting and cerebral ischemia while in the upright position, and myocardial ischemia from reduced coronary perfusion pressure. However as previously discussed, in patients with impaired ventricular contractility, substantial increase in cardiac output can usually be achieved with only modest decrease in arterial pressure; such hazards therefore have not proved as serious as originally feared.

Reduction in arterial distensibility with vasodilator therapy has been demonstrated clearly by Pepine et al (1977) and by Levenson et al (1979). However it is not certain how much of this effect is attributable to decrease in mean arterial pressure, and how much is due to direct effect of the drug on the arterial wall. Pepine et al attempted to assess this by measuring characteristic impedance in the aorta under control conditions, then during nitroprusside infusion with mean pressure low, and again during nitroprusside infusion but with mean pressure restored to near normal through infusion of phenylephrine. Characteristic impedance was substantially reduced during nitroprusside infusion but was increased again, almost to the control value (no significant difference was apparent) with infusion of phenylephrine. This is not necessarily a good test for effects of vasodilator drugs on arterial muscular tone and distensibility, since phenylephrine may itself stimulate arterial muscle relaxed by nitroprusside.

At present the pharmaceutical industry is actively investigating the possibility that specific vasodilator agents can be produced which have preferential effects on arterial smooth muscle tone and so on arterial distensibility. Such drugs, by reducing pulse pressure, could confer the advantage of arteriolar vasodilation (decreased pressure during systole) without its disadvantages (decreased mean and diastolic pressures). The effects of smooth muscle on arterial distensibility are complex and variable; these are discussed on page 30.

Recent research on arterial pulse contour in man, and discussed on page 144, has emphasised the importance of wave reflection in determining left ventricular load and the potential benefits of vasodilator therapy in altering intensity and timing of wave reflection. It has been shown by Murgo et al (1980), and quite convincingly, that wave reflection in apparently normal human adults returns during systole and contributes substantially to left ventricular afterload. In early life – and in most experimental animals – wave reflection is beneficial to the heart through reducing aortic systolic pressure and augmenting pressure in the early part of diastole (McDonald and Taylor 1959, Taylor 1964, O'Rourke 1971). Arterial degeneration with advancing years increases pulse wave velocity and causes this favourable relationship to be reversed, so that even in apparently normal adults, early return of wave reflection increases ventricular afterload and reduces coronary perfusion pressure. Vasodilator therapy under these conditions would be expected to have two beneficial effects. Reduction in arteriolar tone, through reducing peripheral reflection coefficient (p. 88) would be expected to reduce wave reflection, and so, late systolic augmentation of the ascending aortic and left ventricular pressure pulse. The second beneficial effect is a consequence of decrease in mean pressure and pulse wave velocity. Decreased wave velocity would cause wave reflection from arterial terminations to be delayed. The most favourable effect would be achieved if the reflected wave from the lower body were to return after the aortic valve had closed. If vasodilator therapy could achieve this, it would have the effect of reversing (functionally) the ill effects of arterial degeneration and temporarily restoring the favourable relationship of wave reflection

to ventricular ejection that is seen in childhood (p. 144).

Vasodilator therapy in acute myocardial infarction

Vasodilator agents have been investigated extensively in animals with experimentally induced coronary artery obstruction and in patients with acute infarction. Hemodynamic benefit – decrease in left ventricular filling pressure and increase in cardiac output – have been observed consistently in animals and patients with cardiac failure (Gold et al 1972, Kelly et al 1973, Chatterjee et al 1973, Epstein et al 1975, Franciosa et al 1978). Changes in cardiac output are small or absent however in patients without cardiac failure (Gold et al 1972, Chatterjee et al 1973), as might be predicted from consideration of ventricular function curves (Fig. 16.5). Despite these hemodynamic differences, however, vasodilator agents appear also to be beneficial in reducing myocardial ischemia, infarct size, and arrhythmic complications of acute infarction in animals and in patients irrespective of the presence or absence of cardiac failure (Reid et al 1973, Maroko and Braunwald 1973, Shell and Sobel 1974, Epstein et al 1975, Muller et al 1979), especially when reflex tachycardia from undue hypotension is obviated (Epstein et al 1975).

Reduction in myocardial ischemic injury in acute infarction through use of vasodilator therapy can be attributed to a number of factors – reduction in ventricular dimensions as a result of decreased preload (and afterload), coronary vasodilation and relief of coronary artery spasm (Maseri et al 1978, Epstein et al 1975, Alpert and Cohn 1979) – as well as to alteration in arterial pressure.

If all other factors remained constant – heart rate, heart size, coronary artery calibre, right atrial pressure, left ventricular end diastolic pressure – one might expect that a decrease in mean arterial pressure would decrease pressure during systole, and pressure during diastole to the same degree, and so cause no difference in the relationship between ventricular oxygen demand and ventricular oxygen supply (p. 166). However, as just discussed, decrease in arterial compliance and delay in wave reflection and reduction in wave reflection lead to a greater fall in systolic than in diastolic pressure (Fig. 16.9). Thus the change in pressure wave contour which accompanies vasodilation and hypotension can in itself account for a favourable alteration in the balance between myocardial oxygen demand and supply. Obviously, decrease in oxygen demand is augmented by decrease in ventricular dimensions, and increase in coronary perfusion pressure by decrease in right ventricular and left ventricular end-diastolic pressure as well.

Details of treatment of acute infarction, and of heart failure with vasodilator agents are given in many recent reviews and textbooks (e.g. Zeilis et al 1979, Alpert and Cohn 1979, Smith and Braunwald 1980). Emphasis here is on mechanism of action and effects of afterload alone on the left ventricle. It goes without saying that vasodilator agents are powerful drugs with capacity for causing as much (if not more) harm as benefit. Acute treatment should be given with careful monitoring of systemic and pulmonary artery pressures, and if

possible, cardiac oupput as well. Chronic therapy is best introduced gradually and preferably commenced when the patient is hospitalised.

ARTERIAL COUNTERPULSATION

Description, history, physiological principles

Arterial counterpulsation is a technique of mechanical heart assistance whereby ascending aortic pressure is artificially decreased during systole and increased during diastole. As currently applied, counterpulsation is achieved by rhythmic inflation and deflation of a sausage shaped balloon inserted into the descending thoracic aorta from the femoral artery (Fig. 16.10); the pump is synchronised with the patient's electrocardiogram and inflation and deflation timed to create the maximal possible increase and decrease respectively in pressure during diastole and during systole (Fig. 16.11).

The beneficial effects of arterial counterpulsation are a consequence of alteration in aortic pres-

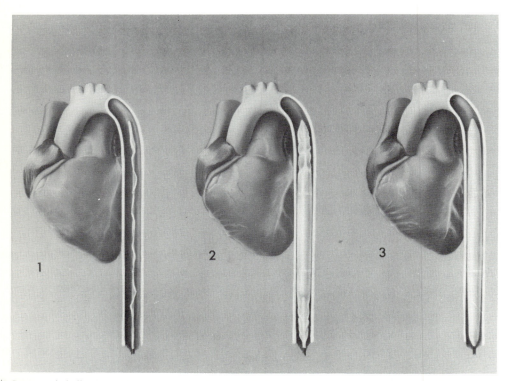

Fig. 16.10 Intra aortic balloon counterpulsation, showing the balloon completely deflated at the end of systole (left), completely inflated at the end of diastole (right) and at an intermediate stage (centre). Figure by courtesy of Avco Corp

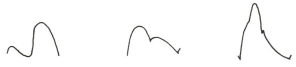

Fig. 16.11 Diagrammatic representation of ascending aortic pressure waves during counterpulsation (left) and under control conditions in a young human without arterial degeneration (centre), and a human with arterial degeneration (right). Counterpulsation decreases pressure during systole and increases pressure during diastole; arterial degeneration has the opposite effect, increasing pressure during systole and decreasing pressure during diastole

sure wave contour. This mechanical form of heart support can be viewed as exaggerating and reinforcing normal physiological processes which lower systolic pressure and elevate pressure in diastole. Counterpulsation is thus very relevant to "arterial function", and so warrants discussion in detail.

The concept of altering the aortic pulse mechanically to the heart's advantage was first conceived by the Kantrowitz brothers in 1953, and first applied in experimental animals during the late 1950s (Clauss et al 1959). At that time, counterpulsation was achieved by withdrawal and reinfusion of blood with each beat of the heart. Such a technique proved impracticable for clinical use because of mechanical problems and hemolysis as blood was pumped at high velocity over short periods through narrow tubing. Introduction of the intra-aortic balloon by Moulopoulos et al (1962) made clinical application a practical possibility. With the intra-aortic balloon, counterpulsation is achieved by pumping a gas into and out of a balloon instead of blood into and out of the aorta. Initial experience with balloon counterpulsation was reported by Adrian Kantrowitz and colleagues in 1968, and the largest clinical evaluation has been reported by Buckley, Gold and colleagues at the Massachusetts General Hospital (e.g. Dunkman et al 1972, Sanders et al 1972, Leinbach et al 1973, Mundth 1976, Levine et al 1978, 1979). At present, intra-aortic balloon counterpulsation is widely used throughout the world on thousands of patients annually, for three principal indications:— unstable angina pectoris refractory to conventional medical therapy, cardiogenic shock complicating acute myocardial infarction, and low output heart failure following heart surgery. A technique of external counterpulsation has been introduced (Soroff et al 1974) which involves rhythmic inflation and deflation of a pressure suit over the lower part of the body. This has not gained popularity because counterpulsation achieved is less effective than with the intra-aortic balloon, and harder to time accurately, while the device is uncomfortable to the patient, and cumbersome for its operators.

The beneficial physiological effects of arterial counterpulsation are readily apparent – decrease in pressure during ventricular systole with consequent increase in cardiac output and decrease in myocardial oxygen demands (p. 164), and increase in pressure during diastole with capacity for greater myocardial blood flow (p. 166). Counterpulsation achieves the same benefit as vasodilator therapy – reduction in systolic pressure – while increasing instead of decreasing coronary perfusion pressure.

While counterpulsation is obviously an artificial phenomenom, with energy added to the circulation by a pump in series with the heart, its effects are the same as those normally achieved by pressure pulse wave reflection. Under normal circumstances (i.e. in the absence of arterial degeneration), wave reflection augments pressure during diastole after the aortic valve has closed, and slightly decreases pressure during the next ventricular contraction (p. 162). As described on page 193, arterial degeneration with advancing years leads to earlier return of wave reflection, and disturbance of this favourable relationship. Counterpulsation can be looked upon as an artificial means of exaggerating a normally-occurring phenomenom (wave reflection); i.e. counterpulsation is an unnatural technique with a natural function. The comparison with wave reflection can be taken further; if counterpulsation is not appropriately timed, it can increase systolic pressure and decrease diastolic pressure, as does early wave reflection in arteriosclerosis (p. 189). Figure 16.11 contrasts ascending aortic pressure waves (drawn diagrammatically) during counterpulsation (left), under control conditions (center), and in a patient with arteriosclerosis (right).

When counterpulsation was initially introduced, the direct and immediate beneficial effects of reduced afterload on ventricular performance were not generally acknowledged. Benefit was attributed to relief of myocardial ischemia through reduction in tension-time index and so in left ventricular myocardial blood need, with concurrent increase in coronary perfusion pressure and so in coronary flow (Ch. 10). It is now acknowledged that hemodynamic benefit is partly a direct effect of afterload reduction on the failing ventricle, and partly a consequence of decreased myocardial ischemia.

Experimental results and pathophysiological principles in acute coronary occlusion

Prior to clinical application, exhaustive studies with counterpulsation were performed on experimental animals with ligated or embolised coronary arteries (Jacobey et al 1962, 1963, Brown et al 1967, Goldfarb et al 1968, Goldfarb et al 1969, Gundel et al 1970, Braunwald et al 1969, Spotnitz et al 1969, Powell et al 1970). Results were as predicted from physiological principles, consistent, and exciting. Cardiac output was increased substantially, and ventricular filling pressure, decreased. Coronary blood flow was increased with flow passing through collateral vessels into the ischemic area; evidence of myocardial ischemia was decreased, and, following standardised occlusion, infarct size was decreased considerably compared to control animals. In animals allowed to recover from standardised coronary occlusion, 24 hour survival was increased three fold in Jacobey's series (Jacobey et al 1963, Harken 1974), and six fold in Goldfarb's (Goldfarb 1969).

Unfortunately these excellent results in experimental animals with severe heart failure following coronary obstruction have not been reproduced in man. In dogs subjected to arterial counterpulsation, this was instituted within minutes of onset of myocardial ischemia. In patients, counterpulsation has usually been delayed for many hours, and sometimes days, after onset of clinical symptoms of infarction. This one factor – *time* – can explain the difference between the extremely good results of arterial counterpulsation in experimental coronary occlusion, and the depressingly bad results in acute myocardial infarction in man. Clinicians are apt to see this matter differently, and to attribute poor results to inefficiency of the technique, rather than to the stage at

which this was applied. Abundant experimental evidence supports this contention.

Experimental myocardial infarction has been studied extensively, especially in dogs. After coronary artery occlusion in a dog, the area of muscle supplied becomes cyanotic, ceases to contract, then bulges paradoxically. These changes, first described by Tennant and Wiggers (1935), are seen within 1–2 minutes. If occlusion is released within 20 minutes, myocardial blood flow is restored and reactive hyperemia is seen; the electrocardiogram, characterised during occlusion by marked ST segment elevation, returns to normal within minutes, but myocardial contractility returns much more slowly, with normal function delayed for up to 3 hours or more after a 5 minute occlusion, and for 6 hours or more after a 15 minute occlusion (Jennings et al 1975, Heyndrickxx et al 1975). During this period of depressed myocardial function, reversibility may be uncovered by post extrasystolic potentiation (Cohn 1980). No irreversible changes are usually seen histologically in myocardial cells if reperfusion occurs within 20 minutes (Jennings and Ganote 1974, Muller et al 1979).

If occlusion in dogs is continued for over 20 minutes, signs of irreversible damage are noted in myocardial cells within the ischemia area. However for periods up to 3–4 hours in dogs, and up to 2 hours in monkeys, myocardial viability is retained in some parts of the ischemia area. Within this time, reperfusion can salvage some myocardial tissue, but after 4 hours, myocardial reperfusion usually has no apparent effect on the size of evolving infarction (Maroko et al 1972, Ginks et al 1972, Constantini et al 1975, Smith et al 1974, Baughman et al 1981). Indeed, reperfusion after 4 hours in dogs has often led to hemorrhage into and spread of infarction (Bresnahan et al 1974, Muller et al 1979, McIntosh and Buccino 1979). Beta blocking drugs administered to limit infarct size have been effective when initiated within 4 hours of coronary occlusion in dogs (Miura et al 1979), but no benefit has been evident after this time.

After onset of symptoms of myocardial infarction in man, enzymes are released from necrotic cells into blood over 24 – 48 hours. This was initially considered to parallel the time course of infarction (Shell and Sobel 1974), so that relief of ischemia and limitation of infarction were considered possible with interventions (including coronary bypass surgery and counterpulsation) introduced more than 4 hours after the onset of symptoms. The early findings of Shell and Sobel have not been reproduced with beta blocking agents (Peter et al 1978) nor with counterpulsation (O'Rourke et al 1979), when initiated more than 4 hours after onset of symptoms. The progression of myocardial ischemia to irreversible necrosis in man appears to be much the same as in dogs (McIntosh amd Buccino 1979). Limitation of infarction might only be expected after 4 hours if the process of critical coronary occlusion is recurrent (and so the infarction process 'stuttering') or if some complication supervenes (such as an arrhythmia, cardiac failure or shock) that increases blood demand or decreases blood or oxygen supply, and so potentiates ischemia.

This subject – progression of reversible to irreversible myocardial damage in man following onset of the clinical syndrome of infarction – is of extreme practical importance in relation to modern coronary care, but is still highly controversial. It has been proposed that acute myocardial infarction be regarded as an acute surgical emergency – like acute obstruction of a peripheral artery – and that revascularisation or recanalisation be performed before irreversible damage has occurred (or at least before all ischemic damage has become irreversible) (Berg et al 1975, Phillips et al 1979 Rentrop et al 1979, 1981 Ganz et al 1981). Benefit has been claimed up to 25 hours after onset of symptoms (Phillips et al 1979). Cardiologists remain sceptical (McIntosh and Buccino 1979). In cardiogenic shock following infarction, coronary artery bypass has been considered an important factor for improving survival, even when performed 48 hours or more after onset of infarction (Dunkman et al 1972, Mundth 1976). The benefit of this, however has been challenged (Hagermeijer et al 1977, O'Rourke et al 1979). Hemorrhage into infarction with infarct extension (as seen in animals) has always been a concern with coronary bypass surgery in acute infarction, but the Massachusetts General Hospital group, who have had a vast experience, have found little or no evidence of this (Levine et al 1978).

Clinical experience

It is possible with hindsight to criticise the clinical application of counterpulsation as deviating from pathophysiological principles established in experimental animals, and to suggest more logical application. Short of correcting coronary obstruction (through surgical bypass or drug therapy for spasm or for clot lysis), counterpulsation is the most effective method known for relief of myocardial ischemia. As with bypass surgery, counterpulsation must be initiated when ischemic damage is still reversible for maximal benefit to be realised. Yet in man it has not. Counterpulsation has usually been reserved until all other conventional measures have proved unavailing, and so applied when reversible damage had become minimal and irreversible damage, maximal.

Clinical application of arterial counterpulsation over the last thirteen years follows the usual pattern for any new unusual therapeutic technique. Treatment was reserved initially for desperately ill patients in whom all else had failed. Depressing results remained depressing. Too much was expected of the new treatment. Further, clinical scientific interest was on hemodynamic indices for characterising severity of disease and assessing improvement. Time taken to determine these before initiation of therapy further delayed its initiation. Extreme concern was properly shown in the hazards of treatment, but the incidence of these hazards was exaggerated by the severity of the patients' illness. When the treatment (counterpulsation) was not promptly successful (i.e. within 24–48 hours), another variable (coronary artery bypass surgery) was introduced, making independent assessment of either an even greater problem.

At present there is no consensus on the value of counterpulsation in acute coronary artery disease. It has come to be employed as an adjunct to coronary artery bypass surgery at the two extremes of the clinical spectrum of acute coronary artery disease – unstable angina at the one end and cardiogenic shock on the other. There has been little clinical application between these two extremes, and little use of counterpulsation as a therapeutic technique in its own right. Physiological principles, experimental results, and pathophysiological studies argue that this is illogical. The current practice with counterpulsation is outlined below.

Cardiogenic shock. Counterpulsation was initially evaluated in patients with cardiogenic shock following acute myocardial infarction. This is still the most common indication for its use. The initial clinical experience reported by Kantrowitz et al (1968) was good, and similar to that reported recently in patients with severe left ventricular failure (in or apparently just short of shock) and in whom coronary artery surgery was not employed routinely (Hagermeijer et al 1977, O'Rourke et al 1979). Kantrowitz and colleagues were however criticised for their selection of patients on the basis of clinical criteria alone, and their work was discounted by many. There followed a phase when it was considered essential to document cardiogenic shock precisely through invasive measurements of systemic and pulmonary artery pressure and cardiac output, with careful trials of medical therapy before proceeding to counterpulsation. Though scientifically proper in evaluating a new therapeutic technique, this made little sense if myocardial ischemic damage was progressing to irreversibility during catheterisation and clinical evaluation. Measurements in man showed that counterpulsation has the same salutary acute hemodynamic and metabolic effects in patients with cardiogenic shock as in experimental animals (Mueller et al 1971, Sanders et al 1972, Schidt et al 1973, Dilley et al 1973); Ultimate outcome however was quite different; survival in man was far lower than in dogs – but the timing of intervention was totally different.

Early results of counterpulsation alone in cardiogenic shock were poor:–Dunkman et al (1972) reported survival of 12 percent, Scheidt et al (1973), 9 percent, Willerson et al (1975) 10 percent, and Bardet et al (1977), 12 percent. These figures were very depressing and were considered to be little better than with continued medical therapy alone. In an attempt to improve survival, the Massachusetts General Hospital group suggested that patients who could not be weaned from balloon pumping after 24–48 hours be evaluated for coronary artery bypass surgery. Results improved with this therapy (Dunkman et al 1972) and at present the Massachusetts General Hospital has hospital survival rate of about 45 percent in patients with cardiogenic shock undergoing counterpulsation and coronary bypass surgery (see Mundth 1976).

Treatment of cardiogenic shock with counterpulsation and coronary artery bypass surgery is practiced widely at this time (see Boolooki 1977, Alpert and Cohn 1979). However groups in Rotterdam (Hagermeijer et al 1977) and in Sydney (O'Rourke et al 1975, 1979) have obtained similar results with counterpulsation alone continued for 1–4 weeks, with coronary artery bypass reserved for patients who develop evidence of further ischemia during or after the weaning period. These results appear to conflict with the early results and interpretations of Dunkman, Scheidt, Willerson and Bardet, quoted above. Similar criteria were used for definition of cardiogenic shock (the original U.S. MIRU definition of cardiogenic shock has in the interests of expediency been relaxed in virtually all centres) so it is hardly possible to explain differences on this basis. Apparent benefit of coronary artery bypass is based on historical controls, identification of 'pump dependence' at 24–48 hours, secondary deterioration of patients during continuation of counterpulsation alone (Dilley et al 1973, Erich et al 1977), and on patient selection for revascularisation surgery. With a decade of experience of arterial counterpulsation, and relaxation of criteria for its initiation, it is hardly fair to compare results obtained now with those achieved when this therapy was in its infancy. It might be said that better results are still obtained now in patients selected for bypass surgery than in those undergoing counterpulsation alone; however patients rejected for surgery often have other undesirable features in coronary anatomy, ventricular performance, or elsewhere, which mitigate against a favourable result. 'Pump dependence' is usually quoted as the indication for bypass surgery. But 'pump dependence' varies with time. We (O'Rourke et al 1975, 1979) have often found that a patient who was 'pump dependent' at 2 days was not so dependent at 4 or 7 days, or that a patient, dependent at 7 days was not dependent at 14 days. Indeed with continued counterpulsation, we have usually seen progressive improvement for up to 21 days. (We have not observed further improvement beyond this time). Secondary deterioration on counterpulsation has been reported as a reason for coronary bypass. We have seen this only in patients desperately ill (and unusually in complete renal failure) at the time counterpulsation was initiated. Our mortality rate for patients on counterpulsation (Fig. 16.12) has shown decrease after initiation of counterpulsation. We attribute continued improvement on counterpulsation alone to gradual recovery of reversibly damaged myocardium (Heyndrickxx et al 1955) and to growth of collateral vessels. Gradual improvement of myocardial performance after infarction is well established (Russell et al 1970). It is interesting that the average duration of counterpulsation in our series (O'Rourke et al 1979) i.e. 7.0 days is similar to the average duration of vasodilator therapy chosen by Chatterjee et al (1976) i.e. 7.6 days on the basis of stabilisation of hemodynamics and clinical improvement. The reason for secondary deterioration as reported by Dilley et al, and by Erich et al is not clear. It may have been related to the strains of angiographic investigation and trials of weaning.

Other reasons for avoiding early bypass surgery relate to the uncertain role that this has in myocardial infarction generally (McIntosh and Buccino 1979), the disruption of routine services when patients proceed to urgent angiography and urgent surgery in addition to counterpulsation, and our own results with early revascularisation surgery. On the basis of experimental studies, discussed earlier, I see little logic in coronary bypass surgery when a patient is stable, albeit temporarily

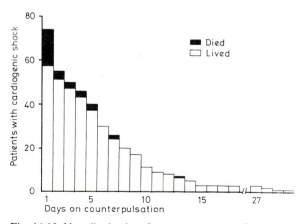

Fig. 16.12 Mortality by day after commencement of counterpulsation in a group of 74 patients with cardiogenic shock. From O'Rourke et al (1979)

dependent on counterpulsation. I see little hope of limiting the present infarct by coronary bypass performed 24–48 hours (or more) after onset of symptoms; I do however see the prospect of preventing later ischemia or infarction through coronary bypass, but believe that this matter can best be approached when the patient has recovered from the initial insult. Urgent angiography and bypass surgery can be handled with ease in some major centres but in most (including our own) where there is already a heavy load on facilities and a long waiting list for elective surgery, this can pose a heavy and unfair burden on staff and patients. Our own results for early urgent revascularisation surgery show no benefit over treatment with counterpulsation alone (O'Rourke et al 1979).

Many patients with cardiogenic shock have mechanical complications of infarction, often a consequence of myocardial disruption. These include hemopericardium (from subacute heart rupture or hemorrhagic pericarditis), severe mitral valve incompetence (from papillary muscle rupture), ventricular septal defect (from septal rupture) and subacute aneurysm formation (often a pseudoaneurysm associated with subacute rupture). Septal defect and mitral incompetence are usually obvious on clinical grounds, and can be diagnosed using monitoring catheters. Hemopericardium and aneurysm should be considered and excluded in all patients. These are discussed elsewhere (Leinbach et al 1973, O'Rourke 1973, Mundth 1976, Bardet et al 1977, Boolooki 1977, Alpert and Cohn 1979). It is generally agreed that these complications warrant urgent surgical correction. Results – especially long term – are far better than in patients whose cardiogenic shock is due completely to poor myocardial contraction.

Our personal experience at St. Vincent's Hospital, Sydney has been reported in a series of papers (O'Rourke 1972, 1973, Windsor et al 1973, O'Rourke et al 1975, 1979). Our first 100 patients with acute infarction who underwent arterial counterpulsation included 76 with cardiogenic shock. Twenty five of these were hospital survivors (33 percent) but late survival was poor. Actuarial curves are shown in Figures 16.13, 16.14 and 16.15. The best results were seen in patients with mechanical lesions, corrected surgically, and in patients undergoing counterpulsation

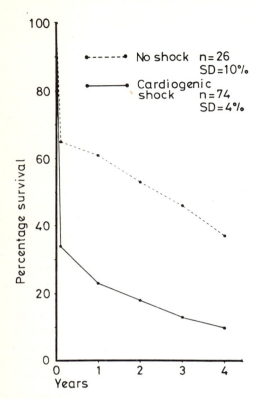

Fig. 16.13 Life tables of 100 patients with acute myocardial infarction and severe refractory heart failure, treated with arterial counterpulsation. Dashed line: patients not in cardiogenic shock. Solid line: patients in cardiogenic shock. From O'Rourke et al (1979)

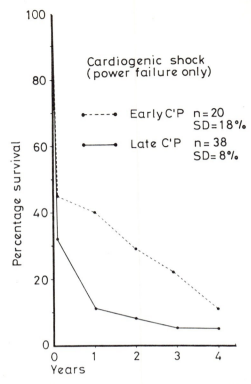

Fig. 16.14 Life tables: 58 patients with acute myocardial infarction and cardiogenic shock, but without myocardial disruption causing septal defect, mitral incompetence or hemopericardium. Dashed line: 'early' counterpulsation – commenced within 8 hours of the apparent onset of shock. Solid line: late counterpulsation – commenced 8 hours or more after apparent onset of shock. From O'Rourke et al (1979)

early – i.e. within 8 hours of the onset of cardiogenic shock. Worst results were seen (survival rate 6 percent at 4 years, 6/58 alive at the time of follow up) in patients without mechanical lesions. Functional status was good in patients with corrected mechanical defects (all in N.Y.H.A. class 1 or 2) but generally poor in those without mechanical lesions (4 of 6 in N.Y.H.A. class 3 or 4); all limited by dyspnoea).

Complications of counterpulsation occurred in 17 of the 74 patients with cardiogenic shock (and in only 2 of another 26 without shock). Complications are listed on Table 16.1. None directly caused death. Thirteen of the 19 complications occurred on the first day, 4 subsequently during counterpulsation, and two on removal of the balloon catheter. Contrary to other views (Pace et al 1976), we believe that complications are largely a consequence of the insertion procedure in a des-

Table 16.1 Complications of counterpulsation in 100 patients

Ischemia of leg (1 with gangrene)	10
Arterial dissection	3
Bleeding (1 with infection)	3
Balloon damage	2
Embolism	1
TOTAL:	19

perately ill patient. Once counterpulsation is established and the patient responding, the chance of late complication appears to be remote; we believe that fear of complications should not dictate early termination in a patient who is responding well.

Our experience with counterpulsation in cardiogenic shock is in line with what one might pre-

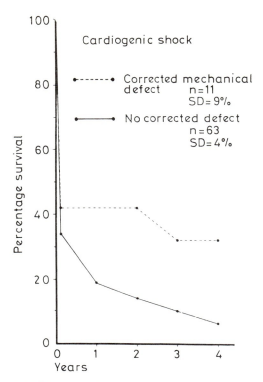

Fig. 16.15 Life tables: 74 patients with acute myocardial infarction and cardiogenic shock, treated with arterial counterpulsation. Dashed line: – patients with mechanical defects corrected surgically. Solid line: – all other patients. From O'Rourke et al (1979)

dict from physiological principles, and only as good as one might realistically expect in patients undergoing treatment many hours or even days after onset of infarction. Our present approach to a patient with suspected cardiogenic shock in acute infarction can be summarised as follows:-

1. Confirmation of severe medically refractory left ventricular failure and shock on clinical and radiological grounds. Specific exclusion of hypovolemia and of other medically correctable factors – acidosis, arrhythmia etc
2. Exclude contraindications
3. Initiate counterpulsation promptly: insert systemic and pulmonary catheters during balloon insertion procedure in order to avoid additive delays
4. Exclude mechanical lesions; if present, urgent surgery indicated
5. Continue counterpulsation for one week before first trial of weaning

6. Discontinue counterpulsation between 1–3 weeks, when completely stable
7. Angiography and possible coronary artery bypass if signs of ischemia reappear during or after weaning.

Severe Heart Failure without Shock, following acute myocardial infarction. Vasodilator therapy has proved more popular than counterpulsation in treatment of severe left ventricular failure without shock. Use in failure without shock is a logical extension of use in cardiogenic shock, especially in patients refractory to all medical therapy, including vasodilators. Hagermeijer (1975) reported 75 percent (6/8) long term (average 20 months) survival in such patients. We (O'Rourke et al 1979, Sammel and O'Rourke 1979) had hospital survival 65 percent (17/26) and four year survival 37 percent in a similar group. Our results were far better than predicted on the basis of Peel and Norris prognostic indices. Our best results were obtained in a subgroup of these patients (determined retrospectively) with continuing ischemic pain and ST segment elevation (Sammel and O'Rourke 1979) In 12 such patients, there was only one hospital death, compared to 8 deaths in 14 patients without continuing pain. These results were consistent with the thesis that counterpulsation is most effective in acute infarction through relief of myocardial ischemia and limitation of infarction.

These encouraging results led us to undertake a randomised controlled trial of counterpulsation in patients with early (within 15 hours of symptom onset) infarction and acute heart failure (O'Rourke et al 1980). A 25 percent reduction in hospital mortality was sought. The trial was terminated after entry of 30 patients when such a mortality reduction was shown to be improbable (at 5 percent confidence level), and with no difference apparent in infarct size between the two groups. A smaller reduction in mortality was possible but would have required more patients to prove. These results were hard to reconcile with earlier uncontrolled studies. In this trial, counterpulsation was introduced 4.8–13.7 hours after onset of symptoms. It is likely that all ischemic damage had become irreversible by this time. Propranolol has been found effective in decreasing enzyme release (and so presumably in limiting infarct size) when administered less than 4 hours after onset of

248 ARTERIAL FUNCTION IN HEALTH AND DISEASE

symptoms, but not later. I believe that the trial of counterpulsation should be repeated, with entry less than 4 hours after onset of symptoms.

Unstable Angina The Massachusetts General Hospital group pioneered the use of counterpulsation in medically–refractory unstable angina pectoris. This is generally regarded as a pre-infarctional condition, warranting the same early management in a coronary care ward as acute infarction. Indeed it is often difficult except in retrospect to know whether or not myocardial infarction is occurring. Nonetheless this condition represents the opposite end of the clinical spectrum from cardiogenic shock in that recovery is the rule rather than the exception with conventional treatment (Co-Operative Unstable Angina Study Group 1978, 1980). However relapse is common (45 percent of medically treated patients in the later co-operative study required bypass surgery within 3.5 years for unacceptable angina), and infarction frequent both in medically treated patients, and in surgically treated patients about the time of urgent revascularisation.

Gold and colleagues (1973) introduced counterpulsation in patients requiring urgent coronary artery bypass surgery as a means to stabilise and prevent deterioration during angiography and preparation for surgery. Effects were prompt, with over 80 percent of patients having complete relief of anginal pain; no patient developed cardiac complications during angiography. In the latest report from the Massachusetts General Hospital, Levine et al (1978) reported 3.3 percent hospital mortality and 1.6 percent perioperative infarction rate in 60 patients with medically refractory angina pectoris who underwent counterpulsation, angiography, and coronary artery bypass. Mortality rate was similar but infarction rate markedly less than in the cooperative studies, where counterpulsation was not used routinely.

The effects of counterpulsation in unstable angina are predictable on the basis of physiological principles. Treatment is applied to relieve myocardial ischemia and its complications and to prevent the prolonged imbalance between myocardial supply and demand that results in myocardial infarction. One's only concern relates to the potential hazards of the therapy itself in relatively good risk patients. The M.G.H. experience is reassuring; virtually no complications of counterpulsation have occurred in these patients.

Low output heart failure following cardiac surgery. Low output heart failure is a serious problem following cardiac surgery and is the most common cause of post-operative death. The cause of impaired myocardial contractility is not fully established, but is related to myocardial ischemia, mechanical handling, and to the technique of bypass and of cardiac arrest. Modern techniques of cardioplegia have reduced the incidence of this as a serious problem following surgery. Impaired contractility following bypass appears to have the same time course as that following brief experimental coronary occlusion (Heyndrickxx et al 1975) – i.e. taking hours or days to recover. Buckley et al (1972) were the first to report use of counterpulsation in this condition. Their results were good. Our group's initial experience with this indication were indifferent, but counterpulsation was at first delayed until all other measures had proved ineffective. With greater confidence and willingness to commence balloon pumping earlier, results have improved. Currently (O'Rourke et al 1980) we have 59 percent hospital survival and 35 percent four year survival in 34 patients who could not readily be weaned from cardiopulmonary bypass. In the largest series to date, Sturm et al (1980) reported 45 percent hospital survival in 419 patients with low output syndrome following surgery.

These good results with counterpulsation are easily understood. Counterpulsation acts as an effective afterload reducing technique for the temporarily depressed heart, while maintaining coronary blood flow. The treatment is introduced within one or two hours of the cardiac insult, and is not delayed (as following infarction) for hours or days by a patient's reluctance to seek medical attention, and by his cardiologist's conservatism. The temporary nature of the underlying problem usually enables counterpulsation to be withdrawn after 1–2 days.

REFERENCES

Alpert JS, Cohn L 1979 Medical/Surgical treatment of acute myocardial infarction. In: Cohn L (ed) the Treatment of Acute Myocardial Ischemia Futura Mt Kisco p 127–171

Awan NA, Miller RR, deMaria AN, Maxwell KS, Neumann A, Mason DT 1977 Efficacy of ambulatory systemic vasodilator therapy with oral prazosin in chronic refractory heart failure. Circulation 56: 346–354

Bardet J, Masquet C, Kahn JC, Gourgon R, Bourdarias JP, Mathivat A, Bouvrain Y 1977 Clinical and hemodynamic results of intra-aortic balloon counterpulsation and surgery for cardiogenic shock. American Heart Journal 93: 280–288

Baughman KL, Maroko PR, Vatner SF 1981 Effect of coronary artery reperfusion on myocardial infarct size and survival in conscious dogs. Circulation 63: 317–323

Berg R Jr., Kendall RW, Dvvoisin GE, Ganji JH, Rudy LW, Everhart FJ 1975 Acute myocardial infarction, a surgical emergency. Journal of Thoracic and Cardiovascular Surgery 70: 432–439

Boolooki H 1977 Clinical application of intra-aortic balloon pump. Mt Kisco Futura

Braunwald E 1974 Regulation of the circulation. New England Journal of Medicine 290; 1124–1129; 1420–1425

Braunwald E, Ross J Jr. 1979 Control of cardiac performance. In: Handbook of Physiology. Section 2 The Cardiovascular System Volume 1 The Heart Berne RM (ed) American Physiological Society Maryland p. 533–580.

Braunwald E, Covell JW, Maroko P, Ross J Jr 1969 Effects of drugs and of counterpulsation on myocardial oxygen consumption Circulation 39: Supplement 4 220–230

Braunwald E, Ross J Jr, Sonnenblick EH 1967 Mechanisms of contraction of the normal and failing heart.

Little Brown Boston

Bresnahan GF, Roberts R, Shell WE, Ross J Jr, Sobel B 1974 Deletirious effects due to hemorrhage after myocardial reperfusion. American Journal of Cardiology 33: 82–86

Brown BG, Goldfarb D, Topaz SR, Gott VL 1967 Diastolic augmentation by intra-aortic balloon. Circulatory hemodynamics and treatment of severe acute left ventricular failure in dogs. Journal of Thoracic and Cardiovascular Surgery 53: 789–804

Brutsaert DL, De Clerk NM, Goethals MA, Housmans PR 1978 Relaxation of ventricular cardiac muscle. Journal of Physiology, (London) 283: 469–480

Buckley MJ, Graver JM, Gold HK, Mundth ED, Daggett WM, Austen WG 1972 Intra-aortic balloon pump assist for cardiogenic shock after cardiopulmonary bypass. Circulation 47: Supplement 3 90–94

Bussmann WD, Schupp 1978 Effect of sublingual nitroglycerine in emergency treatment of severe pulmonary oedema. 1978 American Journal of Cardiology 41: 931–936

Chatterjee K, Swan HJC, Kaushik VS, Jobin G, Magnusson P, Forrester JS 1976 Effects of vasodilator therapy for severe pump failure in acute myocardial infarction on short-term and late prognosis. Circulation 53: 797–802

Chatterjee K, Parmley WW 1977 The role of vasodilator therapy in heart failure. Progress in Cardiovascular Diseases 19: 301–325

Chatterjee K, Parmley WW, Ganz W, Forrester J, Walinsky P, Crexells C, Swan HJC 1973 Hemodynamic and metabolic responses to vasodilator therapy in acute myocardial infarction. Circulation 48: 1183–1193

Chatterjee K, Parmley WW, Massie B, Greenberg B, Werner J, Klausner S, Norman A 1976 Oral hydralazine therapy for chronic refractory heart failure. Circulation 54: 879–883

Chatterjee K, Swan HJC 1974 Vasodilator therapy in acute myocardial infarction. Modern Concepts of Cardiovascular Disease 43: 119–124

Clauss RH, Birtwell WC, Albertal G, Lunzer S, Taylor W, Fosberg A, Harken D 1961 Assisted Circulation 1. The arterial counterpulsator Journal of Thoracic and Cardiovascular Surgery 41: 447–458

Cohn J 1974 Vasodilator therapy of myocardial infarction. New England Journal of Medicine 290: 1433–1434

Cohn JN 1980 Vasodilators in congestive heart failure. Circulation 61: 661–663

Cohn JN, Franciosa JA 1977 Vasodilator therapy of cardiac failure. New England Journal of Medicine 297: 254–258

Cohn LH 1979 The treatment of acute myocardial ischemia; an integrated medical/surgical approach. Futura Mt. Kisco

Cohn PF 1980 Editorial: Evaluation of inotrophic contractile reserve in ischemic heart disease using postextrasystolic potentiation. Circulation 61: 1071–1075

Cohn PF, Cohn LH 1979 Medical/surgical treatment of unstable angina. In: Cohn LH (ed) The treatment of acute myocardial ischemia Futura Mt Kisco p 93–126

Cooperative Unstable Angina Study Group 1978 Unstable Angina pectoris: national cooperative study group to compare surgical and medical therapy 11. In-hospital experience and initial follow-up results in patients with one, two, and three vessel disease. American Journal of Cardiology 42: 839–848

Cooperative Unstable Angina Study Group 1980 Unstable angina pectoris: National Cooperative Study Group to compare surgical and medical therapy 111. Results in patients with S-T segment elevation during pain. American Journal of Cardiology 45: 819–824

Dilley RB, Ross J Jr, Bernstein EF 1973 Serial hemodynamics during intra-aortic balloon counterpulsation for cardiogenic shock. Circulation 47 and 48 Suppl 3 99–104

Dunkman WB, Leinbach RC, Buckley MJ, Mundth ED, Kantrowitz AR, Austen WG, Sanders C 1972 Clinical and hemodynamic results of intra-aortic balloon pumping and surgery for cardiogenic shock. Circulation 46: 465–477

Elzinga G, Westerhof N 1974 End diastolic volume and source impedance of the heart. In: The physiological basis of starling's law of the heart Ciba Foundation Symposium 24 Excerpta Medica Amsterdam p 242–255

Elzinga G, Westerhof N 1978 The effect of an increase in inotropic state and end-diastolic volume on the pumping ability of the feline left heart. Circulation Research 42: 620–628

Elzinga G, Westerhof N 1979 How to quantify pump function of the heart. The value of variables derived from measurements on isolated muscle. Circulation Research 44: 303–308

Epstein S, Kent KM, Goldstein RE, Borer JS, Redwood DR 1975 Reduction of ischemic injury by nitroglycerin during acute myocardial infarction. New England Journal of Medicine 292: 29–35

Erich DA, Biddle TL, Kronenberg MW, Yu PN 1977 The hemodynamic response to intra-aortic balloon counterpulsation in patients with cardiogenic shock complicating acute myocardial infarction. American Heart Journal 93: 274–279

Franciosa JA, Cohn JN 1978 Hemodynamic responsiveness to vasodilators in left ventricular failure. American Journal of Medicine 65: 126–133

Franciosa JA, Notargiacomo AV, Cohn JN 1978 Comparative hemodynamic and metabolic effects of vasodilator and inotropic agents in experimental myocardial infarction. Cardiovascular Research 12: 294–302

Ganz W, Buchbinder N, Marcus H, Mondkar A, Maddahi J, Charuzi Y, O'Connor L, Shell W, Fishbein M, Kass R, Miyamoto A, Swan HJC 1981 Intra-coronary thrombolysis in evolving myocardial infarction. American Heart Journal 101: 4–13

Ginks WR, Sybers HD, Maroko PR, Covell JW, Sobel BE, Ross J Jr 1972 Coronary artery reperfusion 11. Reduction of myocardial infarct size at one week after the coronary occlusion. Journal of Clinical Investigation 51: 2717–2723

Gold HK, Leinbach RC, Sanders CA 1972 Use of sublingual nitroglycerin in congestive failure following acute myocardial infarction. Circulation 46: 839–845

Gold HK, Leinbach RC, Sanders CA 1973 Intra-aortic balloon pumping for control of recurrent myocardial ischemia. Circulation 47: 1197–1203

Goldfarb D, Brown BG, Conti CR, Gott VL 1968 Cardiovascular responses to diastolic augmentation in the intact canine circulation and after ligation of the anterior descending coronary artery. Journal of Thoracic and Cardiovascular Surgery 55: 243–254

Goldfarb D 1969 Mechanical circulatory assistance in the treatment of cardiac failure. Progress in Cardiovascular Disease 12: 221–242

Gould KL 1981 New technology for coronary heart disease. Journal of the American Medical Association 245: 689–694

Gould L, Zahir M, Ettinger S 1969 Phentolamine and cardiovascular performance. British Heart Journal 31: 154–162

Gundel WD, Brown BG, Gott VL 1970 Coronary collateral flow studies during variable aortic root pressure waveforms. Journal of Applied Physiology 29: 579–586

Hagemeijer F, Laird JD, Haalebos MMP, Hugenholtz PG 1977 Effectiveness of intra-aortic balloon pumping without cardiac surgery for patients with severe heart failure secondary to a recent myocardial infarct. American Journal of Cardiology 40: 951–956

Harken DE 1974 Achievements and potential of counterpulsation in coronary artery disease. In: Russek H (ed) Cardiovascular disease: new concepts in diagnosis and therapy. University Park Baltimore p 159–165

Henderson Y 1906 The volume curve of the ventricles of the mammalian heart and the significance of this curve in respect to the mechanics of the heart beat and filling of the ventricles. American Journal of Physiology 16: 325–367

Heydrickxx GR, Millard RW, McRitchie RJ, Maroko PR, Vatner SF 1975 Regional myocardial functional and electrophysiological alterations after brief coronary artery occlusion in conscious dogs. Journal of Clinical Investigation 56: 978–985

Hill AV 1938 Heat of shortening and dynamic constants of muscle. Proceedings of the Royal Society of London (Biology) 126: 136–195

Jacobey JA, Tayolr WJ, Smith GT, Gorlin R, Harken DE 1962 A new therapeutic approach to acute coronary occlusion 1. Production of standardised coronary artery occlusion with microspheres. American Journal of Cardiology 9: 60–73

Jacobey JA, Taylor WJ, Smith GT, Gorlin R, Harken DE 1963 A new therapeutic approach to acute coronary occlusion 11. Opening dormant coronary collateral channels by counterpulsation. American Journal of Cardiology 11: 218–227

Jennings RB, Ganote CE 1974 Structural changes in myocardium during acute ischemia. Circulation Research 34 and 35: Supplement 3 156–172

Jennings RB, Ganote CE, Reimer KA 1975 Ischemic tissue injury. American Journal of Pathology 81: 179–194

Kantrowitz A, Kantrowitz A 1953 Experimental augmentation of coronary flow by retardation of the arterial pressure pulse. Surgery 34: 678–687

Kantrowitz A, Tjonneland S, Freed PS 1968 Intial clinical experience with intra-aortic balloon pumping in cardiogenic shock. Journal of the American Medical Association 203: 113–118

Kelly DT, Delgado CE, Taylor DR, Pitt B, Ross RS 1973 Use of phentolamine in acute myocardial infarction associated with hypertension and left ventricular failure. Circulation 47: 729–735

Leinbach RC, Gold HK, Dinsmore RE, Mundth ED, Buckley MJ, Austen WG, Sanders CA 1973 The role of angiography in cardiogenic shock. Circulation 47: Supplement 3 95–98

Leinbach RC, Gold HK, Buckley MJ, Austen WG 1976 Identifying features of survivors from cardiogenic shock treated with intra-aortic balloon pumping. American Journal of Cardiology 37: p 151

Levenson J, Cheli J, Payen D, Simon A, Safar M 1979 Vasodilating anti hypertensive drugs: effect on arterial compliance. Proceedings Symposium International Alpha – Bloquants Specia Paris p 41

Levine FH, Gold HK, Leinbach RC, Daggett WM, Austen WG, Buckley MJ 1977 Management of acute myocardial ischemia with intra-aortic balloon pumping and coronary artery bypass surgery. Circulation 55 and 56 Supplement 3 p. 61

Levine FH, Gold HK, Leinbach RC, Dasggett WM, Austen WG, Buckley MJ 1978 Safe early revascularisation for continuing ischemia after acute myocardial infarction. Circulation 57 and 58: Supplement 2 p. 17

McDonald DA, Taylor MG 1959 The hydrodynamics of the arterial circulation. Progress in Biophysics and Biophysical Chemistry 9: 107–173

McIntosh HD, Buccino RA 1979 Emergency coronary artery revascularisation of patients with acute myocardial infarction: you can . . . . .but should you? Circulation 60: 247–250

Maroko PR, Braunwald E 1973 Modification of myocardial infarction size after coronary occlusion. Annals of Internal Medicine 79: 720–733

Maroko P, Kjekshus JK, Sobel BE, Watanabe T, Covell JW, Ross J Jr, Braunwald E 1971 Factors influencing infarct size following experimental coronary artery occlusion. Circulation 43: 67–82

Maroko PR, Libby P, Ginks WR, Bloor CM, Shell WE, Sobel BE, Ross J Jr 1972 Coronary artery reperfusion 1. Early effects on local myocardial function and the extent of myocardial necrosis. Journal of Clinical Investigation 51: 2710–2716

Maseri A, L'Abbate A, Baroldi G, Chierchia S, Marzilli M, Ballestra AM, Severi S, Parodi O, Biagini A, Distante A, Pesola A, 1978 Coronary vasospasm as a possible cause of myocardial infarction; a conclusion derived from the study of 'preinfarction' angina. New England Journal of Medicine 299: 1271–1277

Mehta J, Iacona M, Feldman RL, Pepine CJ, Conti CR 1978 Comparative hemodynamic effects of intravenous nitroprusside and oral prazosin in refractory heart failure. American Journal of Cardiology 41: 925–930

Merillon JP, Motte G, Fruchaud J, Masquet C, Gourgon R 1978 Evaluation of the elasticity and characteristic impedance of the ascending aorta in man. Cardiovascular Research 12: 401–406

Merillon JP, Motte G, Aumont MC, Prasquier R, Gourgon R 1979 Study of left vetricular pressure-volume relations during nitroprusside infusion in human subjects without coronary artery disease. British Heart Journal 41 : 325–330

Merillon JP, Fontenier J, Chastre JF, Lerallut JF, Jaffrin MY, Gourgon R 1980 Etude du spectre d'impedance chez l'homme normal et hypertendu. Effects de l'accroissement de frequence cardiaque et des drogues vasomotrices. Archives Des Maladies du Coeur 73: 83–90

Moulopoulos SD, Topaz S, Kolff WJ 1962 Diastolic balloon pumping (with carbon dioxide) in the aorta; a mechanical assistance to the failing circulation. American Heart Journal 63: 669–675

Mueller H, Ayres SM, Conklin EF, Giannelli S, Mazzara JT, Grace WT, Nealon TF 1971 The effects of intra-aortic counterpulsation on cardiac performance and metabolism in shock associated with acute myocardial infarction. Journal of Clinical Investigation 50: 1885–1900

Muller JE, Maroko PR, Braunwald E 1979 The pathophysiology of acute myocardial infarction and modification of infarct size. In: Cohn L (ed) The treatment of acute myocardial ischemia. Futura Mt. Kisco p. 49–76

Mundth E 1976 Mechanical and surgical interventions for the reduction of myocardial ischemia Circulation 53: Supplement 1 176–182

Murgo JP, Westerhof N, Giolma JP, Altobelli SA 1980 Aortic input impedance in normal man: relationship to pressure waveshapes Circulation 62: 105–116

Opie LH 1980 Drugs and the heart. VI Vasodilating drugs Lancet 1: 966–972

O'Rourke MF 1970 Influence of ventricular ejection on the relationship between central aortic and brachial pressure pulse in man. Cardiovascular Research 4: 291–300

O'Rourke MF 1971 The arterial pulse in health and disease. American Heart Journal 82: 687–702

O'Rourke MF 1972 Arterial counterpulsation in treatment of cardiogenic shock. Medical Journal of Australia 1: 1258–1261

O'Rourke MF 1973 Subacute heart rupture following myocardial infarction. Clinical features of a correctable condition. Lancet 2: 124–126

O'Rourke MF, Chang VP, Windsor HM, Shanahan MX, Hickie JB, Morgan JJ, Gunning JF, Seldon WA, Hall GV, Michell G, Goldfarb D, Harrison DG 1975 Acute severe heart failure complicating myocardial infarction. Experience with 100 patients referred for consideration of mechanical left ventricular assistance. British Heart Journal 37: 169–181

O'Rourke MF, Norris RM, Campbell TC, Chang VP, Sammel NL 1981 Randomised controlled trial of intraaortic balloon counterpulsation in early myocardial infarction with acute heart failure. American Journal of Cardiology 47: 815–820

O'Rourke MF, Sammel NL, Campbell TC, Chang VP 1980 Long-term results of intra aortic balloon counterpulsation for medically refractory heart failure complication acute myocardial infarction and open heart surgery. Proceedings European Congress of Cardiology Paris p 113

O'Rourke MF, Sammel N, Chang VP 1979 Arterial counterpulsation in severe refractory heart failure complicating acute myocardial infarction. British Heart Journal 41: 308–316

Pace P, Tilney N, Couch N, Lesch M 1976 Peripheral arterial complications of intra-aortic balloon counterpulsation. Circulation 53 and 54: Supplement 2 p 13

Packer M, Meller J 1978 Oral vasodilator therapy for chronic heart failure; a plea for caution. American Journal of Cardiology 42: 686–689

Pepine CJ, Nichols WW, Curry RCJr, Conti CR 1979 Aortic input impedance during nitroprusside infusion. A reconsideration of afterload reduction and beneficial action. Journal of Clinical Investigation 64: 643–654

Phillips SJ, Kongtahworn C, Zeff RH, Benson M, Iannone PL, Brown T, Gordon DF 1979 Emergency coronary artery revascularisation; a possible therapy for acute myocardial infarction. Circulation 60: 241–246

Pickering GW 1968 High blood pressure. Churchill London

Powell WJ, Daggett WM, Magro AE, Bianco JA, Buckley MJ, Sanders CA, Kantrowitz AR, Austen WG 1970 Effects of intra-aortic balloon counterpulsation on cardiac performance, oxygen consumption and coronary blood flow in dogs. Circulation Research 26: 753–764

Reichel H, Baumann K 1979 The effect of systolic rise in arterial pressure on stroke volume and aortic flow. In: Bauer RD, Busse R (eds) The arterial system Springer Berlin p 227–235

Reid P, Flaherty J, Taylor D 1973 Effect of nitroglycerin on ST segments in acute myocardial infarction. Circulation 48: Supplement 4 p 207

Rentrop P, Blanke H, Karsh K 1979 Limitation of myocardial injury by transluminal recannulisation in acute myocardial infarction. Circulation Volume 59, 60, Supplement 2, p 162

Rentrop P, Blanke H, Karsch KR, Kaiser H, Kostering H, Leitz K 1981 Selective intracoronary thrombolysis in acute myocardial infarction and unstable angina pectoris. Circulation 63: 307–317

Ross J Jr, Covell JW, Sonnenblick EH 1966 Contractile state of the heart characterised by force-velocity relations in variably afterloaded and isovolumic beats. Circulation Research 18: 149–163

Rowell LB, Brengelmann GL, Blackmon JR, Bruce RA, Murray JA 1968 Disparity between aortic and peripheral pulse pressure induced by upright exercise and vasomotor changes in man. Circulation 37: 954–964

Russell RO Jr, Rackley CE, Pombo J, Hunt D, Potanin C, Dodge HT, 1970 Effect of increasing left ventricular filling pressure in patients with acute myocardial infarction. Journal of Clinical Investigation 49: 1539–1550

Sagawa K 1978 The ventricular pressure-volume diagram revisited. Circulation Research 43: 678–687

Sammel NL, O'Rourke MF 1979 Arterial counterpulsation in continuing myocardial ischemia after acute myocardial infarction. British Health Journal 42: 579–582

Sanders CA, Buckley MJ, Leinbach RC, Mundth ED, Austen WG 1972 Mechanical circulatory assistance. Current status and experience with combining circulatory assistence, emergency coronary angiography, and acute myocardial revascularisation. Circulation 45: 1292–1313

Scheidt S, Ascheim R, Killip T 1900 Shock after myocardial infarction. American Journal of Cardiology 26: 556–564

Scheidt S, Wilner G, Mueller H 1973 Intra-aortic balloon counterpulsation in cardiogenic shock. Report of a cooperative clinical trial. New England Journal of Medicine 288: 979–984

Shell WE, Sobel BE 1974 Protection of jeopardised ischemic myocardium by reduction of ventricular afterload. New England Journal of Medicine 291: 481–486

Smirk H, Alstad KS 1951 Treatment of arterial hypertension by penta–and hexa-methonium salts, based on 150 tests on hypertensives of varied aetiology and 53 patients treated for periods of two to fourteen months. British Medical Journal 1: 1217–1228

Smith GT, Soeter JR, Haston HH, McNamara JJ 1974 Coronary reperfusion in primates. Serial electrocardiographic and histological assessment. Journal of Clinical Investigation 54: 1420–1427

Smith TW, Braunwald E. 1980 The management of heart failure. In: Braunwald E (ed) Heart Disease Saunders Philadelphia p 509–570

Sonnenblick EH 1966 Mechanics of myocardial contraction. In: Briller SA, Cohn HL (eds) The myocardial cell: structure, function and modifications. University of Pennsylvania Philadelphia p. 173–250

Sonnenblick EH, Downing SE 1963 Afterload as a primary determinant of ventricular performance. American Journal of Physiology 204: 604–610

Soroff HS, Cloutier CT, Birtwell WC 1974 External counterpulsation: management of cardiogenic shock after myocardial infarction. Journal of the American Medical Association 229: 1441–1450

Spotnitz HM, Covell JW, Ross J Jr, Braunwald E. 1969 Left ventricular mechanics and oxygen consumption during arterial counterpulsation. American Journal of Physiology 217: 1352–1358

Sturm JT, McGee MG, Fuhrman TM, Davis GL, Turner SA, Edelman SK, Norman JC 1980 Treatment of postoperative low output syndrome with intra-aortic balloon pumping; experience with 419 patients. American Journal of Cardiology 45: 1033–1036

Suga H, Sagawa K, Demer L 1980 Determinants of instantaneous pressure in canine left ventricle; time and volume specifications. Circulation Research 46: 256–263

Taylor MG 1964 Wave travel in arteries and the design of the cardiovascular system. In: Attinger EO (ed) Pulsatile blood flow. McGraw New York p. 343–372

Tennant R, Wiggers CJ 1935 The effect of coronary occlusion on myocardial contraction. American Journal of Physiology 112: 351–361

Wiggers CJ 1950 Physiology in health and disease. 5th ed Lea and Febiger Philadelphia

Wilcken DEL, Charlier AA, Hoffmann JIE, Guz A 1964 Effects of alterations in aortic impedance on the performance of the ventricles. Circulation Research 14: 283–293

Willerson JT, Curry GC, Watson JT, Leshin SJ, Ecker RR, Mullins CB, Platt MR, Sugg WL 1975 Intra-aortic balloon counterpulsation in patients in cardiogenic shock, medically refractory left ventricular failure and/or recurrent ventricular tachycardia. American Journal of Medicine 58: 183–191

Windsor HM, O'Rourke MF, Shanahan MX, Chang VP 1973 Surgery and counterpulsation in cardiogenic shock. Medical Journal of Australia 2: 841–846.

Zelis R, Flaim SF, Moskowitz RM, Nellis SH 1979 How much can we expect from vasodilator therapy in congestive cardiac failure? Circulation 59: 1092–1097

Zobel LR, Finkelstein SM, Carlyle PF, Cohn JN 1980 Pressure pulse contour analysis in determining the effect of vasodilator drugs on vascular hemodynamic impedance characteristics in dogs. American Heart Journal 100: 81–87

17

Nomenclature and interpretation of the arterial pulse

PERSPECTIVE

There is in clinical medicine no physical sign more basic or important than the arterial pulse. From ancient times the pulse has been recognised as the most fundamental sign of life; disturbances in the pulse were noted in disease, and absence of the pulse in death. Before the birth of Christ, and even before any association was known between it and the heart, examination of the pulse had become an important part of Chinese, Indian and Greek medicine. Examination of the pulse (Fig. 17.1) took the form of some mystic rite, and by itself (without any other examination or interrogation) enabled the physician to make a diagnosis (even of pregnancy), offer a prognosis (even as to the sex of the child) and order treatment. Things were little better in Galen's day (the second century A.D.). Galen wrote voluminously on the pulse and described over one hundred different forms of pulse all of which he claimed could be distinguished and classified by careful examination. His full writings on the pulse (17 books) are only available in Latin or Greek but are reviewed by Broadbent (1890), Bedford (1951) and Harris (1973). Galen's teachings were so subtle, so difficult to challenge, so overpowering, and so authoritative that they were accepted for sixteen centuries, until well after Harvey's description of the circulation established a sound basis for interpretation of the pulse. Galen's concepts and descriptions of the pulse (some of which are still in use) were based on the erroneous notion that arterial movement was due to some inherent property rather than to passive expansion from cardiac contraction. Galen confused the physicians of his time and for centuries after. One suspects his influence is still apparent.

The modern approach to the pulse commenced with the work of Harvey and Hales and was further advanced by Marey's introduction of the sphygmogram (Fig. 17.2). This and its refinements led to careful descriptions of the pulse and characterisation of the changes seen in different

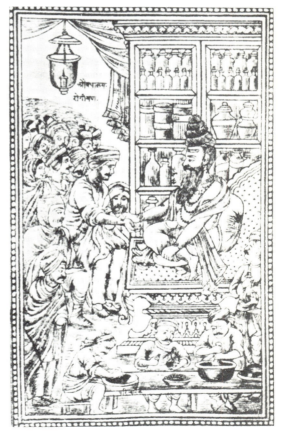

Fig. 17.1 Consultation with the Hindu physician Susruta, who is shown feeling the pulse. From Castiglioni's L'Histoire de la Medecine, Editions Payot, Paris, and Bedford (1951)

diseases by Sanderson (1867), Mahomed (1872), Roy and Adami (1890), and Broadbent (1890) in Britain, but most of all by James Mackenzie (1902) whose classic monograph was written from his general practice in the north of England. Despite the many advances that have taken place in cardiovascular physiology and cardiology since this time, modern textbooks show little improvement in description and analysis of the pulse as felt at the bedside, when compared to the works of Broadbent and of Mackenzie. There appear to have been two obstacles to progress, the first being understanding of factors responsible for pulse contour under normal circumstances and in disease, and the second being the terminology employed, much of which is a Galenic legacy. On the basis of experimental studies, reported earlier, explanations can be given for pulse contour as determined clinically under different conditions.

Form of the pulse

It is generally thought that the arterial pulse, as perceived by the finger, and as recorded by the sphygmograph, polygraph, or other external device, is the same as the pressure wave that one would record from within the artery. This is in general true (Dontas 1960), and the pressure wave

and diameter expansion wave are virtually identical in all arteries (Ch. 2). But there are a few *caveats*, stressed by Broadbent (1890), Mackenzie (1902) and Bramwell (1937).

The first consideration (Broadbent 1890, Bramwell 1937) is that one does not merely appreciate a minute expansion in an artery when feeling the pulse. Rather, one needs to compress the artery over a bone (usually the end of the radius) to detect its systolic expansion and diastolic decay. The apparent strength of the pulse will depend on the degree of compression, and so (in arteries of similar size) on the arterial pressure within (Fig. 17.3). For arteries of the same size, the pulse may feel stronger (greater amplitude of expansion) when blood pressure is low, than when pressure is high. This would apply if the finger were sensitive to movement and vessel expansion underneath (as are externally recording devices) but if it were sensitive to pressure change in an artery compressed throughout the cardiac cycle, the finger might register a stronger pulse in the patient with higher systolic pressure. (It is not really known what the finger senses but it is probably a mixture of movement and of force). Amplitude of the externally recorded pulse depends on the pressure applied; likewise the character of the pulse as felt depends on the pressure applied. The clinician should feel

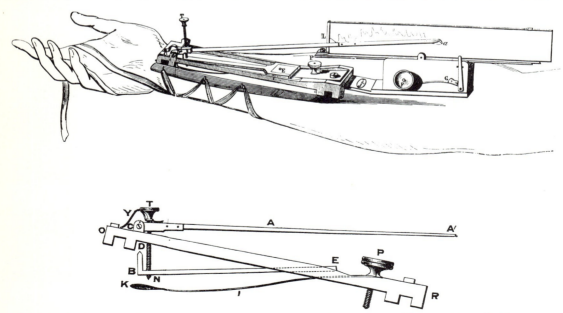

Fig. 17.2 Marey's sphygmograph in profile (below), and as applied to the forearm (above). From Sanderson (1867)

the pulse with the fingers just resting over the artery, and with different degrees of compression. By standardising his own technique, he comes to recognise different characteristics of the pulse in different patients. Usually (Broadbent 1890), a diastolic wave will be felt with very light pressure, a twice beating systolic or 'bisferiens' pulse with heavy pressure. The size (diameter) of the artery also determines the apparent strength of the pulse (Fig. 17.3) On palpating the pulse, one appears to sense volume displacement and force (pressure × area), and both are greater in the larger than in the smaller artery.

The second consideration relates to the position of the fingers or external transducer. Both must be placed directly over the artery. If the transducer is placed to one side, and the artery angulates laterally in the other direction during systole, one will record a distorted pulse, and the wave may even be inverted (Mackenzie 1902). The last consideration relates to frequency response of external transducers (Ch. 2). This is usually low. The early mechanical transducers also were markedly underdamped, and so exaggerated sharp movements such as the upstroke of the pulse and the foot of the diastolic wave. Mackenzie was aware of these problems in his tracings, and because of them was reluctant to distinguish between an 'anacrotic' and 'bisferiens' pulse.

Description of the pulse

Figure 17.4 shows (at top) the pressure waves recorded by Mackenzie in two normal subjects, the second with lower arterial pressure (and apparently younger). The subsidiary waves p, s, and d are marked. Confusing names are given to these waves. The first (p) is sometimes called the 'percussion' wave (Mahomed 1872), 'papillary' wave (Roy and Adami 1890), or 'anacrotic' wave, the second (s), the 'tidal' wave (Mahomed 1872) or 'outflow remainder' wave (Roy and Adami 1890) or predicrotic wave, and the third (d) the dicrotic or diastolic wave. Dicrotic is derived from Greek, and means 'twice beating'; this is the second wave in the lower trace, but the third wave in the upper. The notch (n) is sometimes referred to as the incisura (implying that it results from aortic valve closure) and sometimes as the 'dicrotic notch' (implying that it represents the foot of the diastolic wave). These terms are so confusing that one would have expected them to have been discarded years ago, but most are still in common use (Feinstein et al 1971 Hurst and Schlant 1978). I would like to see all discarded, and replaced by some standard and simple terminology – i.e. first systolic wave, second systolic wave, diatolic wave, etc.

Further confusion exists in the names given to different pulses. The most frequent confusion relates to the terms 'dicrotic' and 'bisferiens' and to the difference between 'anacrotic', 'bisferiens' and normal pulses. The first is quickly settled. Both 'dicrotic' and 'bisferiens' mean literally 'twice beating' with the former derived from Greek, and the latter from Latin. 'Dicrotic' is only used to

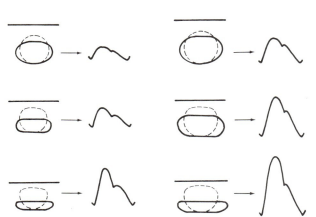

Fig. 17.3 Diagrammatic representation of the pulse one might expect to feel in two different sized arteries (left and right) with increasing pressure (from above down), if the sensation of the pulse were caused by different degrees of force sensed by the finger during the cardiac cycle. Broken line indicates cross section of the artery during systole, continuous line, cross section of the artery during diastole

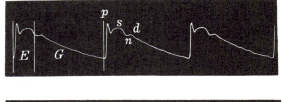

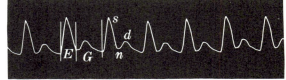

Fig. 17.4 Sphygmographs recorded by Mackenzie (1902) from the radial artery in two normal human subjects

describe a second wave in diastole, 'bisferiens' only for a second wave in systole; i.e. the Latin is for the surge of flow, the Greek for its ebb. There is no logic to this, but then both are Galenic descriptions.

The second matter is harder to settle, since there is so much confusion and varied opinion in the literature. The normal pulse shown by Wiggers (1952) in his textbook seems identical to the anacrotic pulse illustrated by Wood (1968) in his (Fig. 17.5). The anacrotic pulse in Hurst's (1978)

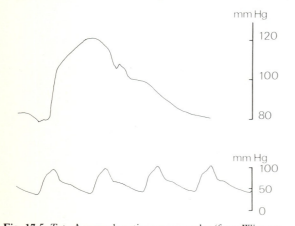

Fig. 17.5 *Top*: A normal aortic pressure pulse (from Wiggers 1952)
Bottom: The 'anacrotic' pulse of aortic stenosis (from Wood 1968) From O'Rourke (1971)

textbook looks like the bisferiens pulse in Mackenzie's text (Fig. 17.6), the normal pulse in Mackenzie's text (Fig. 17.6) like the bisferiens pulse in Hurst's. The term 'anacrotic' really means 'ana di crotic' or 'twice beating on the upstroke'. The usual distinction with 'bisferiens' is that the first systolic wave is larger in the 'bisferiens' pulse, but the matter is only one of degree. As currently used 'anacrotic' is usually used to describe a slow rising pulse of low amplitude as occurs in aortic stenosis. Hurst and Schlant (1978) use this term interchangeably with 'pulsus parvus et tardus' (a better descriptive term). In the past, Mackenzie (1902) used the term 'anacrotic' to describe the pulse in hypertension where there was a late systolic peak, but high amplitude of the wave.

This confusion will I believe only be settled when mechanisms involved in arterial pulse contour are fully understood, and a new, simpler terminology adopted. The following explanations are based on the material presented earlier in this book.

Explanation of pulse contour

Normal pulse

There is a wide range to the normal contour of the arterial pulse. Figure 17.4(b) represents the pulse

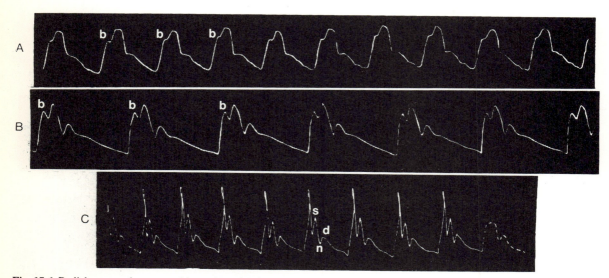

Fig. 17.6 Radial artery sphygmographic tracings showing an 'anacrotic' pulse A; a 'bisferiens' pulse B; and a normal pulse distorted by sphygmographic resonance C. From Mackenzie (1902). In the bottom panel is shown what Mackenzie considered to be the undistorted pulse contour in the normal subject. Mackenzie's figures as rearranged by O'Rourke (1971)

one would expect to feel in a peripheral artery of a child (p. 146). The pulse rises to a single peak, and there is a secondary wave in diastole. This diastolic wave is not artifact, but it can rarely be appreciated, and then only when the pulse is felt very lightly. It is the echo of the initial wave retraversing the arterial system after reflection at arterial terminations in the upper and lower parts of the body (p. 90). Figure 17.4(a) is the type of pulse one would expect in an adult. The pulse is different to that in the child as a result of arterial degeneration which increases pulse wave velocity and causes the reflected waves to return earlier, and to fuse with the systolic part of the wave (Fig. 9.5). The initial wave (p) is a sygmograph artifact, as Mackenzie correctly inferred. (See also Fig. 17.6c) It is not felt by the finger, nor is it recorded by an intra-arterial catheter or transducer. The finger senses a single peak, and a gradual diastolic decay.

Hypertension

In hypertension (Fig. 17.7) arterial pressure rises more slowly than usual to a peak in late systole. No diastolic wave is apparent. An anacrotic shoulder or first systolic wave may be seen in sphygmographs but is not apparent on palpation; when present on external pulse recordings, this is probably artifact. These features are just what one sees in pressure tracings recorded directly from within the artery (Fig. 9.5). These features are attribut-

able to increased pulse wave velocity and fusion of the reflected waves with the systolic part of the pulse. The pulse appears just the same as in an adult with unsuspected arterial degeneration

Hypotension

In hypotension, pulse pressure is low, the artery is small, and the pulse feels soft. The externally recorded pulse is often however of good amplitude (Fig. 17.8). Sphygmographs often show a diastolic wave, and this may be apparent clinically, especially when the pulse is palpated softly. The genesis of the diastolic wave and its significance have been discussed at length in clinical texts on the pulse. In the presence of hypotension associated with infectious fevers, presence of a diastolic wave was considered to be a favourable prognostic sign (Broadbent 1890, Mackenzie 1902, Osler 1905). Broadbent considered this to be an indication of vasodilation, and this view has been echoed in recent textbooks (e.g. Wood 1968). It is now clear that the reverse is the case:– that the diastolic wave is the echo of the systolic wave after its reflection at upper and lower parts of the body (Ch. 9). The diastolic wave is thus dependent on high arteriolar tone (p. 88), and it disappears when arteriolar tone is low. This specific subject was investigated by Hamilton (1944) who showed that the cause of hypotension can be inferred from the contour of the pulse – with a small or absent diastolic wave indicating arteriolar relaxation (as

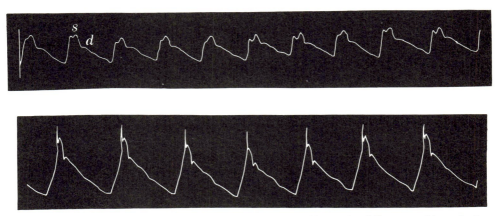

Fig. 17.7 Mackenzie's illustration of the pulse in hypertension, in the same subject under different conditions. In the top panel an 'anacrotic' wave was identified, whereas in the bottom panel pressure rose gradually to its peak. Peak pressure in both cases was in late systole, and there was little or no diastolic fluctuation

often seen in the terminal stage of hemorrhagic shock) and a prominent diastolic wave, compensatory vasoconstriction. This explanation can be applied to the tracings a and b in Figure 17.8. The first (a) was taken in a man who had fainted and in whom the pulse had just become perceptible; the very small diastolic wave is attributable to vasodilation – doubtless the cause of the faint. The second (b) was taken when the patient had regained consciousness, but was still hypotensive, with intense sweating indicative of sympathetic discharge. The prominent diastolic wave here is attributable to vasoconstriction and strong wave reflection.

Augmentation of the diastolic wave is discussed on page 134. It was pointed out that this is most obvious when hypotension and vasoconstriction are combined with short duration of ejection, so that the diastolic wave is completely separated from the systolic wave. This explains the tracing in Figure 17.8(c) where, during an arrhythmia, the diastolic wave is most prominent after the beats with the shortest systolic period. When systole is relatively long, the diastolic wave merges with the systolic part of the pulse. Figure 17.8(d) illustrates the phenomenom of 'hyperdicrotism'. This is a simple consequence of rate, and manifests as apparent exaggeration of the diastolic wave when rate is sufficiently fast for the duration of ejection to be short, and for successive pulses to commence right at the end of the diastolic wave. It is thus seen in the presence of hypotension, vasoconstriction, and tachycardia, with heart rate around half the resonant frequency (p. 146) of the arterial system.

Aortic incompetence

In aortic incompetence, amplitude of the ventricular ejection wave is increased (Brawley et al 1967)

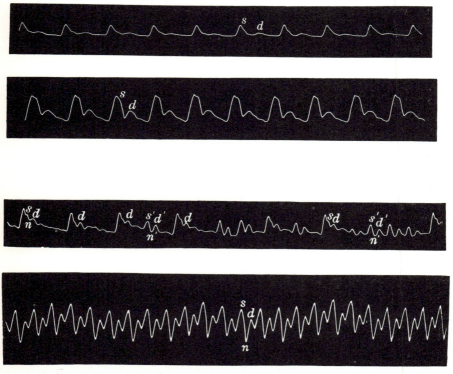

Fig. 17.8 Top two panels: Sphygmographs of the radial pulse in the same patient during (above) and after (below) recovery from a hypotensive faint. The small diastolic wave in the panel above is attributable to the effects of peripheral vasodilation, the prominent diastolic wave in the lower panel to return of vasoconstrictor tone Bottom two panels: Sphygmographs illustrating exaggeration of the diastolic wave under different conditions – (above), during atrial fibrillation following abbreviated systolic contractions, and (below) when tachycardia is associated with hypotension, as in clinical shock. From Mackenzie (1902)

but aortic impedance is normal. Ventricular ejection thus generates a pressure wave of high amplitude. This rises quickly because of rapid ventricular ejection, but falls quickly too because of backflow through the aortic valve during diastole. The pulse has been given many names – 'collapsing pulse', 'waterhammer pulse', 'Corrigan's pulse', but the best description is Corrigan's own simple statement 'The pulse is invariably full . . . at each diastole, the subclavian, carotid, temporal, brachial and is some cases, even the palmar arteries are suddenly thrown from their bed, bounding up under the skin.' Would that Corrigan's predecessors – and followers – had used the same simple language.'

In pure aortic incompetence, aortic flow velocity is considerably lower than in the presence of aortic stenosis. Hence any Venturi effect is small and unlikely to alter the arterial pressure pulse.

Aortic incompetence with stenosis (the 'bisferiens' pulse)

When aortic incompetence is combined with stenosis, peak aortic velocity is considerably higher than in the presence of incompetence alone. The jet of blood creates a Venturi effect in the aorta such that lateral pressure is reduced relative to the pressure that would be registered if the blood had no kinetic energy (Fig. 17.9). Studies on this phenomenom (Katz et al 1928, Fleming 1957, O'Rourke 1971) are discussed on page 118. Since the peak effect is seen at peak forward flow, the Venturi is associated with an initial rise in pressure, then a slight fall, then a second rise – i.e. with a 'bisferiens' pulse. Thus the 'bisferiens' pulse in this condition can be attributed to a normal wave with a 'bite' taken out of its systolic portion. Such an explanation has previously been advanced by Katz el al (1928) and by Fleming (1957). Dow (1941) showed that the distorted pressure wave in aortic stenosis is transmitted unchanged to peripheral arteries. This was confirmed for mixed aortic stenosis and incompetence as well as for pure stenosis by O'Rourke (1970).

Aortic stenosis (the 'Anacrotic' pulse)

In aortic stenosis, a similar phenomenom exists as in combined stenosis and incompetence – a Venturi effect in the aorta at the time of peak forward flow. The only difference between stenosis and the combined lesion is that the theoretic systolic pressure wave is smaller (because volume ejected during systole is less). Thus the 'bite' of the Venturi is take out of a smaller pressure wave. The effect of this is that pressure during systole rises slowly, instead of to an early peak (i.e. the pulse has an 'anacrotic' configuration) (Fig. 17.9).

There has in the past been much debate on the difference between the 'anacrotic' and 'bisferiens' pulse. It is apparent that in aortic valve disease, this type of debate is of academic significance only. The two pulses are manifestations of the same

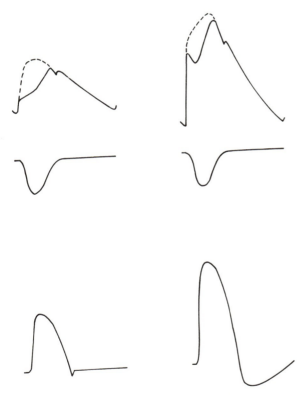

Fig. 17.9 Explanation of the anacrotic (left) and bisferious (right) pulse in aortic valve disease. The pressure wave is shown above, with the dotted line indicating what the pressure wave would be in the absence of a Venturi effect. The middle wave represents the timing and magnitude of a Venturi effect in the two cases, if peak flow velocity were the same in each. The bottom trace represents aortic flow (in volumetric terms). The anacrotic and bisferious pulses appear to be a manifestation of the same phenomenon – a relative decrease in lateral pressure with high peak flow velocity (see p. 45, 118)

phenomenom, and so in the presence of mixed aortic valve disease, one would expect to see a continuous spectrum between one and the other.

This explanation accounts for another feature of aortic stenosis – disappearance of the 'anacrotic' pulse contour in the presence of tachycardia (Steell 1894). This is attributable to fall in stroke volume and in peak aortic flow velocity. The fall in lateral pressure depends on velocity squared, so that a modest reduction in peak flow velocity may cause the Venturi effect to become inapparent. (p. 118).

*Hypertrophic obstructive cardiomyopathy –
('Bisferiens' pulse)*

A 'bisferiens' or twice beating systolic pulse is a frequent feature of hypertrophic cardiomyopathy. The pulse is usually different to that observed in mixed aortic stenosis and incompetence, in that the first systolic wave is usually wider and of greater amplitude; in addition the trough between the two systolic waves corresponds in time with the falling limb of the aortic flow wave rather than with its peak. The mechanism of genesis of this characteristic pulse thus appears to be completely different to that in organic aortic valve disease.

This pulse contour can however readily be explained on the basis of the unusual aortic flow wave seen in this condition (Hernandez et al 1964, Murgo et al 1981).

In hypertrophic obstructive cardiomyopathy, the aortic flow wave has a curious biphasic pattern (Fig. 17.10), with an initial narrow systolic peak, and a shoulder on the wave in the latter part of systole. The second systolic pressure peak corresponds with the second period of late systolic flow. This second wave appears to represent the reflected wave from the first systolic peak, superimposed on a second pressure wave generated by late systolic flow. This type of explanation has previously been offered to explain the late systolic peak of the pressure wave in the presence of high pulse wave velocity. Such subjects usually do not have two obvious pressure peaks during systole, doubtless because ventricular ejection is more prolonged. Murgo et al (1980) however have shown that with high frequency manometry, two separate systolic pressure waves can be distinguished in apparently normal adults. In hypertrophic cardiomyopathy, the dip between these two waves is exaggerated by the early fall in flow.

This explanation is consistent with the timing of the two systolic pressure waves in relation to ven-

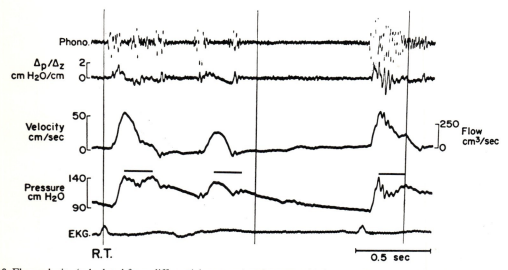

Fig. 17.10 Flow velocity (calculated from differential pressure) and pressure in the ascending aorta of a patient with hypertrophic obstructive cardiomyopathy, from Hermandez et al (1964). The time interval between the two systolic peaks of a full pulse (indicated by the horizontal line) is the same as the time interval between the systolic and diastolic peaks of an abbreviated pulse. The 'bisferious' pulse in this condition appears to be due to rapid early ejection, with wave reflection from the early pressure peak returning during the latter part of systole when flow is markedly reduced

tricular ejection. It also accounts for another feature (Fig. 17.10). When, during an extrasystole, the duration of ejection is short, and the flow contour, normal, the pressure wave is completely normal, and the peak of the diastolic wave occurs at the same interval after peak flow as the peak of the second systolic pressure wave after peak flow during the normal beat.

REFERENCES

Bedford DE 1951 The ancient art of feeling the pulse. British Heart Journal 13: 423–437

Bramwell C 1937 The arterial pulse in health and disease. Lancet 1: 239–247; 301–305; 366–371.

Brawley RK, Morrow AG 1967 Direct determinations of aortic blood flow in patients with aortic regurgitation. Circulation 35: 32–45

Broadbent W 1890 The pulse. Lea Philadelphia

Broadbent W 1899 Pulsus bisferiens. British Medical Journal 1: 75–77

Corrigan DJ 1832 On permanent patency of the mouth of the aorta, or inadequacy of the aortic valves. Edinburgh Medical and Surgical Journal 37: 225–245

Dontas AS 1960 Comparison of simultaneously – recorded intra-arterial and extra-arterial pressure pulses in man. American Heart Journal 59: 576–590

Dow P 1941 The development of the anacrotic and tardus pulse of aortic stenosis. American Journal of Physiology 131: 432–436

Feinstein AR, Hochstein E, Luisada AA, Perloff JK, Rosner S, Schlant RC, Segal B, Soffer AL 1971 Glossary of cardiologic terms related to physical diagnosis: Part 4 Arterial pulses. American Journal of Cardiology 27: 708–709

Fleming PR 1957 The mechanism of pulsus bisferiens. British Heart Journal 19: 519–524

Hamilton WF 1944 The patterns of the arterial pressure pulse. American Journal of Physiology 141: 235–241

Harris CRS 1973 The heart and vascular system in ancient Greek medicine. Oxford London p 397–431

Hernandez RR, Greenfield JC, McCall BW 1964 Pressure-flow studies in hypertrophic subaortic stenosis. Journal of Clinical Investigation 43: 401–407

Hurst JW, Schlant RC 1978 Examination of the arteries and their pulsations. In: Hurst JW (ed) The Heart McGraw New York p. 183–192

Katz LN, Ralli EP, Cheer S 1928 The cardiodynamic changes in the aorta and left ventricle due to stenosis of the aorta. Journal of Clinical Investigation 5: 205–227

Mackenzie J 1902 The study of the pulse. MacMillan Edinburgh

Mahomed FA 1892 The physiology and clinical use of the sphygmograph. Medical Times and Gazette 1: 62–64, 128–130, 220–222

Murgo JP, Alter BR, Dorethy JF, Altobelli SA, McGranahan GM 1981 The dynamics of left ventricular ejection in 'obstruction' and 'non obstructive' hypertrophic cardiomyopathy. Journal of Clinical Investigation 66: 1369–1382

O'Rourke MF 1968 Impact pressure, lateral pressure and impedance in the proximal aorta and pulmonary artery. Journal of Applied Physiology 25: 533–541

O'Rourke MF 1970 Influence of ventricular ejection on the relationship between central aortic and brachial pressure pulse in man. Cardiovascular Research 4: 291–300

O'Rourke MF 1971 The arterial pulse in health and disease. American Heart Journal 82: 687–702

Osler W 1905 The principles and practice of medicine. Appleton Century Crofts New York

Roy CS, Adami JG 1890 Heart beat and pulse wave. Practicioner London 44: 81–94, 161–177, 241–253, 347–361, 412–425

Sabban HN, Blick EF, Anbe DT, Stein PD, 1980 Effect of turbulent blood flow on systolic pressure contour in the ventricles and great vessels: significance related to anacrotic and bisferiens pulses. American Journal of Cardiology 45: 1139–1147

Sanderson B 1867 The handbook of the sphygmograph. Hardwicke London

Schwartz CJ, Wethessen NT, Wolf S 1980 Structure and function of the Circulation. New York Plenum

Steell G 1894 The pulse in aortic stenosis. Lancet 2: 1206–1210

Wiggers CJ 1952 Circulatory dynamics. Grune and Stratton New York

Wood P 1968 Diseases of the heart and circulation. Eyre and Spottiswoode London

Glossary

Intended as a guide to the neophyte in a difficult interdisciplinary area, not as a comprehensive list of authoritative definitions. More complete explanation on the page indicated

Amplification (of a pulse)
Increase in amplitude of the pressure pulse between a central and a peripheral artery. This is largely attributable to summation of incident and reflected waves (p. 73, 86, 145)

Anacrotic (pulse)
Twice beating on the upstroke with amplitude of the first systolic wave smaller than that of the second. This is usually due to a Venturi effect in the ascending aorta (p. 255, 259)

Antinode
A site of maximal pressure or flow oscillation (p. 83–86)

Arterial termination
Junction of distributing artery and high resistance arteriole. Mean pressure and pulse pressure fall precipitously immediately beyond the arterial termination. The pressure wave is reflected strongly at the termination and travels backwards towards the heart (p. 7–9)

Arteries
Blood vessels which receive blood from the ventricles of the heart and terminate in arterioles of diameter approximately 200 μm (p. 7)

Arterioles
Muscular walled vessels in which the arterial system terminates, and which provide most of the resistance to steady flow through a vascular bed. Diameter is usually less than 200 μm (p. 7)

Attenuation (of a pulse)
Decrease in amplitude of a travelling wave, usually due to viscosity of blood and of blood vessel walls (p. 135)

Bisferiens (pulse)
Twice beating on the upstroke with amplitude of the first systolic wave similar to that of the second. Often due to a Venturi effect in the ascending aorta (p. 255, 259)

Compliance
Synonomous with DISTENSIBILITY (p. 27)

Compound Wave
Wave which is made up of more than one harmonic component. All pulse waves are examples of compound waves (p. 67–69)

Damped natural frequency
Resonant frequency of a complete manometer system as used in an experiment (p. 18, Appendix 1)

Damping
Attenuation (p. 135)

Dicrotic notch
The foot of the dicrotic or diastolic wave. Due to peripheral wave reflection but often confused with the incisura which is caused by aortic valve closure (p. 90, 135)

Dicrotic wave
(From The Greek di – twice, crotos – beat) An obvious diastolic wave following the systolic peak. This is the echo of the first wave following its reflection in the peripheral vasculature (p. 90, 135)

Differential pressure
See PRESSURE (DIFFERENTIAL)

Distensibility
A measure of the ease with which a hollow structure can change its volume or diameter. The inverse is elasticity (p. 27)

Dynamic accuracy (of recording system)
Ability of a system to measure pulsatile events accurately and with minimal distortion at different frequencies (p. 18–20)

Elasticity
A measure of resistance to deformation. Inverse of distensibility or compliance. Usually expressed as Young's modulus or pressure/strain modulus (Ch. 3)

Energy
Work (p. 46, 157)

External Ventricular Work
Energy imparted to blood by the contracting ventricle. Measured as two components:–
Steady Work – Work lost as blood flows forward through resistance vessels
Pulsatile work – work lost in arterial pulsations (Both have pressure and kinetic components, but both these are measured together if pressure is recorded end-on to the direction of flow when velocity profile is flat) (p. 46, 157)

Fourier analysis
The mathematical technique of separating a compound wave into component harmonics. See Appendix 2, p. 67

Frequency response
See DYNAMIC ACCURACY. Characterisation of the degree of distortion of input signals produced by a recording system at different frequencies (p. 18–20)

Hertz (Hz)
Cycle sec^{-1} (p. 67–75)

Ideal fluid
A fluid without viscosity (or internal friction) (p. 23, 45)

Incisura
The high frequency wavelet on an arterial pulse wave due to sudden closure of the aortic or pulmonary valve. To be distinguished from the dicrotic notch (p. 134)

Inertia
The property of blood due to its mass, which opposes its acceleration or deceleration (p. 27, 36)

'In-phase'
Occurring simultaneously, without delay (p. 154)

Impedance (characteristic)
Vascular or input impedance in the absence of wave reflection (p. 116)

Impedance ('in phase')
An expression of vascular input impedance, describing the relationship between pulsatile flow and the component of pulsatile pressure which is 'in phase' with flow. Displayed as Modulus × cosine of phase at different frequencies (p. 154)

Impedance (input)
Synonomous with VASCULAR IMPEDANCE (p. 70, Ch. 8)

Impedance (longitudinal)
Different from all others in that it is the relationship of flow in an artery to *differential pressure* between two points in the artery. Determined by the properties of the arterial segment, not by the properties of the vascular bed. Displayed as modulus and phase as a function of frequency (p. 72)

Impedance (vascular)
Opposition to pulsatile as well as steady flow through a vascular bed. Measured by relating mean values and corresponding harmonics of pressure and flow waves at the input of the vascular bed. Displayed as modulus (amplitude of pressure ÷ amplitude of flow) and phase (delay of flow after pressure), both as a function of frequency. Similar to electrical, acoustic and hydraulic impedance. (p. 70, Ch. 8)

Kinetic Energy
Energy associated with velocity:– measured as ½ mass × velocity^2 (p. 46)

Laminar flow
Flow of concentric laminae in a tube, each sliding over the other. Contrasted with turbulent flow (p. 43)

Linearity
Direct relationship between two variables or their corresponding components. A single frequency component of one variable produces a single frequency component of a second variable (p. 35)

Lumped
Appearing to be located at one site (p. 88)

Modulus (of pressure or flow)
Amplitude of sinusoidal pressure or flow at a particular frequency

Modulus (of elasticity)
Measure of elasticity as force required to produce a certain extension (p. 29)

Modulus (of impedance)
Amplitude of pressure component ÷ flow component (Ch. 8)

Neper
A measure of attenuation. If a wave attenuates as $e^{-\alpha L}$ with distance travelled L, the attenuation is α nepers/unit length

Node
A site of minimal pressure or flow fluctuation (opposite of antinode) (p. 83–86)

Non-linearity
Lack of direct relationship between two variables or their corresponding components. A single frequency component of one variable produces multiple frequencies of a second variable (p. 35)

Newtonian fluid
A fluid whose viscosity is constant in different sized tubes and at different rates of shear (p. 23–27)

Peripheral resistance
The ratio of mean pressure drop across a vascular bed to mean flow through it. Analogous with modulus of vascular impedance at zero frequency (p. 7–9, Ch. 8)

Phase
Delay (i.e. for impedance, the delay between corresponding pressure and flow components). Usually expressed in terms of circular frequency – as degrees or radians rather than in milliseconds (p. 67–73, Ch. 8)

Pressure (lateral)
Pressure exerted at right angles to the direction of flow – i.e. pressure exerted on the arterial wall (p. 11, 118)

Pressure (impact)
Pressure measured end-on to the direction of flow. The technique of measurement causes kinetic energy to be converted into pressure energy (p. 11, 118)

Pressure (differential)
Pressure between two points in an artery, both usually at right angles to the direction of flow (p. 13)

Pressure gradient
Synonomous with DIFFERENTIAL PRESSURE

Pulse
Fluctuation in pressure, flow or diameter caused by cardiac contraction

Pulse wave velocity
See WAVE VELOCITY

Radian

A measure of phase. One cycle sec^{-1} (or Hertz) = 6.2832 radians sec^{-1}

Reflection

Return of a (pressure) wave which passes down a tube or along an artery. An echo (Ch. 7)

Reflection coefficient

The ratio of the amplitude of reflected/incident waves (p. 88)

Resonance

Abnormally large oscillation produced by multiple reflections (p. 91)

Reynold's number

A non-dimensional number determined by diameter, flow rate, viscosity and density. When exceeded in a long straight tube, laminar flow is likely to become turbulent (p. 43)

Sinusoidal (pressure, flow, diameter etc)

Components of a compound wave in simple harmonic motion (p. 68, 70)

Standing waves

A phenomenon seen in the presence of resonance. Waves appear to have simultaneous peaks between reflecting site and nearest node (p. 91, 136)

Strain

Deformation in length (tensile) or volume (volumetric)

Stress

Deforming force per unit area (p. 29)

Turbulent flow

Opposite of laminar flow. Particles move in a radial and a circumferential as well as in a longitudinal direction (p. 43)

Velocity profile

Rate of longitudinal flow of different particles at different points across the diameter of a vessel. For steady flow in a long tube the velocity profile takes the form of a parabola. For pulsatile flow, the profile is more flattened, especially in large vessels (p. 34–35)

Viscosity

Internal friction of a fluid (p. 23–27)

Viscosity (Newtonian)

Constant viscosity with different rates of shear and in different sized vessels (p. 23–27)

Viscosity (anomalous)

Viscosity is dependent on rate of shear and on size of vessel (p. 23–27)

Wave velocity

Velocity of travel of a disturbance along an artery. Principally determined by distensibilitly of the arterial wall (p. 41–43)

Wave Velocity (foot-to-foot)

As measured from the distance between two recording sites, divided by the delay of the foot of the wave between the two sites (p. 41–43)

Wave Velocity (regional)

Foot-to-foot velocity in a particular region (p. 41–43)

Wave Velocity (apparent)

A complicated concept relating to wave velocity as modified by effects of wave reflection. Essentially, distance between two sites divided by delay of different harmonics of the pressure pulse between the two sites (p. 43)

Windkessel

The inverted air filled dome in old fire engines which converted intermittent injection from a pump into steady flow from the firemans nozzle. The cushioning function of arteries is likened to this (p. 3)

CONVERSION TABLE

Conventional Units		SI Units
	1 cm H_2O	= .098 kPa
Pressure	1 mmHg	= 0.133 kPa (kilopascal)
Flow	1 ml/sec	= 1×10^{-3} L/s
	1 cm/sec	= 1×10^{-2} m/s
Resistance	1 dyne sec cm^{-3}	= .01 $kPa.s.m^{-1}$
Impedance	1 dyne sec cm^{-5}	= 100 $kPa.s.m^{-3}$
Viscosity	I cP	= 1×10^{-3} Pa.s
Power	1 Watt	= 1 Watt

Reference: Kappagoda CT, Linden RJ 1976. The use of SI units in cardiovascular studies. Cardiovascular Research 10: 141–148.

APPENDIX 1:
Determination of frequency response of a manometer system

After completion of an experiment or clinical procedure, the catheter, still attached to its manometer is inserted through a Tuohy-Borst adaptor into the bottom of a rigid chamber having a side opening and open top (Figure A1.1). Over the open top a rubber membrane is laid (surgical glove is quite satisfactory) and held in place with a rubber band. A sphygmomanometer bulb is attached to the side opening and the chamber is pressurized through this, causing the rubber membrane to stretch and balloon outwards. The membrane is then suddenly ruptured with a lighted match or scalpel blade, causing pressure to fall suddenly to atmospheric. Dynamic response is determined from the frequency of oscillations induced and their exponential decay (Figure A1.2) as follows:

If T_D = period between successive oscillations
then $1/T_D$ = damped natural frequency.

If θ_1 and θ_2 are amplitude of successive oscillations
then θ_1/θ_2 = ratio of damping
and Λ, the logarithmic decrement = $\ln(\theta_1/\theta_2)$

From T_d and logarithmic decrement Λ one calculates

Relative damping $\beta = \dfrac{\Lambda}{\sqrt{4\pi^2 + \Lambda^2}}$

and

Undamped natural frequency ω_o

$= \dfrac{\sqrt{4\pi^2 + \Lambda^2}}{T_D}$ (radians/sec)

These are the general properties of the manometer system, and the manometer characteristics are described in terms of β and ω_o.

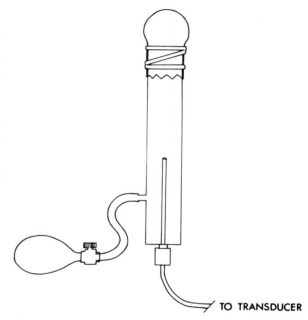

Fig. A1.1 Method for determination of manometer frequency response. For details, see text.

However, the amplitude and phase distortion will be different at different frequencies. The distortion at any frequency f radians/sec is calculated as follows, using γ as a term describing the ratio of driving frequency f to undamped natural frequency ω_o (i.e. $\gamma = f/\omega_o$).

Amplitude distortion (D) at frequency f

$D = \dfrac{1}{\sqrt{(1 - \gamma^2)^2 + 4\beta^2\gamma^2}}$

Phase delay (Ψ) at frequency f

$\Psi = \tan^{-1}\dfrac{2\beta\gamma}{1 - \gamma^2}$

Appropriate corrections for modulus and phase of pressure can readily be incorporated in a computer programme calculating the Fourier components of a compound wave. (See Appendix 2)

In practice one always endeavours to have natural frequency as high as possible so that γ is as small as possible.

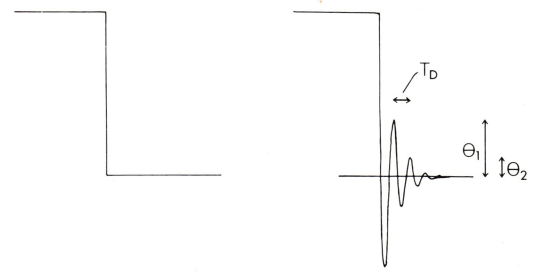

Fig. A1.2 Pressure step induced (left) and recorded (right). Manometer frequency response is determined from the natural frequency (T_D) and decay (θ_1/θ_2) of oscillations induced.

APPENDIX 2:
Fourier Analysis of a Compound Wave

Fourier analysis is the mathematical technique whereby the harmonic components of a compound wave are determined. The basic technique is simple in concept, but the repetitive calculations can only be performed realistically on a computer or sophisticated pocket calculator.

1. For the first harmonic

The amplitude Y_r of N points regularly spaced along the compound wave are multiplied at each point by the corresponding values of a sinusoidal wave which begins and ends at the same time as the compound wave. From this one determines B, the amplitude of the sinusoidal component of the compound wave at the fundamental frequency as

$$B = \frac{2}{N} \cdot \sum_{r=1}^{r=N} Y_r \cdot \sin\left\{r \cdot \left(\frac{360°}{N}\right)\right\}$$

Likewise one can determine A, the amplitude of the cosine component of the compound wave which begins and ends at the same time as

$$A = \frac{2}{N} \cdot \sum_{r=1}^{r=N} Y_r \cdot \cos\left\{r \cdot \left(\frac{360°}{N}\right)\right\}$$

From the independent amplitude of these sine and cosine components, one can determine the modulus M of the resultant sine waves

as $M = \sqrt{A^2 + B^2}$

and the phase delay ϕ

as $\phi = \tan^{-1} \dfrac{B}{A}$

2. For subsequent harmonics

This calculation gives only the amplitude and phase of the first harmonic of the compound wave. Amplitude and phase of subsequent harmonics are determined in similar fashion — for the second harmonic by multiplying data points by the sine and cosine waves which have two complete oscillations within the period of the compound wave, for the third harmonic by sine and cosine waves having three complete oscillations, and so on.

The general formula for the nth Harmonic is:

$$B_n = \frac{2}{N} \cdot \sum_{r=1}^{r=N} Y_r \cdot \sin\left\{r \cdot \left(\frac{n \cdot 360°}{N}\right)\right\}$$

$$A_n = \frac{2}{N} \cdot \sum_{r=1}^{r=N} Y_r \cdot \cos\left\{r \cdot \left(\frac{n \cdot 360°}{N}\right)\right\}$$

A useful programme for a Texas Instruments Calculator (T1–59) is given below. Similar programmes are readily available for other calculators and computers, or can easily be written.

loc	cd	key	loc	cd	key	loc	cd	key	loc	cd	key
000	29	CP	053	89	π	106	22	INV	159	43	RCL
001	70	RAD	054	95	=	107	67	EQ	160	03	03
002	01	1	055	42	STO	108	10	E'	161	22	INV
003	01	1	056	00	00	109	43	RCL	162	44	SUM
004	42	STO	057	43	RCL	110	05	05	163	03	03
005	01	01	058	02	02	111	65	×	164	43	RCL
006	32	X:T	059	32	X:T	112	02	2	165	10	10
007	00	0	060	43	RCL	113	95	=	166	22	INV
008	42	STO	061	04	04	114	55	÷	167	49	PRD
009	02	02	062	91	R/S	115	43	RCL	168	00	00
010	42	STO	063	76	LBL	116	02	02	169	43	RCL
011	03	03	064	15	E	117	95	=	170	10	10
012	42	STO	065	42	STO	118	42	STO	171	91	R/S
013	04	04	066	10	10	119	05	05	172	76	LBL
014	43	RCL	067	49	PRD	120	43	RCL	173	11	A
015	01	01	068	00	00	121	06	06	174	43	RCL
016	91	R/S	069	00	0	122	65	×	175	05	05
017	76	LBL	070	42	STO	123	02	2	176	91	R/S
018	14	D	071	05	05	124	95	=	177	76	LBL
019	72	ST*	072	42	STO	125	55	÷	178	12	B
020	01	01	073	06	06	126	43	RCL	179	43	RCL
021	69	OP	074	76	LBL	127	02	02	180	06	06
022	21	21	075	10	E'	128	95	=	181	91	R/S
023	69	OP	076	43	RCL	129	42	STO	182	76	LBL
024	22	22	077	00	00	130	06	06	183	13	C
025	43	RCL	078	65	×	131	43	RCL	184	43	RCL
026	02	02	079	43	RCL	132	05	05	185	04	04
027	91	R/S	080	03	03	133	33	X²	186	91	R/S
028	76	LBL	081	95	=	134	85	+	187	76	LBL
029	18	C'	082	42	STO	135	53	(	188	16	A'
030	69	OP	083	09	09	136	43	RCL	189	43	RCL
031	31	31	084	39	COS	137	06	06	190	07	07
032	73	RC*	085	65	×	138	33	X²	191	91	R/S
033	01	01	086	73	RC*	139	54	)	192	76	LBL
034	44	SUM	087	01	01	140	95	=	193	17	B'
035	04	04	088	95	=	141	34	√X	194	43	RCL
036	43	RCL	089	44	SUM	142	42	STO	195	08	08
037	01	01	090	05	05	143	07	07	196	91	R/S
038	22	INV	091	43	RCL	144	43	RCL	197	76	LBL
039	67	EQ	092	09	09	145	05	05	198	19	D'
040	18	C'	093	38	SIN	146	55	÷	199	43	RCL
041	43	RCL	094	65	×	147	43	RCL	200	08	08
042	02	02	095	73	RC*	148	06	06	201	65	×
043	22	INV	096	01	01	149	95	=	202	01	1
044	49	PRD	097	95	=	150	22	INV	203	08	8
045	04	04	098	44	SUM	151	30	TAN	204	00	0
046	43	RCL	099	06	06	152	42	STO	205	95	=
047	02	02	100	69	OP	153	08	08	206	55	÷
048	35	1/X	101	21	21	154	43	RCL	207	89	π
049	65	×	102	69	OP	155	03	03	208	95	=
050	02	2	103	23	23	156	22	INV	209	91	R/S
051	95	=	104	43	RCL	157	44	SUM			
052	65	×	105	03	03	158	01	01			

Fourier Analysis Programme for Texas Instruments Calculator TI-59.

Fig. A2.1 Fourier analysis programme for Texas Instruments Calculator

USER INSTRUCTIONS

Step	Procedure	Enter	Press	Display
1	Start program and initialise registers		RST R/S	11
2*	Enter data (repeat this step for each datum)	x	D	N**
3	Calculate mean value A_o		C'	A_o
4	Calculate Fourier coefficients' modulus and phase for specified harmonic ($H_n = 1, 2, 3 \ldots$)	H_n	E	H_n
5	Display cosine coefficients (A_n)		A	A_n
6	Display sine coefficient (B_n)		B	B_n
7	Display modulus (M_n)		A'	M_n
8	Display phase (radians) (ϕ_r)		B'	ϕ_r
9	Display phase (degrees) (ϕ_d)		D'	ϕ_d
10	Display mean value (A_o)		C	A_o
11	For further harmonics go to Step 4			

Note

* If data is read in from cards, *Step* 2 is omitted, and the following steps substituted:
  i. The value of the total number of data points (N) to be stored in R_{02} (register 02)
  ii. The value of $11 + N$ to be stored in R_{01} (register 01)
Steps 1–4 must be followed in that order
Steps 5–10 may be executed in any order
** $N_{max} = 49$ with normal partition of 459.59
  Minimum partition possible is 239.89
  $\therefore N_{max}$ (absolute) $= 79$

Index